Register Now for Online Access to Your Book!

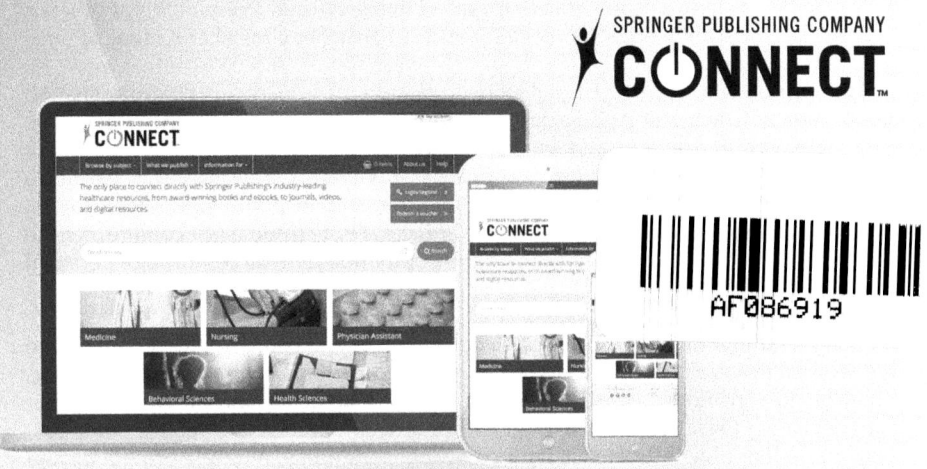

Your print purchase of *Pharmacological Considerations in Gerontology* **includes online access to the contents of your book—increasing accessibility, portability, and searchability!**

Access today at:

http://connect.springerpub.com/content/book/978-0-8261-2772-3
or scan the QR code at the right with your smartphone
and enter the access code below.

81AXL9PN

Scan here for quick access.

If you are experiencing problems accessing the digital component of this product, please contact our customer service department at cs@springerpub.com

The online access with your print purchase is available at the publisher's discretion and may be removed at any time without notice.

Publisher's Note: New and used products purchased from third-party sellers are not guaranteed for quality, authenticity, or access to any included digital components.

SPRINGER PUBLISHING COMPANY

View all our products at springerpub.com

Abimbola Farinde, PhD, PharmD, is a healthcare professional and professor experienced in the field and practice of mental health, geriatrics, and pharmacy. In particular, her work includes medication therapy and disease state management for active duty soldiers with a dual diagnoses of traumatic brain injury and psychiatric disorders, and she has also worked with intellectually challenged and developmentally disabled individuals in a state-supported living setting. These different practice experiences have allowed her to develop and enhance her clinical and medical writing skills over the years.

Dr. Farinde is a Fellow of the American Society of Consultant Pharmacists and the American College of Apothecaries. She is the associate editor of several healthcare and scientific journals, and she has served as an exam committee development member for the Commission for Certification in Geriatric Pharmacy. Dr. Farinde's research interests focus on cognitive decline, the veteran population, older adults, neuropsychiatric disturbances, and mental illness. Dr. Farinde has a commitment to providing increasingly enhanced care to the populations she serves through personal and professional growth.

Megan Hebdon, PhD, DNP, RN, NP-C, is a professor and primary care provider who has worked in a variety of clinical settings with older adults including long-term care, home health, oncology, pain management, internal medicine, and primary care. Her experiences in these settings have given her a deep appreciation for the complexities of care that older adults face with comorbid conditions, multiple providers, and varied clinical care settings. She has endeavored to include these important aspects of aging into her teaching in undergraduate and graduate nursing courses.

Dr. Hebdon is actively involved in research focused on cancer survivorship, palliative care, cancer caregiver needs, and rural caregiving. She is passionate about supporting patients and informal caregivers in wellness, management of chronic conditions, and end-of-life care. She believes in the importance of approaching teaching and nursing practice with loving kindness. She emphasizes this and wellness in her own life through nutrition, mindfulness, exercise, and community engagement.

Pharmacological Considerations in Gerontology

A Patient-Centered Guide for Advanced Practice Registered Nurses and Related Health Professions

Abimbola Farinde, PhD, PharmD
Megan Hebdon, PhD, DNP, RN, NP-C

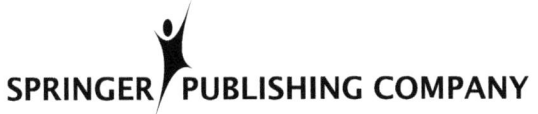

SPRINGER PUBLISHING COMPANY

Copyright © 2020 Springer Publishing Company, LLC

All rights reserved.

No part of this publication may be reproduced, stored in a retrieval system, or transmitted in any form or by any means, electronic, mechanical, photocopying, recording, or otherwise, without the prior permission of Springer Publishing Company, LLC, or authorization through payment of the appropriate fees to the Copyright Clearance Center, Inc., 222 Rosewood Drive, Danvers, MA 01923, 978-750-8400, fax 978-646-8600, info@copyright.com or on the Web at www.copyright.com.

Springer Publishing Company, LLC
11 West 42nd Street
New York, NY 10036
www.springerpub.com
http://connect.springerpub.com

Acquisitions Editor: Elizabeth Nieginski
Compositor: Exeter Premedia Services Private Ltd.

ISBN: 978-0-8261-2769-3
ebook ISBN: 978-0-8261-2772-3
DOI: 10.1891/9780826127723

19 20 21 22 / 5 4 3 2 1

The author and the publisher of this Work have made every effort to use sources believed to be reliable to provide information that is accurate and compatible with the standards generally accepted at the time of publication. Because medical science is continually advancing, our knowledge base continues to expand. Therefore, as new information becomes available, changes in procedures become necessary. We recommend that the reader always consult current research and specific institutional policies before performing any clinical procedure. The author and publisher shall not be liable for any special, consequential, or exemplary damages resulting, in whole or in part, from the readers' use of, or reliance on, the information contained in this book. The publisher has no responsibility for the persistence or accuracy of URLs for external or third-party Internet websites referred to in this publication and does not guarantee that any content on such websites is, or will remain, accurate or appropriate.

Library of Congress Cataloging-in-Publication Data

Names: Farinde, Abimbola, author. | Hebdon, Megan, author.
Title: Pharmacological considerations in gerontology : a patient-centered guide for advanced practice registered nurses and related health professions / Abimbola Farinde, Megan Hebdon.
Description: New York, NY : Springer Publishing Company, LLC [2020] | Includes bibliographical references and index.
Identifiers: LCCN 2019043407 (print) | LCCN 2019043408 (ebook) | ISBN 9780826127693 (paperback) | ISBN 9780826127723 (ebook)
Subjects: MESH: Drug Therapy | Aged | Pharmacokinetics | Pharmacological Phenomena—physiology | Aging—physiology | Advanced Practice Nursing | Case Reports
Classification: LCC RS55.2 (print) | LCC RS55.2 (ebook) | NLM WT 166 | DDC 615.1—dc23
LC record available at https://lccn.loc.gov/2019043407
LC ebook record available at https://lccn.loc.gov/2019043408

Contact us to receive discount rates on bulk purchases.
We can also customize our books to meet your needs.
For more information please contact: sales@springerpub.com

Abimbola Farinde: https://orcid.org/0000-0002-6782-6523
Megan Hebdon: https://orcid.org/0000-0003-1916-5043

Publisher's Note: New and used products purchased from third-party sellers are not guaranteed for quality, authenticity, or access to any included digital components.

Printed in the United States of America.

The development of this book is dedicated to my loving family and friends who provided me with the motivation to begin and finish this process. It is with their unwavering support that I dedicate this publication to them all.
—*Abimbola Farinde*

I dedicate this work to my husband and children who help me remember the important things in life.
—*Megan Hebdon*

Contents

Contributors   *xi*
Preface   *xiii*
Acknowledgments   *xv*

SECTION I: INTRODUCTION TO THE GERIATRIC PATIENT

1. Physiologic Changes That Occur in Geriatric Patients   3
   Megan Hebdon

2. The Examination of the Geriatric Patient   11
   Megan Hebdon

SECTION II: INTRODUCTION TO PHARMACOKINETICS AND PHARMACODYNAMICS OF THE GERIATRIC PATIENT

3. Pharmacokinetics/Pharmacodynamics of the Geriatric Patient   21
   Abimbola Farinde

4. Aging and Pharmacokinetic Impact   27
   Abimbola Farinde

5. Available Guidelines for Therapeutic Drug Selections in Geriatric Patients   31
   Abimbola Farinde

6. Drug–Drug Interactions   35
   Abimbola Farinde

7. Drug–Food Interactions   39
   Abimbola Farinde

8. Common Medications for Comorbidities and Side Effects   43
   Abimbola Farinde

9. Available Drug Therapies Utilized in Geriatric Patients   45
   Abimbola Farinde

SECTION III: GUIDELINES FOR DOSING GERIATRIC PATIENTS BY DISORDERS/BODY SYSTEMS

10. Guidelines for Dosing Geriatric Patients   51
    Abimbola Farinde
    Interprofessional Case Study: *Megan Hebdon*

11. **Auditory Disorders** *59*
    Abimbola Farinde
    Interprofessional Case Study: *Megan Hebdon*

12. **Neurologic Disorders** *67*
    Abimbola Farinde
    Interprofessional Case Study: *Megan Hebdon*

13. **Hematologic Disorders** *73*
    Abimbola Farinde
    Interprofessional Case Study: *Megan Hebdon*

14. **Nutritional Issues** *79*
    Abimbola Farinde
    Interprofessional Case Study: *Megan Hebdon*

15. **Endocrine Disorders** *89*
    Megan Hebdon
    Interprofessional Case Study: *Megan Hebdon*

16. **Hyperlipidemia** *107*
    Megan Hebdon
    Interprofessional Case Study: *Katie R. Katz*

17. **Cardiovascular Disorders** *119*
    Abimbola Farinde
    Interprofessional Case Study: *Wendy R. Downey*

18. **Respiratory Disorders** *127*
    Abimbola Farinde
    Interprofessional Case Study: *Megan Hebdon*

19. **Gastrointestinal Disorders** *143*
    Megan Hebdon
    Interprofessional Case Study: *Megan Hebdon*

20. **Central Nervous System Impairments** *161*
    Lisa C. Hutchison
    Interprofessional Case Study: *Megan Hebdon*

21. **Mental Disorders** *179*
    Megan Hebdon
    Interprofessional Case Study: *Jerusalem Walker*

22. **Musculoskeletal Disorders** *197*
    Amanda M. Bellile
    Interprofessional Case Study: *Megan Hebdon*

23. **Pain Management** *211*
    Amanda M. Bellile
    Interprofessional Case Study: *Phyllis Brown Whitehead*

24. **Renal Impairments** *227*
    Abimbola Farinde and Megan Hebdon
    Interprofessional Case Study: *Megan Hebdon*

25. **Genitourinary Pharmacotherapy, Urinary Tract Infections, and Sexual Health** *247*
    Madeline Burke
    Interprofessional Case Study: *Marjorie Young*

SECTION IV: PRESCRIBING CONSIDERATIONS UNIQUE TO THE GERIATRIC POPULATION

26. The Beers Criteria for Inappropriate Medication Use in Older Adults 277
    Megan Hebdon

27. Examples of Inappropriate Medication Prescribing 297
    Madeline Burke

28. Polypharmacy and Nonadherence/Patient Education Tips 305
    Megan Hebdon

Index 311

Contributors

Amanda M. Bellile, PharmD, BCPS, PGY2 Pain and Palliative Care Pharmacy Resident, Central Arkansas Veterans Healthcare System, Little Rock, Arkansas

Madeline Burke, PharmD, PGY2 Geriatrics Pharmacy Resident, Central Arkansas Veterans Healthcare System, Little Rock, Arkansas

Wendy R. Downey, DNP, MSEd, RN, CNE, Assistant Professor, Radford University College of Health and Human Services, School of Nursing, Radford, Virginia

Abimbola Farinde, PhD, PharmD, Professor, Columbia Southern University, Phoenix, Arizona

Megan Hebdon, PhD, DNP, RN, NP-C, T-32 Postdoctoral Fellow in Cancer, Caregiving, and Palliative Care, University of Utah College of Nursing, Salt Lake City, Utah

Lisa C. Hutchison, PharmD, MPH, BCPS, BCGP, FCCP, Professor, University of Arkansas for Department of Pharmacy Practice, University of Arkansas for Medical Sciences, Little Rock, Arkansas

Katie R. Katz, DNP, RN, FNP-BC, Assistant Professor, Radford University College of Health and Human Services, School of Nursing, Radford, Virginia

Jerusalem Walker, DNP, BA, FNP-BC, CNE, Assistant Professor, Radford University College of Health and Human Services, School of Nursing, Radford, Virginia

Phyllis Brown Whitehead, PhD, APRN/CNS, ACHPN, RN-BC, Palliative Medicine/Pain Management Clinical Nurse Specialist, Carilion Roanoke Memorial Hospital, Roanoke, Virginia and Associate Professor, Virginia Tech Carilion School of Medicine, Roanoke, Virginia

Marjorie Young, DNP, RN, IBCLC, FNP-BC, Assistant Professor, Radford University College of Health and Human Services, School of Nursing, Radford, Virginia

Preface

Dr. Farinde recognized the need for a reference book that emphasized pharmacologic considerations in older adults for the primary care nurse practitioner. As a pharmacist, she recognized the complexity that is encountered when caring for aging patients with multiple chronic conditions, polypharmacy, and aging changes that can complicate seemingly simple prescribing decisions. Dr. Hebdon was immediately drawn to this idea because she had encountered these issues in every day clinical practice. Both editors identified the importance of having relevant clinical examples for nurse practitioners with interprofessional care considerations. This book is an effort to combine the presentation of chronic health conditions experienced by aging patients with pharmacologic considerations that are unique to this population. Nurse practitioners are increasingly responsible for delivering care to elderly patients in primary care who present with complex conditions, medication regimens, and numerous specialty providers. This reference will provide a "big picture" look at how to approach pharmacotherapy and present principles to guide decision-making so that adverse drug events may be prevented.

Abimbola Farinde
Megan Hebdon

Acknowledgments

Abimbola Farinde

I would like to acknowledge the coauthor (Dr. Hebdon) and contributors of this publication who were instrumental in the creation and finalization of this book. You are all amazing!

Megan Hebdon

I would like to acknowledge Dr. Farinde for her creativity, persistence, and expertise in moving this project forward. She is a rock star!

Introduction to the Geriatric Patient

1 Physiologic Changes That Occur in Geriatric Patients

Megan Hebdon

OBJECTIVES
1. Describe physiologic changes with aging
2. Identify geriatric syndromes that are not part of the normal aging process
3. Discuss aging theories
4. Review goals of care in the aging population including an emphasis on quality of life and functionality

INTRODUCTION
For an advanced practice nurse (APRN), the goals of care should always emphasize patient well-being and functionality. Geriatric care is a setting when these goals are brought into sharper focus due to functional decline, increased prevalence of illness, and the reality of end of life. A foundational issue to geriatric care is understanding the difference between disorders, illness, and normal aging processes (Chaudhry, Wang, Gill, & Krumholz, 2010). Often, "normal aging" changes are related to disorders rather than the actual aging process (Daley-Placide, n.d.; Taffet, 2019). In fact, a Danish twin study (Hjelmborg et al., 2006) demonstrated that about 25% of variation in longevity was attributed to genetics while about 50% was related to environment and lifestyle factors. The influence of genetics became more significant past the age of 60 (Hjelmborg et al., 2006).

Understanding both the normal process of aging and aberrancies in aging is essential for appropriate assessment, diagnosis, and treatment of the geriatric patient. This chapter delineates theories of aging, overall aging changes within the body, aging changes by organ system, and geriatric syndromes.

THEORIES OF AGING
There are numerous theories addressing aging, but they generally fall into two main categories—aging as a programmed state and aging resulting from an accumulation of damage (Sergiev, Dontsova, & Berezkin, 2015). Some aging researchers emphasize that aging as a deterioration of survival rather than a programmed part of development helps clarify the process (American Federation for Aging Research [AFAR], 2011). Programmed senescence and aging as a result of cellular damage are not mutually exclusive and may both address the why and how of aging (AFAR, 2011; Sergiev et al., 2015). Buildup of damage and decreased capacity to repair damage may be affected by programmed senescence, so the complex interplay of environment and genetic predisposition may result in aging. Proposed sources of cellular damage in aging include reactive oxygen species, although these may be protective

in some pathways, accumulation of metabolic waste, disruption of regulatory pathways such as the hypothalamus–pituitary–adrenal axis, telomere length and telomerase activity, and biologic clocks and metabolic activity (AFAR, 2011). Programmed senescence occurs in other species, and researchers have argued over aging as a consequence or side effect of genetic pathways (Sergiev et al., 2015). Genetic mutations may contribute favorably to longevity, but further research is needed to understand the genetic mechanisms affecting the aging process (Sergiev et al., 2015). Aging is an ever-evolving area of research, but aging, itself, continues to be inevitable. Acknowledging the consequences of aging is crucial to supporting patients in both health and illness.

AGING CHANGES WITHIN THE BODY

General aging changes in the body are related to loss of complexity in physiologic function such as cardiac, neurologic, and stress responses (Taffet, 2019). The phenomenon of homeostenosis occurs with body maturity and senescence, where there are fewer physiologic reserves to meet homeostasis. Body processes such as the circadian rhythm of body temperature, plasma cortisol, and sleep are affected. The end point is system inflexibility where small challenges overwhelm available reserves (Taffet, 2019). The process of aging can be attenuated by activities such as exercise or mental stimulation (Taffet, 2019).

Aging Changes of the Cardiovascular System

The cardiovascular system changes center around decreased system flexibility. In addition to genetics and lifestyle, older individuals are at increased risk for elevated blood pressure, heart attack, stroke, and other cardiovascular diseases as a result of the following changes:

- Decreased mechanical and contractile efficiency
- Arterial wall thickening and stiffening of the veins
- Increased elastolytic and collagenolytic activity
- Increased smooth muscle tone
- Elevated systolic arterial pressures due to stiffening of vessels
- Increased preload and afterload
- Left ventricular hypertrophy
- Decreased plasma renin and aldosterone activity including decreased reactivity to upright posture or response to sodium restriction
- Cardiac hypertrophy, which may lead to diastolic dysfunction
- Conduction defects and rhythm disturbances, such as increased risk of atrial fibrillation
- Fall in stroke volume and then cardiac output, so cardiac output may not be as efficient with exercise (Navaratnarajah & Jackson, 2013)

Aging Changes of the Respiratory System

Similar to changes in the cardiovascular system, respiratory system changes occur due to loss of tissue elasticity and blunting of responses to internal or external environmental changes. Individuals without underlying lung disease may still have issues related to pulmonary decline at the end of life. Changes in the respiratory system include:

- Loss of elasticity in airways and bony thorax
- Loss of muscle and weakening of respiratory musculature, contributing to poor lung expansion
- Ventilation–perfusion mismatch
- Reduced arterial oxygen tension
- Blunted ventilator response to hypoxia or hypercapnia (Navaratnarajah & Jackson, 2013)

Aging Changes of the Gastrointestinal System

As individuals age, the smooth muscle activity and absorption may change in the gastrointestinal system. This may result in more issues with constipation, appetite, and nutritional imbalances. Other changes with aging include:

- Decreased saliva production
- Desynchronization of contraction and relaxation of smooth muscle and sphincter control, making deglutition less effective
- Altered protein metabolism and nutrient absorption
- Prolonged transit time
- Atrophy of gastrointestinal mucosa
- Decreased strength of colonic muscle
- Decrease in liver and pancreas size (Navaratnarajah & Jackson, 2013; Rughwani, 2011)

Aging Changes of the Urologic System

Changes in the urologic system occur from the kidneys down to the bladder. Renal changes may affect drug metabolism, fluid balance, and blood pressure. Changes in elimination, such as retention or incontinence, may occur due to structural changes in the bladder and reproductive organs. Overall changes include:

- Loss of cortical renal mass, sclerosis of glomeruli, and reduced surface area for filtration, which can cause a decrease in glomerular filtration rate (GFR)
- Increase in basement membrane permeability leading to albuminuria and proteinuria even in the absence of diabetes, hypertension (HTN), and *chronic kidney disease* (CKD)
- Decreased renal blood flow and decreased ability to vasodilate the renal artery
- Loss of muscular tone in the bladder, ureters, and urethra
- Reduced bladder capacity (Daley-Placide, n.d.; Navaratnarajah & Jackson, 2013)

Aging Changes of Musculoskeletal System

Structural changes in the musculoskeletal system may place aging patients at increased risk for weakness, immobility, falls, musculoskeletal injuries, and pain syndromes. Selected aging changes include:

- Cartilage degeneration and loss of tissue elasticity in the joints
- Decreased muscle mass and contractility
- Increased muscular fat, causing reduced muscle quality
- Loss of bone mass (Besdine, 2019; Daley-Placide, n.d.; Taffet, 2019)

Aging Changes of the Neurologic System

The neurologic system may experience an overall decline in production of neurohormones, response to nervous system signaling centrally and peripherally, as well as a decrease in neural density. Individuals experience 30% loss of brain mass, especially gray matter, by age 80. As is clear in other systems, a blunting of response to hormone activity occurs with aging, which affects both brain and body-wide functioning. Individuals are at greater risk of cognitive decline with age, although lifestyle and genetics are important predictors of neurologic disease. Aging changes may include:

- Reduced production of neurotransmitters such as catecholamines, serotonin, and acetylcholine
- Reduced dopamine uptake sites and transporters
- Depleted gamma-aminobutyric acid (GABA) binding sites
- Decreased motor, sensory, and autonomic nerve fibers
- Decreased nerve conduction velocity
- Decline of signal transduction rate of brainstem and spinal cord
- Denervation and muscular atrophy
- Blunted response to beta-adrenergic stimulation
- Decreased aortic arch and carotid sinus baroreceptors
- Weakened heart rate response to arterial pressure changes
- Autonomic dysregulation, which may cause increased risk of syncope (Navaratnarajah & Jackson, 2013)

Aging Changes of the Integumentary System

The aging changes of the integumentary system are the most readily observed including hair distribution, color and quality, nail thickness and color, and skin thinning, decreased elasticity, reduced subcutaneous tissues, and prolonged healing time (Daley-Placide, n.d.). These changes can place elderly individuals at greater risk for infection, temperature dysregulation, soft tissue injury, and longer recovery from soft tissue injuries.

Aging Changes of the Endocrine System

Due to the complexity of the endocrine system, determining the effects of aging on specific glands beyond atrophy and decreased secretion is difficult. The clinical implications of these changes are uncertain. Hormonal action may be the most apparent change in aging. These changes in function are most apparent in glucose maintenance, reproductive functioning, and calcium metabolism and less clear in adrenal and thyroid function (Daley-Placide, n.d.).

Aging Changes of the Hematologic and Immune Systems

The hematologic and immune systems are affected by aging in multiple ways, which can increase risk of infection and delay recovery from illness. Total body water decreases with age, thus reducing blood volume (Daley-Placide, n.d.). Bone marrow mass decreases and fat in bone marrow increases, so functional reserves of bone marrow are reduced with age (Navaratnarajah & Jackson, 2013). Blood disorders such as anemia, clotting, and bleeding in older adults may also occur at higher rates.

These changes include:

- Impaired macrophage function, blunted response of complement pathway
- Blunted B- and T-cell function
- Thymic involution, which reaches 90% at 60

- Reduced capacity to generate mediators such as TNF-alpha, interleukin-1, and nitric oxide
- Increased autoimmunity (Navaratnarajah & Jackson, 2013)

AGING VERSUS ILLNESS

Caring for the geriatric population requires a precise understanding of aging versus illness. Disorders are the primary source of functional loss in aging (Besdine, 2019). With a change in health status or report of new symptoms, health conditions must first be ruled out before these alterations can be attributed to the aging process (Besdine, 2019). This can be extremely challenging, because elderly patients often have six or more chronic health conditions (Besdine, 2019). As noted earlier, older patients have increased susceptibility to certain conditions such as heart disease, diabetes, and cancer with age, compounding the difficulty in understanding decline related to aging versus disease (Taffet, 2019).

Geriatric Syndromes

Geriatric syndromes are conditions that occur more often in older adults and are a major factor in morbidity and poor outcomes in aging patients (Inouye, Studenski, Tinnetti, & Kuchel, 2007). Generally multifactorial, geriatric syndromes cannot be directly attributed to an organ-based disease and are best evaluated with a comprehensive geriatric examination (Ward, 2019). The Fulmer SPICES tool provides information on six conditions that coincide with geriatrics syndromes such as sleep disturbances, problems with eating and feeding, incontinence, confusion, evidence of falls, and skin breakdown (Brown-O'Hara, 2013). Four risk factors have been proposed as contributory to geriatric syndromes: older age, baseline cognitive impairment, baseline functional impairment, and impaired mobility (Brown-O'Hara, 2013; Inouye et al., 2007).

These syndromes have been presented as a core five: pressure injuries, incontinence, falls, functional decline, and delirium (Brown-O'Hara, 2013). However, other experts have expanded the list to include general skin breakdown, changes in sleep, gait disorders, sensory deficits, weight loss and nutrient imbalances, fatigue, dizziness, and frailty (Health in Aging Foundation, 2017; Ward, 2019). Osteoporosis, anemia, and mild cognitive impairment have also been described as geriatric syndromes (American Society of Clinical Oncology, n.d.). Table 1.1 provides an overview of select syndromes.

KEEPERS OF THE MEANING

An important aspect of caring for aging individuals is remembering to look at aging as a holistic experience. Especially in the Western world, health is synonymous with youth, and aging is viewed in terms of deficits. A different perspective is to look at aging as a complex experience with aging potentially resulting in decline, change, and development (Vaillant & Mukamal, 2001). Holland and Greenstein (2015) discuss the U-bend paradox where well-being is high in early adulthood, hits a nadir in midlife, and then starts climbing again through later life. A positive psychology approach to aging balances the challenges that may come with aging with the growth and increased character resilience that may coincide with older age (Holland & Greenstein, 2015). Older individuals may be "keepers of meaning" when they preserve and share their collected wisdom (Holland & Greenstein, 2015; Nolan & Kadavil, 2003). In addition, older age often brings into sharp focus the values and priorities that matter most to individuals, allowing them to be more present in their lives (Holland & Greenstein, 2015).

TABLE 1.1 Geriatric Syndromes Overview

Syndrome	Description
Urinary incontinence	Urinary continence may be classified as functional, urge, stress, or a combination of categories. This condition can lead to falls, social isolation, and skin breakdown.
Sleep disorders	May be due to physiologic changes in the body, medications, chronic health conditions, pain, decreased mobility, and increased napping during the day.
Delirium	An acute change in condition that primarily affects attention. The most common causes of delirium are illness, medications, and fluid and electrolyte imbalances.
Falls	Falls are a predictor of increased mortality in elderly patients. Falls can result from a host of issues including medication side effects, hydration, nutrition, environmental barriers, balance disorders, muscle weakness, neuromuscular conditions, and sensory disorders.
Weight loss and nutrient imbalances	Weight loss and nutrient imbalances can contribute to other geriatric syndromes such as skin breakdown, frailty, and falls. Weight and nutritional alterations may occur due to taste changes with aging, medication side effects, chronic health conditions, and functional and financial barriers to obtaining food.
Skin breakdown and pressure injuries	Skin breakdown may place patients at greater risk for infection, functional decline, social isolation, decreased well-being, and increased mortality. Factors contributing to skin breakdown and pressure injuries include decreased nutrition, circulatory and dermatologic aging changes, fecal and urinary incontinence, decreased mobility, and chronic health conditions, such as diabetes.
Functional decline	Functional decline occurs as aging individuals are less able to independently carry out personal care and functional activities. This may occur acutely or gradually and may be related to chronic conditions and other geriatric syndromes.
Frailty	Characterized by decreased reserve and resistance to stressors, decline across multiple systems, and increased vulnerability to poor health outcomes. Aging changes, multiple chronic conditions, and other geriatric syndromes contribute to the development of frailty.
Gait disorders	Gait disorders are widely variable in presentation, but can all contribute to falls, decreased mobility, functional decline, skin alterations, and frailty. Gait disorders may occur due to injury, structural defects, or sensory deficits.
Sensory deficits	Sensory deficits such as hearing loss, decreased visual acuity, alterations in smell and taste, and decreased sensation may put geriatric patients at greater risk for injury, nutritional decline, and decreased independence.

(continued)

TABLE 1.1   Geriatric Syndromes Overview (*continued*)

Syndrome	Description
Fatigue	The perception of fatigue is a common issue experienced by aging individuals, and the causes are diverse. Factors such as decreased nutrition, deconditioning, aging changes in the musculoskeletal system, sleep disorders, medication side effects, anemia, and other chronic health conditions all contribute to fatigue.
Dizziness	Dizziness is a vague symptom that ranges from true vertigo to light-headedness. Dizziness may increase fall risk and contribute to functional decline. It may be caused by fluid and electrolyte imbalances, medication side effects, chronic health conditions, sensory deficits, inadequate nutrition, and deconditioning.

Source: Data from American Society of Clinical Oncology. (n.d.). *Geriatric syndromes.* Retrieved from https://www.asco.org/practice-guidelines/cancer-care-initiatives/geriatric-oncology/geriatric-syndromes; Brown-O'Hara, T. (2013). Geriatric syndromes and their implications for nursing. *Nursing, 43*(1), 1–3. doi:10.1097/01.NURSE.0000423097.95416.50; Fried, L. P., Tangen, C. M., Walston, J., Newman, A. B., Hirsch, C., Gottdiener, J., . . . McBurnie, M. A. (2001). Frailty in older adults: Evidence for a phenotype. *The Journals of Gerontology: Series A: Biological Sciences and Medical Sciences, 56*(3), M146–M157. doi:10.1093/gerona/56.3.m146; Health in Aging Foundation. (2017). *A guide to geriatric syndromes.* Retrieved from https://www.healthinaging.org/tools-and-tips/guide-geriatric-syndromes-common-and-often-related-medical-conditions-older-adults; Huang, J. (2018). Delirium. In R. S. Porter (Ed.), *Merck manual professional version.* Kenilworth, NJ: Merck. Retrieved from https://www.merckmanuals.com/professional/neurologic-disorders/delirium-and-dementia/delirium; Inouye, S. K., Studenski, S., Tinetti, M. E., & Kuchel, G. A. (2007). Geriatric syndromes: Clinical, research, & policy implications of a core geriatric concept. *Journal of the American Geriatric Society, 55*(5), 780–791. doi:10.1111/j.1532-5415.2007.01156.x; Kirman, C. N. (2018). What is the mortality rate for pressure injuries (pressure ulcers)? In J. Geibel (Ed.), *Medscape.* Retrieved from https://www.medscape.com/answers/190115-82434/what-is-the-mortality-rate-for-pressure-injuries-pressure-ulcers; Mangram, A., Dzandu, J., Harootunian, G., Zhou, N., Sohn, J., Corneille, M., . . . Johnson, W. G. (2016). Why elderly patients with ground level falls die within 30 days and beyond? *Journal of Gerontology & Geriatric Research, 5*(2), 289. doi:10.4172/2167-7182.1000289

SUMMARY

Aging is a significant life experience, and one that is an inevitable progression of life for geriatric patients. Recognizing the risks related to the aging process, the differences between disorders and aging, and acknowledging the challenges of geriatric syndromes is an essential part of the nurse practitioner role. Additionally, recognizing the holistic experience of aging with both challenges and resilience factors allows nurse practitioners to see their patients fully. Through recognizing and responding to aging issues appropriately, nurse practitioners can be key members of the geriatric healthcare team.

REFERENCES

American Federation for Aging Research. (2011). *Theories of aging.* New York, NY: Author. Retrieved from https://www.afar.org/docs/AFAR_INFOAGING_GUIDE_THEORIES_OF_AGING_2016.pdf

American Society of Clinical Oncology. (n.d.). *Geriatric syndromes.* Retrieved from https://www.asco.org/practice-guidelines/cancer-care-initiatives/geriatric-oncology/geriatric-syndromes

Besdine, R. W. (2019). Physical changes with aging. In R. S. Porter (Ed.), *Merck manual professional version*. Kenilworth, NJ: Merck. Retrieved from https://www.merckmanuals.com/professional/geriatrics/approach-to-the-geriatric-patient/physical-changes-with-aging?query=physical%20changes%20with%20aging

Brown-O'Hara, T. (2013). Geriatric syndromes and their implications for nursing. *Nursing, 43*(1), 1–3. doi:10.1097/01.NURSE.0000423097.95416.50

Chaudhry, S. I., Wang, Y., Gill, T. M., & Krumholz, H. M. (2010). Geriatric conditions and subsequent mortality in older patients with heart failure. *Journal of the American College of Cardiology, 55*(4), 309–316. doi:10.1016/j.jacc.2009.07.066

Daley-Placide, R. (n.d.). Physical changes with aging: Observations regarding senescence [PowerPoint]. University of North Carolina Chapel Hill.

Fried, L. P., Tangen, C. M., Walston, J., Newman, A. B., Hirsch, C., Gottdiener, J., . . . McBurnie, M. A. (2001). Frailty in older adults: Evidence for a phenotype. *The Journals of Gerontology: Series A: Biological Sciences and Medical Sciences, 56*(3), M146–M157. doi:10.1093/gerona/56.3.m146

Health in Aging Foundation. (2017). *A guide to geriatric syndromes*. Retrieved from https://www.healthinaging.org/tools-and-tips/guide-geriatric-syndromes-common-and-often-related-medical-conditions-older-adults

Hjelmborg, J., Iachine, I., Skytthe, A., Vaupel, J., McGue, M., Koskenvuo, M., . . . Christensen, K., (2006). Genetic influence on human lifespan and longevity. *Human Genetics, 119*(3), 312–321. doi:10.1007/s00439-006-0144-y

Holland, J., & Greenstein, M. (2015). Changing how we view aging. *Journal of Geriatric Oncology, 6*(3), 175–177. doi:10.1016/j.jgo.2015.03.002

Huang, J. (2018). Delirium. In R. S. Porter (Ed.), Merck manual professional version. Kenilworth, NJ: Merck. Retrieved from https://www.merckmanuals.com/professional/neurologic-disorders/delirium-and-dementia/delirium

Inouye, S. K., Studenski, S., Tinetti, M. E., & Kuchel, G. A. (2007). Geriatric syndromes: Clinical, research, & policy implications of a core geriatric concept. *Journal of the American Geriatric Society, 55*(5), 780–791. doi:10.1111/j.1532-5415.2007.01156.x

Kirman, C. N. (2018). What is the mortality rate for pressure injuries (pressure ulcers)? In J. Geibel (Ed.), *Medscape*. Retrieved from https://www.medscape.com/answers/190115-82434/what-is-the-mortality-rate-for-pressure-injuries-pressure-ulcers

Mangram, A., Dzandu, J., Harootunian, G., Zhou, N., Sohn, J., Corneille, M., . . . Johnson, W. G. (2016). Why elderly patients with ground level falls die within 30 days and beyond? *Journal of Gerontology & Geriatric Research, 5*(2), 289. doi:10.4172/2167-7182.1000289

Navaratnarajah, A., & Jackson, S. H. D. (2013). The physiology of aging. *Medicine in Older Adults, 41*(1), 5–8. doi:10.1016/j.mpmed.2012.10.009

Nolan, R. E., & Kadavil, N. (2003, October). *Valliant's contribution to research and theory of adult development*. Paper presented at 2003 Midwest Research to Practice Conference in Adult, Continuing, and Community Education, Columbus, OH. Retrieved from https://scholarworks.iupui.edu/bitstream/handle/1805/341/Nolan%20%26%20Kadavil.pdf?sequence=1

Rughwani, N. (2011). Normal anatomic and physiologic changes with aging and related disease outcomes: A refresher. *Mount Sinai Journal of Medicine, 78*, 509–514. doi:10.1002/msj.20271

Sergiev, P. V., Dontsova, O. A., & Berezkin, G. V. (2015). Theories of aging: An ever-evolving field. *Acta Naturae, 7*(1), 9–18. doi:10.32607/20758251-2015-7-1-9-18

Taffet, G. E. (2019). Normal aging. In K. E. Schmader (Ed.), *UpToDate*. Retrieved from https://www.uptodate.com/contents/normal-aging

Vaillant, G. E., & Mukamal, K. (2001). Successful aging. *American Journal of Psychiatry, 158*, 839–847. doi:10.1176/appi.ajp.158.6.839

Ward, K. T. (2019). Comprehensive geriatric assessment. In K. E. Schmader (Ed.), *UpToDate*. Retrieved from https://www.uptodate.com/contents/comprehensive-geriatric-assessment

2 The Examination of the Geriatric Patient

Megan Hebdon

INTRODUCTION

As discussed in Chapter 1, Physiologic Changes That Occur in Geriatric Patients, functional outcomes are of primary importance in the geriatric population. Thus, a comprehensive geriatric assessment is focused on wellness, independence, and physical performance as well as the complexity of multiple chronic health conditions encountered in the elderly population (Gill & Moore, n.d.; Tufts University, 2017). Often, the need for a geriatric assessment is triggered by a decline in an individual's health or functional status (Ward, 2019). The assessment should be broad enough to address the full scope of health concerns but specific enough to address specific patient concerns (Tufts University, 2017).

INTERPROFESSIONAL TEAM

A thorough exam is best performed with an interprofessional team with the goal of coordinated and patient-centered care (Gill & Moore, n.d.; Ward, 2019). The core team usually includes a clinician, nurse, and social worker. Other disciplines, such as physical and occupational therapy, nutrition, pharmacy, psychology and psychiatry, audiology and speech, and podiatry, will be included in the team based on patient need (Ward, 2019). If multiple professions will be involved in the assessment, then a case manager may be helpful to coordinate the process and communicate with the patient and caregivers (Tufts University, 2017).

GOALS OF GERIATRIC EXAM

The goal of a geriatric assessment is to develop a plan of care that will account for medical concerns, functional status, and psychosocial considerations (Gill & Moore, n.d.). The process is systematic, generally including the following six steps: data gathering, team discussion including patient and caregiver, development of a treatment plan, implementation of the plan, assessing response to the plan, and revising the plan as needed (Ward, 2019). The data-gathering process can be guided by the five I's of geriatrics: immobility, intellectual impairments, incontinence, iatrogenic disorders, and instability (Tufts University, 2017). Using these emphases as a guide, nurse practitioners can successfully address areas that might contribute to further decline of their geriatric patients (Tufts University, 2017).

PREPARATION FOR EXAM

A well-conducted geriatric assessment requires preparation to account for environment, communication, patient needs, and patient–provider rapport (AGS, n.d.). Due to the financial and time constraints that accompany a traditional clinic setting, the patient may be directed to do some preparation with paperwork before the appointment. If able, the patient can fill out questionnaires that address his or her functional status, mental health, quality of life, and disease-related symptoms (Elsawy & Higgins, 2011; Tufts University, 2017). This can be time-saving for the clinician; but this may also provide a clue to the patient's functionality and motivation (Elsawy & Higgins, 2011; Tufts University, 2017).

GERIATRIC EXAM
Starting the Exam

The first step in a geriatric assessment is controlling the environment where the assessment will occur. Attention to details such as lighting, noise, and interruptions will allow the assessment to go smoothly while accommodating for any hearing or visual disturbances (Gill & Moore, n.d.). A provider should first introduce himself or herself, address the patient by his or her last name, and ask how the patient would like to be addressed. The provider should face the patient and sit at eye level. Speech should be slow, deliberate, and in a deep tone (Gill & Moore, n.d.). Open-ended questions such as What concerns would you like to address in visit today? allow the patient to tell his or her story. This directs the provider to specific issues affecting the patient's functioning and well-being. When asking questions, adequate time should be provided for the patient to answer. Also, a polite inquiry regarding any hearing or visual deficits will allow the provider to make patient-specific accommodations that will facilitate communication (AGS, n.d.).

Medical History

After opening the visit with preliminary questions, the provider should then conduct a thorough medical history using the available health records, the patient, and family members if present. The provider should always direct questions to the patient but can allow for input from family members. Often, seeing the family as the unit of care will promote goal setting and assessment that is appropriate for the patient's daily living and care priorities (National Consensus Project [NCP], 2013). A comprehensive geriatric assessment will include all the components of a general medical exam; but it will also include focused assessment on areas of particular importance to geriatric patients (Elsawy & Higgins, 2011). Eliciting information regarding past medical history, surgical history, hospitalizations, chronic health conditions, current sensory impairments, medications, allergies, family history, social history, immunization status, diet and exercise activities, daily functioning, and review of symptoms will provide a background to conduct the rest of the assessment (Tufts University, 2017). Much can be learned from simply asking the patient to describe his or her typical day (Besdine, 2016).

Physical Exam

The physical portion of the assessment should include vital signs and a head-to-toe exam (Tufts University, 2017). Special attention should be paid to functional status, nutrition, vision, and hearing in addition to assessment of the body systems. Providers should be aware that a comprehensive assessment may need to be done in two different sessions or with a rest period, depending on patient stamina (Besdine, 2016).

- Functional status can be assessed using assessment tools such as the Katz Index of Independence in Activities of Daily Living and the Lawton Instrumental

Activities of Daily Living scale (AGS, n.d.; Elsawy & Higgins, 2011). As part of the musculoskeletal exam, the timed "Get Up and Go" test is also helpful (AGS, n.d.). Individuals over 75 years are at high risk for hospitalizations or injury-related death due to falls, so inquiry into the presence and frequency of falls should be made. Assessment of balance through the Tinetti Balance and Gait evaluation tool can be helpful in determining a patient's fall risk (Elsawy & Higgins, 2011). In addition to a fall assessment, understanding an individual's risk for fracture with an osteoporosis screening is advised. Women over the age of 65 should be routinely screened and receive treatment, if needed, for osteoporosis (Elsawy & Higgins, 2011).

- Nutritional status can be assessed through biometrics such as height, weight, and body mass index, visual inspection, and historical weight loss. If weight loss or other signs of poor nutritional status are noted, then assessment regarding medical illnesses, psychiatric concerns, functional decline, or financial difficulties should be completed (AGS, n.d.).
- Vision should be assessed by first asking about difficulties with daily tasks such as driving, watching TV, and reading. Then, performance-based screening can be completed with a Snellen chart or by asking the patient to read from a magazine in the clinic. This would be followed by an eye exam with fundoscopy to identify signs of cataracts, glaucoma, macular degeneration, and diabetic retinopathy (AGS, n.d.; Elsawy & Higgins, 2011).
- Conductive and sensorineural hearing loss should be addressed through questions regarding hearing difficulties, visual inspection of the ear canal and tympanic membrane, and the use of an audioscope. If an audioscope is not available within the clinic, the provider can perform the whisper test. Generally, if there is no evidence of cerumen impaction and the patient is noting hearing difficulties, a referral for a hearing screening would be appropriate (AGS, n.d.; Elsawy & Higgins, 2011).
- Assessment of cognition and memory is an essential aspect of the geriatric exam, because of the increased prevalence of Alzheimer's disease in those over the age of 65 as well as the additional risks to individuals posed by cognitive defects such as accidents, delirium, poor treatment adherence, and disability. Many individuals with dementia will not acknowledge the issue (AGS, n.d.). A Mini-Mental State Exam (MMSE) is a quick and efficient way to determine orientation, registration, recall, attention, calculation, language, and visuospatial skills (AGS, n.d.).
- Urinary incontinence should be thoroughly assessed to understand onset, pattern, strategies to address incontinence, and patient's distress related to incontinence. If it is sudden in onset, an infectious or neurologic source should be investigated. If it is long-standing, assessing for functional, stress, urge, or mixed will allow the clinician to determine the need for referral and develop a plan to address incontinence (Ward, 2019).
- Sexual health is a key aspect of any general health exam. Determining sexual preferences, patterns, and use of safe sex practices will help the nurse practitioner determine if sexually transmitted infection (STI) screening is needed. Additionally, screening for sexual dysfunction allows the provider to intervene with referrals, behavioral strategies, and medications to support patients' sexual health needs (Ward, 2019).
- Mood disorders are growing in recognition in the elderly population and can be associated with poorer health outcomes. Asking a simple question regarding feelings of sadness, depression, anxiety or nervousness, withdrawal, or anhedonia can trigger the provider to pursue further evaluation with validated scales such as the Geriatric Depression Scale and Patient Health Questionnaire-9 (PHQ-9) (AGS, n.d.; Ward, 2019).

- Social assessment is key in crafting a plan of care that will promote ongoing function for the patient in the home. This includes assessing the support system, addressing caregiver burden, identifying financial burdens, and watching for signs of elder mistreatment (AGS, n.d.; NCP, 2013).
  - Social support can be assessed through a social history assessing family and friend networks. Some patients may rely on other networks related to their church, work, or community. In addition, asking patients who is available to take care of them if they become sick helps providers and patients recognize the need for referrals to community agencies if there are fewer than two individuals available for help (Ward, 2019).
  - Caregivers of aging individuals may experience fatigue, health issues of their own, and emotional burnout due to the demands of caregiving (National Cancer Institute, 2017). Due to their significant contributions to the daily care of the aging patient, it is imperative that caregivers' needs are fully addressed. Support services and referrals may need to be included for them as well (Ward, 2019).
  - Elder mistreatment is a serious issue that is often underassessed and underreported. Including an assessment tool for this issue may be an effective approach. The Elder Assessment Instrument has seven sections that assess self-reported complaints related to elder abuse, neglect, exploitation, and abandonment (Fulmer, n.d.).
  - Awareness of financial needs related to housing, transportation, insurance coverage, and medication costs is key to ensuring patient safety and well-being while directing referrals to social services and community programs as needed (Tufts University, 2017).
- Substance use screening is important at any age and should be approached without judgment. Aging individuals should be screened for use of alcohol, tobacco products, and illicit drugs and inappropriate use of prescription drugs. Screening, Brief Intervention, and Referral to Treatment (SBIRT) is a user-friendly and effective approach to assessing for substance abuse and providing referrals when needed (Substance Abuse and Mental Health Services Administration-Health Resources and Services Administration Center for Integrated Health Solutions, n.d.). Understanding substance use patterns allows providers to prescribe more safely and evaluate safety concerns for their patients (Besdine, 2019).
- Driving status is a concern that comes up frequently in the geriatric population due to risks to other drivers when an older driver is impaired as well as risk to the older driver with reduced independence if driving privileges are revoked. State laws regarding impaired drivers should be followed. When in doubt, senior driver safety assessment programs may be offered through local communities or healthcare organizations (AGS, n.d.).
- Medication reconciliation and screening for polypharmacy is an important aspect of caring for aging patients. Due to the complexity of multiple chronic conditions and multiple healthcare providers, patients may be on many medications that have interactions or adverse side effects. One of the most effective ways to accomplish this process is by asking patients to bring in all their medications, including over-the-counter medications and herbal supplements (Ward, 2019).
- A key aspect of any patient encounter is sensitivity to culture, beliefs, and spirituality. Patient health concerns may be attenuated or increased due to cultural and religious health practices. Understanding the geriatric patient's perspectives and beliefs regarding health and illness, quality of life, and death and dying is fundamental to shared decision-making with aging and chronic illness (NCP, 2013).

- Goals of care should be discussed, established, or revised with each geriatric evaluation (Ward, 2019). As aging progresses, diseases worsen, or function declines, patients may change their goals of care to emphasize quality of life and supportive care versus cure of disease (Ward, 2019). Advanced directives are a key part of the Annual Medicare Wellness Visit, but many patients continue without these important legal documents and decisions. Discussion with the patient and key family members should occur regarding the patient's wishes at the end of life. There are many valuable resources to support these discussions including My Five Wishes, which allows patients to identify what they value and what should be emphasized at the end of their lives (Aging With Dignity, n.d.). Many states have approved the use of the Physician's Orders for Life-Sustaining Treatment, which is a portable advanced directive that provides more options for managing acute illness at the end of life (National POLST Paradigm, n.d.).
- The physical exam should be a head-to-toe exam with emphasis on areas that are of particular concern to the patient, family, or clinician during initial history taking and review of systems. Table 2.1 provides an overview of the head-to-toe exam.
- Laboratory and diagnostic testing may be considered and ordered, but the clinician should make decisions about this based on patient and family preferences as well as consideration of long-term outcomes (Elsawy & Higgins, 2011). Treatment of conditions such as diabetes, lipid disorders, hypertension, glaucoma, and certain cancers may promote greater well-being and prevent future illnesses. If a patient has an expected survival of more than 5 years, then screening is warranted if the patient is at risk for the disease and would accept treatment (Elsawy & Higgins, 2011).

TABLE 2.1 Geriatric Head-to-Toe Exam: Exam Components and Areas of Concern

Step	Exam Components	Concerns
Intake	Blood pressure, pulse, respirations, temperature, pulse oximetry, height, and weight	Orthostatic hypotension, low heart rate, increased respirations, sudden weight loss, obesity
HEENT	Head, eyes, ears, nose, mouth and throat, neck	Facial asymmetry, temporal artery tenderness, visual acuity, ocular lens opacification, fundoscopic abnormalities, hearing loss, denture fit, mucosal condition, thyroid enlargement or nodules, carotid bruits
Cardiac	Heart, peripheral pulses, venous appearance, edema, capillary refill	Presence of S4, murmurs, pulse deficit, varicosities, swelling, absent or weak pulses, delayed capillary refill

(*continued*)

TABLE 2.1 Geriatric Head-to-Toe Exam: Exam Components and Areas of Concern (*continued*)

Step	Exam Components	Concerns
Chest and pulmonary	Chest and spine structure, lung sounds, patient effort, breast appearance and character	Barrel chest, dorsal kyphosis, increased respiratory effort, crackles or wheezing, breast changes or nodules
Abdomen	Appearance, pain, organ size, aorta, auscultation of bowel sounds	Bulging, masses, organomegaly, point tenderness, hypo/hyperactive bowel sounds, increased abdominal aorta size
Genitourinary and rectum	External structure, internal examination	Vaginal atrophy, bladder/uterine/rectal prolapse, urinary leakage, increased ovarian size, prostate enlargement or nodularity, rectal bleeding
Musculoskeletal	Gait, muscle character and distribution, joint and spine appearance and range of motion	Joint abnormalities or pain, spinal curvature, muscle wasting, vertebral tenderness or decreased range of motion
Neurologic	Cognition, coordination, balance, strength, sensation, cranial nerves	Movement or strength asymmetry, poor cognitive performance, postural sway, tremor, cranial nerve abnormalities, decreased sensation
Skin	Inspection of skin, hair, and nails	Premalignant or malignant lesions, pressure injuries in immobilized patients, bruising (unexplained, consider elder abuse), nail thickness or discoloration, changes in hair distribution or texture

HEENT, head, eyes, ears, nose, and throat; S4, fourth heart sound.

Source: Data from Besdine, R. W. (2019). *Evaluation of the older adult.* In R. S. Porter (Ed.), *Merck manual professional version.* Kenilworth, N.J: Merck. Retrieved from https://www.merckmanuals.com/professional/geriatrics/approach-to-the-geriatric-patient/evaluation-of-the-older-adult; Tufts University. (2017). *Comprehensive geriatric assessment.* Retrieved from http://ocw.tufts.edu/data/42/499797.pdf

Ongoing Evaluation

Following the initial assessment and treatment plan, ongoing evaluation should occur with sensitivity to changes in health status, patient goals of care, availability of social support, and caregiver status. Developing a trusting relationship with the patient and family from the beginning will help promote effective communication regarding patient and family needs (NCP, 2013; Ward, 2019).

Conclusion

The geriatric examination is fundamental to appropriate treatment decisions, early identification of health and safety issues, and ongoing support for the well-being of aging patients. The environment, assessment approach, and decision-making processes should all focus on the goals of function, well-being, and holistic care.

REFERENCES

Aging with Dignity. (n.d.). Five wishes: Advance care planning. Retrieved from https://fivewishes.org/five-wishes/individuals-families/individuals-and-families/advance-care-planning

Besdine, R. W. (2019). Evaluation of the older adult. In R. S. Porter (Ed.), *Merck manual professional version*. Kenilworth, NJ: Merck. Retrieved from https://www.merckmanuals.com/professional/geriatrics/approach-to-the-geriatric-patient/evaluation-of-the-older-adult

Elsawy, B., & Higgins, K. E. (2011). The geriatric assessment. *American Family Physician, 83*(1), 48–56. Retrieved from https://www.aafp.org/afp/2011/0101/p48.html

Fulmer, T. (n.d.). Elder mistreatment assessment. *ConsultGeri*. Retrieved from https://consultgeri.org/try-this/general-assessment/issue-15

Gill, T. M., & Moore, A. A. (n.d.). Assessment of the older adult [PowerPoint]. In K. Blackstone & E. L. Cobbs (Ed,), *Geriatrics Review Syllabus* (5th ed.). Retrieved from https://geriatricscareonline.org/toc/grs-teaching-slides/S001

National Cancer Institute. (2017). *Family caregivers in cancer: Roles and challenges (PDQ)-Health professional version*. Retrieved from https://www.cancer.gov/about-cancer/coping/family-friends/family-caregivers-hp-pdq#section/_4

National Consensus Project. (2013). *Clinical practice guidelines for quality palliative care* (3rd ed.). Retrieved from https://www.nationalcoalitionhpc.org/wp-content/uploads/2017/04/NCP_Clinical_Practice_Guidelines_3rd_Edition.pdf

National POLST Paradigm. (n.d.). About. Retrieved from https://polst.org/about

Substance Abuse and Mental Health Services Administration-Health Resources and Services Administration Center for Integrated Health Solutions. (n.d.). *Screening tools*. Retrieved from https://www.integration.samhsa.gov/clinical-practice/screening-tools

Tufts University. (2017). Comprehensive geriatric assessment. Retrieved from http://ocw.tufts.edu/data/42/499797.pdf

Ward, K. T. (2019). Comprehensive geriatric assessment. In K. E. Schmader (Ed.), *UpToDate*. Retrieved from https://www.uptodate.com/contents/comprehensive-geriatric-assessment

II Introduction to Pharmacokinetics and Pharmacodynamics of the Geriatric Patient

3 Pharmacokinetics/Pharmacodynamics of the Geriatric Patient

Abimbola Farinde

OBJECTIVES
1. Discuss the principles of pharmacokinetics and pharmacokinetics in the geriatric population
2. Examine how drugs undergo pharmacokinetic and pharmacokinetic processes
3. Discuss the mechanism through which drugs work in older adults and produce their desired effects
4. Therapeutic agents that are used in the management/treatment of the geriatric population

INTRODUCTION
The mechanism by which drugs produce their therapeutic effects in older adults requires the principles of pharmacokinetics and pharmacokinetics. With older adults, this mechanism can be significantly altered when compared to younger adults. The ability to understand the impact that older age can have on pharmacokinetics and pharmacodynamics can help shape drug selection and therapeutic outcomes for this sensitive population.

GENERAL PRINCIPLES OF PHARMACOKINETICS
The concepts of pharmacokinetics focus on the study of the absorption, distribution, biotransformation, and excretion of drugs that can change the drug concentration in tissues and fluids (Davis, 2006; Guy, 2011; Moini, 2013). The acronym LADME describes the pharmacokinetic processes that occur once a drug dose is administered and the drug enters the human body (Figure 3.1):

- Liberation is the release of the drug from its formulation.
- Absorption is the movement of the drug from its site of administration into the bloodstream.
- Distribution is when a drug is diffused and is transferred from the intravascular space to the extravascular space.
- Metabolism is the chemical conversion of the drug into compounds.
- Excretion is the removal of the unchanged drug or metabolite.

All of these processes play an integral role in the mechanism of action of a given drug.

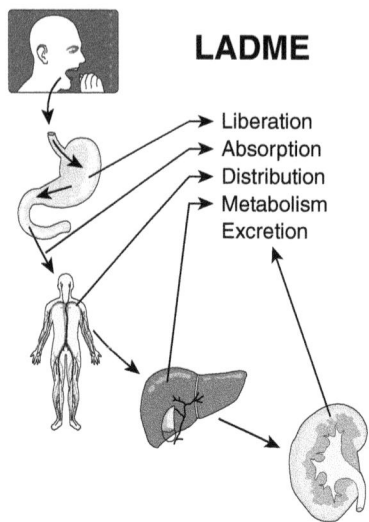

FIGURE 3.1 The LADME scheme.
Source: From RxKinetics. (2009). The LADME scheme. Retrieved from http://www.rxkinetics.com/pktutorial/1_2.html

Once a drug is absorbed, it moves from the site of administration into the bloodstream where it travels throughout the entire body (Guy, 2011). **The process of drug absorption can determine to a great extent how quickly a drug can become available to achieve a desired therapeutic effect.** In general, most drugs that are administered by other routes besides the intravenous route undergo first-order kinetics, where a consistent fraction of the medication is absorbed into the bloodstream (Guy, 2011). Some drugs may have lower absorption rates over an extended period of time while others are much faster, but this can differ from drug to drug. In contrast to first-order kinetics, some drugs do not undergo delayed absorption but rather the immediate availability of the drug in the bloodstream is experienced, which is known as "zero-order kinetics."

After absorption, the next phase is distribution, which is the movement of the drug through the circulatory system and bloodstream to different tissues within the body and eventually to the target area (Turley, 2010). The distribution process can be an uneven one due to variations in tissue binding, blood perfusion, pH, and the permeability of the cell membranes (Le, 2019). There are several factors that can determine how quickly and to what degree a medication can accumulate in any particular tissue. **The distribution equilibrium between the blood and the tissue can be attained more quickly in areas that are richly vascularized.** For instance, the distribution into renal tissue for most drugs can differ from that of adipose tissue. However, drugs can be rapidly distributed to the heart, brain, or liver as a result of the abundance of blood supply (Guy, 2011). The extent to which a drug enters into the tissue can be dependent on blood flow and tissue mass (Le, 2019).

Other compartments that include muscle tissue, fat tissue, and cerebrospinal fluid are less perfused than central compartments (e.g., liver, heart, and kidneys). When drugs enter the blood, they can bind to circulating plasma proteins and they are made pharmacologically inactive as they travel throughout the blood (Turley, 2010). The components of the drug that are not bound to plasma proteins travel through the circulatory system to enter into the body tissues. The drugs that are bound are released by the plasma proteins to maintain an equilibrium of unbound drug in the blood (Turley, 2010). The volume of distribution is the space that the drug is able to occupy, and drugs that tend to be lipid-soluble are able to travel through membranes and into different compartments (Guy, 2011).

The next phase consists of metabolism (or biotransformation), the combination of the chemical and physical changes that can occur within tissues (Moini, 2013). The process of metabolism transforms a drug from its once active form to a less active state where the liver serves as the primary site (Turley, 2010). Drugs can undergo metabolism through the process of oxidation, reduction, hydrolysis, hydration, conjugation, condensation, or isomerization to name a few (Le, 2019). The desired end result of metabolism is to permit the ease of the excretion of the drug once administration occurs (Le, 2019). There are some drugs that undergo rapid metabolism so that the effects of the drug on blood and tissue concentrations are not attained; so the drug must be given through a different route to achieve the desired therapeutic outcome. For example, once administered, nitroglycerin undergoes about a 90% metabolism under first-pass effect when administered through the oral route; hence this is taken into consideration so that an adequate amount is given to remain in the blood to treat a presenting angina (Turley, 2010). The metabolism rates of various drugs can be influenced by a variety of factors, some of which include genetic factors, aging, organ function, and drug interactions. In some individuals, the rate of metabolism can be faster when compared to others, and this can have an impact on the tissue and blood concentration of the drugs.

The last phase of the pharmacokinetic process is excretion, which is an essential process of removing waste products such as inactive drug metabolites from the body and this involves the removal of active drugs that are not necessarily metabolized by the liver (Turley, 2010). The kidneys are recognized as the principle organs for removing drugs that are not metabolized or the by-products of drugs and water-soluble substances. However, there are other drugs that are also involved in the process to a limited degree. Drugs can be excreted through the saliva, sweat, tears, and breast milk, but these can be small in amount. The excretion of drugs is not always an immediate process as this can be determined by whether a drug is bound or unbound to albumin.

PHARMACODYNAMICS

Aside from the altered pharmacokinetics that can occur in the geriatric population, importance is also placed on the changes in pharmacodynamics that can occur as a result of the aging process. Pharmacodynamics is focused on how drugs work within the body and the body's response to the drug (Ruscin & Linnebur, 2018). Having a general understanding of how this occurs within a geriatric patient is vital to the selection of appropriate drug therapies. Whether it is related to associated therapeutic effects or adverse outcomes, the pharmacodynamic process can provide the basics of the elements that can control drug concentration at the site of action (Moini, 2013; Sandhiya & Adithan, 2008).

Drugs have the ability to produce their effects by changing the function of cells and tissues of the body or of an organism (Moini, 2013). The three basic mechanisms by which drugs work include drug/receptor interactions, drug/enzyme interactions, and nonspecific drug interactions (Guy, 2011). A drug/receptor interaction can entail a drug binding to a receptor and the combination allows the drug to act on a target tissue. The binding that occurs can be reversible (drug is able to separate from the receptor) or irreversible (drug cannot separate from receptor) in nature. Many drugs have the ability to produce a desired response.

An agonist is a drug that is able to produce a desired effect by binding to the receptor. However, an antagonist is a drug that has the ability to decrease or remove the physiologic effects of the agonist (Guy, 2011; Moini, 2013). An example of antagonism in action would be the use of several antibiotics that can cause possible antibiotic resistance (Moini, 2013). Pharmacologic antagonism is a process by which the antagonist binds to the receptor and does not allow the biologic effects of an agonist (Guy, 2011). Antagonists can be competitive or noncompetitive in nature. A competitive antagonist binds to the receptor, which can be a reversible process, and a noncompetitive antagonist can irreversibly bind to the receptor (Guy, 2011).

It has been established that drug action can be dependent on many factors, with one being age. In older adults, the pharmacodynamic changes that occur are generally related to those in drug sensitivity and homeostasis. Examples of changes that can occur with drug sensitivity can include responses to benzodiazepines (increased), warfarin (increased), or opioid analgesics (increased) to name a few. The intent of the administration of medication is to achieve a desired physiologic effect or action.

SUMMARY

The effect of a drug can differ in many patients depending on their metabolic rate (Moini, 2013). For older adults, the effect of a comparable drug concentration at the same of action may be more or similar in their younger counterparts (Ruscin & Linnebur, 2018; Teka, Teklay, Ayalew, & Teshome, 2016). In many cases, there is the potential for an increased sensitivity or decreased responsiveness to the effects of the drug in a geriatric individual. The same plasma concentration in a younger patient may be associated with a higher risk of adverse effects in a geriatric individual; so this factor must be taken into consideration when it comes to drug dosing (Midlöv, 2013). In geriatric patients, there is the understanding that there is a trend of greater pharmacodynamic sensitivity, and this must be considered when it comes to drug selection and dosing (Bowie & Slattum, 2007). A clear understanding of pharmacokinetic and pharmacodynamic principles as they relate to older adults can shape the outcomes of therapeutic interventions and whether effects will be adverse or desirable.

REFERENCES

Bowie, M., & Slattum, P. (2007). Pharmacodynamics in older adults: A review. *The American Journal of Geriatric Pharmacotherapy*, 5(3), 263–303. doi:10.1016/j.amjopharm.2007.10.001

Davis, A. (2006). *Medicines by design* (Chapter 1). Retrieved from https://www.nigms.nih.gov/education/Booklets/medicines-by-design/Documents/Booklet-Medicines-by-Design.pdf#page=8

Guy, J. (2011). *Pharmacology for the prehospital professional* (Rev ed.). Burlington, MA: Jones & Bartlett.

Le, J. (2019). Drug distribution to tissues. *MSD manual: Professional version*. Retrieved from http://www.msdmanuals.com/professional/clinical-pharmacology/pharmacokinetics/drug-distribution-to-tissues

Midlöv, P. (2013). Pharmacokinetics and pharmacodynamics in the elderly. *OA Elderly Medicine*, 1(1), 2–5. doi:10.13172/2054-734x-1-1-621

Moini, J. (2013). *Focus on pharmacology: Essentials for health professionals* (2nd ed.). Upper Saddle River, NJ: Prentice Hall.

Ruscin, J. M., & Linnebur, S. (2018). Pharmacodynamics in the elderly. In R. S. Porter (Ed.), *The Merck manual professional version*. Retrieved from http://www.merckmanuals.com/professional/geriatrics/drug-therapy-in-the-elderly/pharmacodynamics-in-the-elderly

RxKinetics. (2009). The LADME scheme. Retrieved from http://www.rxkinetics.com/pktutorial/1_2.html

Sandhiya, S., & Adithan, C. (2008). Drug therapy in elderly. *Journal of the Association of Physicians of India, 56,* 525–531. Retrieved from https://www.researchgate.net/publication/23311191_Drug_therapy_in_elderly

Teka, F., Teklay, G., Ayalew, E., & Teshome, T. (2016). Potential drug–drug interactions among elderly patients admitted to medical ward of Ayder Referral Hospital, Northern Ethiopia: A cross sectional study. *BMC Research Notes, 9,* 431. doi:10.1186/s13104-016-2238-5

Turley, S. (2010). *Understanding pharmacology for health professionals* (4th ed.). Upper Saddle, NJ: Pearson.

4 Aging and Pharmacokinetic Impact

Abimbola Farinde

OBJECTIVES

1. Evaluate the aging process and its impact on pharmacokinetics
2. Discuss specific effects of drugs associated with age-related changes
3. Discuss the formation of a pharmacotherapeutic plan and its effect on therapeutic outcomes in older adults

INTRODUCTION

Pharmacokinetics focuses on how the body is able to process a specific drug once it has been administered (Wooten, 2012). The aging process can involve a progressive decline of the functionality of multiple organs (Klotz, 2008). For individuals who are 65 years of age or older, the basis of pharmacokinetics can be significantly influenced by decline in kidney function rather than the aging process of organs (Aymanns, Keller, Maus, Hartmann, & Czock, 2010). Examples of age-related processes that can occur with diseases in place can include the liver, kidneys, and muscles (Aymanns et al., 2010). The pharmacokinetic changes that occur in any patient are believed to be easier to assess, given the effect that can be had on the plasma concentrations of the drug.

For any given geriatric patient, there can be a variety of disease states, and with these diseases there can be coexisting medication therapies. In the aging patient, the absorption may be decreased, but the absorbed share is generally not impacted (Midlov, 2013). However, with distribution, there can be an observed reduction of the dispersion of hydrophilic drugs and an observed increase in the volume of distribution of lipophilic drugs.

The majority of the information that exists about pharmacokinetics is typically based on studies on younger adults even though it is geriatric patients who will most likely use the medications to manage or treat a variety of conditions (Midlov, 2013). Since the pharmacology of many medications that are used in the geriatric population have not been completely examined, there is great importance placed on making correct predictions regarding pharmacokinetics in this sensitive population, particularly when it comes to the prescribing of medications (Wooten, 2012).

CREATING PHARMACOTHERAPEUTIC PLANS FOR GERIATRIC PATIENTS

The ability to successfully achieve a pharmacotherapeutic plan for a geriatric patient is one that does require a clear understanding of the principles of pharmacokinetics

TABLE 4.1 Age-Related Changes in Pharmacokinetics

Chlormethiazole, labetalol, levodopa, lidocaine, propranolol, verapamil	Increase in bioavailability → F (increase)
Calcium, vitamin B12	Decrease in bioavailability → F (decrease)
Digoxin, edrophonium, ethanol, famotidine, lithium, salicylates	Decrease in volume distribution → V_d (decrease)
Amiodarone, diazepam, fluoroquinolones, daptomycin, linezolid, quinupristin–dalfopristin, teicoplanin, vancomycin, verapamil	Increase in volume of distribution → V_d (increase)
Antipyrine-phenazone	Indicator of cytochrome P450 enzyme activity → Cl (decrease) to 70% by age 70
Acetaminophen-paracetamol, amitriptyline, amlodipine, argatroban, chlormethiazole, citalopram, diltiazem, imipramine, lidocaine, morphine, pethidine, propranolol, rabeprazole, ropinirole, theophylline, verapamil	Decreased hepatic metabolism and reduced drug Cl→ Cl (decrease)
Antiepileptic drugs	Cl (decrease) by 20% to 40%
Lamotrigine	Cl (decrease) → neuropathy, fatigue, and fluid retention
Diazepam, ibuprofen, lorazepam, naproxen, oxaprozin, phenytoin, temazepam, valproate, warfarin	Decreased Cl (free)→ Cl (free) decrease
Docetaxel (oral)	Cl/F (decrease) 1.9 → 1.3 L/min
Lithium, digoxin, hydrochlorothiazide	Renal Cl (decrease)→ Cl (decrease) −36%
Vildagliptin	32% reduced renal Cl→ Cl (decrease)
Enoxaparin	Elevated anti-Xa levels if GFR < 30 ml/min → C_{peak} (increase)
Eptifibatide, tirofiban	Renal Cl (decrease)→ higher bleeding risk
Levofloxacin	T (1/2) increase + 27%
Oxycodone	T(1/2) increase 3.7 hours → 5.7 hours
Cefoxamine	Decreased GFR→T (1/2) increase 1.1 hours→ 2.7 hours

Cl, clearance; GFR, glomerular filtration rate.
Source: From Aymann, C., Keller, F., Maus, S., Hartmann, B., & Czock, D. (2010). Review of pharmacokinetics and pharmacodynamics and the aging kidney. *Clinical Journal of the American Society of Nephrology, 5,* 314–327. doi:10.2215/cjn.03960609

and the impact a drug can have on this population. With the aging process, the gastrointestinal (GI) tract of a geriatric patient can change and this can alter how a specific drug can be absorbed (Table 4.1). A decline in GI blood flow, motility, gastric acid secretion, and an increase in gastric pH can all be witnessed with age, and this can make it more of a challenge for drug absorption. For example, the changes that can be experienced with gastric pH can be the result of drug utilization. **Lipophilic drugs can cause issues in the geriatric patient as the geriatric patient will not be able to clear a fat-soluble drug as quickly as younger counterparts (Hutchinson & Sleeper, 2010).**

SUMMARY

While the majority of information that exists on pharmacokinetics is based on younger individuals, it is important for a clinician to be aware of how these principles can differ with the aging process. The administration of a medication to a younger individual may differ when compared to an older adult due to age-related effects. The aging process can bring about a reduction in physiological effects in older adults or reduced functioning of organs or processes and with this, modifications must be made with drugs that are given to this population.

REFERENCES

Aymann, C., Keller, F., Maus, S., Hartmann, B., & Czock, D. (2010). Review of pharmacokinetics and pharmacodynamics and the aging kidney. *Clinical Journal of the American Society of Nephrology, 5*, 314–327. doi:10.2215/cjn.03960609

Hutchinson, L., & Sleeper, R. (2010). *Fundamentals of geriatric pharmacotherapy* (2nd ed.) Bethesda, MD: American Society of Health-System Pharmacists.

Klotz, U. (2008). Pharmacokinetics and drug metabolism in the elderly. *Drug Metabolism Reviews, 41*(2), 67–76. doi:10.1080/03602530902722679

Midlov, P. (2013) Pharmacokinetics and pharmacodynamics in the elderly. *OA Elderly Medicine, 1*(1), 2–5. doi:10.13172/2054-734x-1-1-621

Wooten, J. (2012). Pharmacotherapy consideration in elderly adults. Medscape. Retrieved from http://www.medscape.com/viewarticle/769412_2

5 Available Guidelines for Therapeutic Drug Selections in Geriatric Patients

Abimbola Farinde

OBJECTIVES
1. Discuss notable guidelines (Beers Criteria and STOPP/START tool) for therapeutic drug selections in geriatric patients
2. Evaluate criteria for specific drug use in geriatric patients
3. Discuss inappropriate drug use and appropriate drug selection in geriatric patients

INTRODUCTION
Given the complexity that can be associated with the geriatric population, it is important for a thorough assessment to be performed when the decision is made to initiate pharmacotherapy (Hutchinson & Sleeper, 2010). With advancing age comes the need for multiple medication use to manage the number of medical conditions that can develop (Halloran, 2013). Medications can be prescribed for a number of reasons in the geriatric population with about one-third of older adults who are 75 years of age or older taking five or more prescribed medications and over a half taking dietary supplements or over-the-counter medications (Hutchinson & Sleeper, 2010). As a result of the potentially inappropriate medication (PIM) uses that can exist with this population, careful consideration must be given with the selection and initiation of medication therapies.

DRUG CRITERIA AND GUIDELINES FOR OLDER ADULTS
Beers Criteria
There are various criteria that have been developed in Canada and the United States, but the most widely used criteria for inappropriate medications are the Beers Criteria. **The first edition of the Beers List was published in 1991 to include medications that should be avoided when treating elderly patients.** To date, the American Geriatrics Society (AGS) Beers Criteria for Potentially Inappropriate Medication Use in Older Adults is recognized as a premier guideline for high-risk drugs that should be avoided in this population, require adjustment for use in this population, or consist of select drug–drug interactions that have been linked to harm in this population (American Geriatrics Society, 2015). The intent of the guideline is to carefully identify medications with risks that can clearly outweigh the benefits of therapy initiation (Halloran, 2013). The prescribing of medication to the geriatric population can present with unique challenges, with a variety of factors contributing to the appropriateness and quality of drug prescribing (Rochon, 2019).

STOPP/START

Another guideline that is utilized to assess the risk versus benefit of medication use in the older population is the Screening Tool of Older Persons' potentially inappropriate Prescriptions/Screening Tool to Alert doctors to the Right Treatment (STOPP/START). The STOPP criteria are designed to be used to avoid medications that can be viewed as potentially inappropriate in this population, which are similar to the Beers Criteria. However, the START criteria are focused on the identification of undertreatment or omissions related to prescribing in elderly patients (Halloran, 2013).

Along with the STOPP criteria, the Assessing Care Of Vulnerable Elders (ACOVE) quality measurement set is used for the comprehensive care of older adults. Alternatively, such implicit approaches as the Assessment of Underutilization of Medication and Medication Appropriateness Index can be used on a case-by-case basis (Shrank, Polinski, & Avorn, 2007).

ADDITIONAL FACTORS REGARDING APPROPRIATE USE OF MEDICATIONS

Some of the factors that should be considered include the avoidance of inappropriate medications, the selection of appropriate use of indicated medications, the monitoring of potential side effects and drug levels when appropriate, and avoidance of drug–drug interactions (Spinewine et al., 2007). The use of PIMs can be associated with negative healthcare outcomes such as falls, confusion, and increased risk of mortality, which is one of the reasons that appropriate medication selections that consider the characteristics of the individual first and foremost are paramount to optimizing drug therapy to achieve desired health outcomes (Rochon, 2019).

SUMMARY

Given the sensitivity of the geriatric population to the administration of medications, the development of guidelines such as the Beers Criteria and STOPP/START tool provides clinicians with guidance on what are viewed as appropriate and inappropriate medications for this population. The Beers Criteria is a widely recognized publication on inappropriate medications and prescribing in older adults while the STOPP/START tool can be used to assess the pros versus cons of administering certain drugs in this unique population. With these resources being utilized, clinicians can move toward making more informed decisions about the care of geriatric patients.

REFERENCES

American Geriatrics Society. (2015). American Geriatrics Society 2015 updated Beers Criteria for potentially inappropriate mediation use in older adults. *Journal of the American Geriatrics Society, 63*(11), 2227–2246. doi:10.1111/jgs.13702

Halloran, L. (2013). Prescribing in the elderly: Practical tips and potential pitfalls. *Journal of Nurse Practitioners, 9*(2), 126–127. doi:10.1016/j.nurpra.2012.11.019

Hutchinson, L., & Sleeper, R. (2010). *Fundamentals of geriatric pharmacotherapy* (2nd ed.). Bethesda, MD: American Society of Health System-Pharmacists.

Rochon, P. (2019). Drug prescribing for older adults. In K. E. Schmader (Ed.), *UpToDate*. Retrieved from https://www.uptodate.com/contents/drug-prescribing-for-older-adults

Shrank, W. H., Polinski, J. M., & Avorn, J. (2007). Quality indicators for medication use in vulnerable elders. *Journal of the American Geriatrics Society, 55*(Suppl. 2), S373–S378. doi:10.1111/j.1532-5415.2007.01345.x

Spinewine, A., Schmader, K. E., Barber, N., Hughes, C., Lapane, K. L., Swine, C., & Hanlon, J. T. (2007). Appropriate prescribing in elderly people: How well can it be measured and optimised. *Lancet, 670*(9582), 173–184. doi:10.1016/S0140-6736(07)61091-5

6

Drug–Drug Interactions

Abimbola Farinde

OBJECTIVES

1. Discuss notable drug–drug interactions (DDIs) that can occur in older adults
2. Discuss potential adverse effects or drug effects that can occur in older adults with the use of specific medications
3. Review common drug interactions that may occur in older adults

INTRODUCTION

Drug-related problems that include drug interactions are considered to be a common occurrence in older adults as the various morbidities of older adults can lead to the need for multiple medications (Hanlon & Schmader, 2005). Many hospital admissions in this sensitive patient population can result from drug toxicity with the administration of a combination of drugs that can cause DDIs (Juurlink, Mamdani, Koop, Laupacis, & Redelmeier, 2003). DDIs are considered to be preventable causes of morbidity and mortality, but the associated consequences may not be well understood by the general public or some within the medical community (Juurlink, Koop, Laupacis, & Redelmeier, 2016). They can occur when one drug changes the absorption character of another drug (Delafuente, 2003). In pharmacokinetics DDI, one DDI, one drug has the ability to influence the absorption, distribution, metabolism, and/or excretion of another drug (Hanlon & Schmader, 2005). **The probability of a DDI increases with the presence of polypharmacy, and a change in pharmacokinetics can contribute to this occurrence.**

While the combination of therapies is typically used to achieve improved therapeutic outcomes, in the geriatric population, this can potentially lead to life-threatening adverse drug reactions (ADRs) or produce a change in the effectiveness of the drugs (Goren, Demirkapu, Acet, Cali, & Oglu, 2017). When a drug interaction occurs, the outcome can either prove to be positive or undesirable (Kondo & Blaschke, 1989).

DDIs COMMON IN OLDER ADULTS

The geriatric population is considered to be a special population as they can differ from their younger adult counterparts in several ways, with one including their vulnerability to DDIs and associated ADRs, which can be the result of many chronic medical conditions that may require multiple drug therapies. In the older population, DDIs are more likely attributed to the use of multiple medications. For example, until 1995, there were only a few oral hypoglycemic agents on the market for diabetes mellitus, but to date this has increased to include several other medication classes that may need to be used in combination with other drugs (Delafuente, 2003). Some of the more common drug classes that can be associated with DDIs that can lead to adverse events include antipsychotics or warfarin therapy. Additional examples of drug interactions that can occur in the geriatric population are listed in Table 6.1.

In the geriatric population, the changes that can occur in the pharmacokinetic properties of drugs can lead to ADRs, and the pharmacodynamics of DDIs can achieve additive, synergistic, or antagonistic effects; the presence of multiple drugs being taken can increase this risk (Goren et al., 2017; Rochon, 2019). For example, the combination of warfarin and nonselective anti-inflammatory drugs can increase the risk of bleeding or the increased risk of digoxin toxicity when combined with clarithromycin (Rochon, 2019).

The development of DDIs among the geriatric population can be viewed by some within the medical community as a common occurrence that can be attributed to inappropriate medication selection and prescribing patterns. The presence of DDIs can be viewed as significant adverse outcomes, and this high risk can be associated with age-related changes in pharmacokinetics or pharmacodynamics.

SUMMARY

In order to effectively reduce the prevalence of potentially inappropriate prescribing, it is important to evaluate the many factors that may be associated with this practice, which can include condition of the patient, prescriber factors, and the work-environment factor (Spinewine et al., 2007). Drug interactions have the ability to reduce the effectiveness of a given drug or can be life-threatening if not immediately identified and addressed. Steps must be taken to ensure that drug interactions are not overlooked in the geriatric population during initiation of drugs or addition of new drugs to the current regimen.

TABLE 6.1 Drug Interactions in the Geriatric Population

Drug Interaction Pair	Drug Toxicity
Continuous added medication	Adverse event
Glyburide trimethoprim–sulfamethoxazole	Hypoglycemia
ACEIs/Angiotensin receptor blockers (ARBs), trimethoprim-sulfamethoxazole	Hyperkalemia
CCBS, macrolide antibiotics Examples: verapamil, diltiazem, nifedipine amlodipine	Hypotension
Spironolactone trimethoprim–sulfamethoxazole/ nitrofurantoin	Hyperkalemia
Warfarin–ciprofloxacin	Hemorrhagic complications

ACEI, angiotensin-converting enzyme inhibitor; ARB, angiotensin receptor blocker; CCBs, calcium channel blockers.

Source: Adapted from Institute of Safe Medication Practices Canada. (2015). Drug–drug interactions in the geriatric patient. Retrieved from https://www.ismp-canada.org/download/DDI/Drug-drug_Interactions_in_the_Geriatric_Population_Summary_Chart.pdf. Reprinted with permission of ISMP Canada.

REFERENCES

Delafuente, J. (2003). Understanding and preventing drug interactions in elderly patients. *Critical Reviews in Oncology/Hematology, 48*(2), 133–143. doi:10.1016/j.critrevonc.2003.04.004

Goren, Z., Demirkapu, M., Acet, G., Cali, S., & Oglu, M. (2017). Potential drug-drug interactions among prescriptions for elderly patients in primary health care. *Turkish Journal of Medical Sciences, 47*, 47–54. doi:10.3906/sag-1509-89

Hanlon, J., & Schmader, K. (2005). Drug-drug interactions in older adults: Which ones matter? *The American Journal of Geriatric Pharmacotherapy, 3*(2), 61–63. doi:10.1016/s1543-5946(05)00030-9

Institute of Safe Medication Practices Canada. (2015). Drug–drug interactions in the geriatric patient. Retrieved from https://www.ismp-canada.org/download/DDI/Drug-drug_Interactions_in_the_Geriatric_Population_Summary_Chart.pdf

Juurlink, D. N., Koop, M. M., Laupacis, A., & Redelmeier, D. A. (2016). *Drug-drug interactions among elderly patients hospitalized for drug toxicity.* Toronto, ON, Canada: Sunnybrook and Women's College Health Sciences Centre. Retrieved from http://biostat.jhsph.edu/courses/bio624/misc/JAMA%20_Example1652.pdf

Juurlink, D. N., Mamdani, M., Koop, A., Laupacis, A., & Redelmeier, D. (2003). Drug-drug interactions among elderly patients hospitalized for drug toxicity. *Journal of American Medical Association, 289*, 1652–1658. doi:10.1001/jama.289.13.1652

Kondo, J. J. L., & Blaschke, T. F. (1989). Drug-drug interactions in geriatric patients. In D. Platt (Ed.), *Gerontology* (pp. 257–269). Berlin, Heidelberg: Springer-Verlag.

Rochon, P. (2019). Drug prescribing for older adults. In K. E. Schmader (Ed.), *UpToDate*. Retrieved from https://www.uptodate.com/contents/drug-prescribing-for-older-adults

Spinewine, A., Schmader, K. E., Barber, N., Hughes, C., Lapane, K. L., Swine, C., & Hanlon, J. T. (2007). Appropriate prescribing in elderly people: How well can it be measured and optimized. *Lancet, 370*(9582), 173–184. doi:10.1016/S0140-6736(07)61091-5

7 Drug–Food Interactions

Abimbola Farinde

OBJECTIVES
1. Discuss notable drug–food interactions that can occur in older adults
2. Examine the severity of drug–food interactions and how this can be addressed

INTRODUCTION
Older adults are known to comprise only about 13% of the population but account for about 34% and 30% of prescription and all over-the-counter (OTC) drugs, respectively, in the United States (Bareuther, 2008). The physiological changes that can occur with the aging process can impact absorption, metabolism, distribution, and excretion of drug as well as food (Bareuther, 2008). Compared to drug–drug interactions, the potential effects of food on the action of drugs may receive less attention but it requires the same level of awareness (Witkamp, 2009). There are a number of drug–food interactions that may occur, but the most significant interactions that affect older adults should be addressed to prevent potentially adverse or even deadly outcomes.

NOTABLE INTERACTIONS
Warfarin and Vitamin K
For instance, the combination of warfarin with high concentrations of vitamin K (e.g., kale, spinach, Brussels sprouts, asparagus) can decrease the ability of warfarin to effectively treat and prevent blood clots. When on warfarin therapy, a geriatric patient should be counseled on the importance of maintaining a consistent intake of vitamin K-containing foods and minimal intake of those foods that are rich in vitamin K.

Oral Diabetic Agents and Alcohol
Another drug–food interaction that both providers and geriatric patients should be aware of involves the combination of oral diabetic agents or insulin therapy with alcohol. This combination can lead to hypoglycemia (sweating, trembling, intense hunger, or confusion) or decreased blood sugar, with alcohol extending the effect of the oral hypoglycemic agent or insulin (Bareuther, 2008). This interaction can be minimized, with approval from physicians, with alcoholic beverages being administered during meals or with a snack. For any geriatric patient who is initiated on an insulin or oral hypoglycemic agent, measures must be taken to identify possible interactions that can occur with alcohol.

Digoxin and Dietary Fiber

The use of digoxin coupled with dietary fiber agents can potentially decrease the absorption or effectiveness of digoxin. Digoxin is designed to aid with the strengthening of the heart muscle and assist with the removal of fluids from the body tissues. Prior to and during the course of treatment with digoxin, the use of dietary fiber should be evaluated for any adverse effects on digoxin therapy.

Reductase Inhibitors/Statins and Grapefruit Juice

The concurrent use of HMG CO-A reductase (3-hydroxy-3-methyl-glutaryl-coenzyme A reductase) inhibitors or statins such as simvastatin, lovastatin, atorvastatin, and pravastatin with grapefruit juice can produce an increase in the amount of statins in the bloodstream to produce toxic effects.

Calcium Channel Blockers and Grapefruit Juice

The combination of calcium channel blockers (e.g., amlodipine, diltiazem) and grapefruit juice (even a small amount) can cause high levels of calcium channel blockers and potentially serious adverse effects. Another interaction that can occur with the use of grapefruit with erectile dysfunction drugs (e.g., sildenafil, tadalafil, and vardenafil) can also increase the blood levels of these drugs and produce headache symptoms or nearly fatal conditions.

Acetaminophen and Alcohol

Acetaminophen is one of the most commonly used OTC pain relievers, and its combination with alcohol can lead to significant problems in geriatric adults because it can increase liver toxicity. With age, the ability of the liver to effectively remove drugs can decrease, and this can be particularly problematic for older adults.

Antibiotics and Dairy Products

The use of antibiotics to treat acute or chronic infections is the mainstay of care for geriatric patients. The concurrent use of antibiotics such as tetracycline and ciprofloxacin with dairy products such as yogurt, cheese, and milk can minimize the absorption and thus decrease the effectiveness of these antibiotics. The resultant interaction comes from the binding of calcium to the antibiotics in the stomach and the upper small intestines to form an insoluble compound. In order to avoid this effect, the recommendation is to take the antibiotics either 1 hour before or 2 hours after the meal. It is not generally recommended to not drink the milk or be exposed to other dairy products with all antibiotics; there are specific instructions that can accompany the administration of most antibiotics.

Antithyroid Drugs and Foods Rich in Iodine

Another potential drug–food interaction that a clinician should be mindful of when working with the geriatric population is the use of antithyroid drugs and foods that are rich in iodine can lead to a decrease in the remission rate for hyperthyroidism (Bareuther, 2008). In the event that a patient has a high-iodine diet, it would be important to adjust the dose of an antithyroid drug to account for this.

Monoamine Oxidase Inhibitors and Smoked Food

A commonly described drug–food interaction but may not be observed as frequently in recent years is the combination of monoamine oxidase inhibitors (e.g., selegiline, isocarboxazid, tranylcypromine) and tyramine containing foods such as smoked fish or cheeses, which can cause hypertensive crisis (extremely high blood pressure). For any patient who is initiated on a monoamine oxidase inhibitor, careful consideration must be given to avoid the consumption of tyramine-containing foods due to this serious adverse effect.

SUMMARY

Similar to the potential for drug–drug interaction that can occur in older adults, the development of drug–food interaction must be assessed with any older adult. Although it is not possible for every single interaction to be identified or avoided, the most significant interactions should be recognized by any clinician who wishes to prescribe to an older adult. Drug–food interactions have the potential to pose serious health risks or even life-threatening outcomes in older adults; so careful monitoring and understanding of these potential effects is imperative to prevent or minimize negative outcomes.

REFERENCES

Bareuther, C. M. (2008). Dangerous food-drug interactions. *Aging Well*, 1(4). Retrieved from https://www.todaysgeriatricmedicine.com/archive/101308pe.shtml

Witkamp, R. (2009). Food–drug interactions in older people. In M. Raats, L. de Groot, & W. van Staveren (Eds.), *Food for the ageing population* (pp. 458–477). Cambridge, United Kingdom: Woodhead. doi:10.1533/9781845695484.2.458

8 Common Medications for Comorbidities and Side Effects

Abimbola Farinde

OBJECTIVES
1. Identify the most commonly used medications for comorbidities and side effects
2. Discuss the impact of chronic conditions on the decision to initiate medication
3. Evaluate the most notable drug classes clinicians should be aware of in prescribing for older adults

INTRODUCTION
The aging process is considered to be a complex process that can be associated with physical, biological, psychological, sociological, and behavioral changes (Moini, 2013). Older adults can typically present with multiple medical conditions, and the coexistence of these conditions can lead to challenges when it comes to diagnosis, treatment, and the natural progression of the individual health conditions in older adults (Karlamangla et al., 2007). Along with these changes, there are other changes that may not be visible but can also have a notable impact on their health. These can be cognitive in nature and can influence whether or not the individual remembers to take medications to manage co-occurring conditions.

CO-OCCURRING CHRONIC CONDITIONS IN THE GERIATRIC POPULATION
For healthcare practitioners who treat geriatric patients, it is important to be aware of these issues and understand the proper steps toward treatment. Chronic conditions exist among the older population with approximately 80% of older adults having at least one and at least half of this population having two (Shah & Hajjar, 2012). Examples of chronic conditions that can be identified in the geriatric population include heart disease, arthritis, diabetes, and cancer, which may require several medications to achieve optimal management.

When evaluating these conditions, heart disease and cancer are considered to be the two leading causes of death among individuals who are 65 years of age or older (Moini, 2013). The incidence of multimorbidity in the older population is estimated to range from 55% to 98% (Nobili, Garattini, & Mannucci, 2011). More than one-third of all deaths in this population are attributed to heart disease and cancer is associated with one-fifth. In the presence of these conditions, management through the use of medication therapies or regimens has become a standard of practice, and this may contribute to polypharmacy. In this case, the appropriateness of medication use should be identified prior to the initiation of therapy. The degree of appropriateness is particularly important for diseases such as heart failure and diabetes, which may require multiple therapies for proper management of these various disease states (Nobili et al., 2011).

MEDICATIONS FOR CO-OCCURRING CHRONIC CONDITIONS IN THE GERIATRIC POPULATION

For the use of medications in the geriatric population, all prescribers should be mindful of the effects of common but specific drugs and classes on older adults. The classes of agents include the vaccines for various infectious diseases, antibiotics in the treatment of pneumonia and other infections, antihypertensives, antihyperglycemic agents, and medications to control pain (Ruscin & Linnebur, 2018).

In addition, medication classes such as aminoglycosides, fluoroquinolones, penicillins, angiotensin-converting enzyme (ACE) inhibitors, and beta-blockers have the ability to decrease renal clearance in geriatric patients; so dosing adjustments must be taken into consideration prior to the administration of any of these medications. On the other hand, calcium channel blockers, phenytoin, lidocaine, theophylline, celecoxib, and isoniazid, have the ability to decrease hepatic clearance in older adults; so consideration must be given when it comes to possible initiation or avoidance of these medications in a specific patient case. Any clinician who is considering medication initiation in any geriatric patient should conduct a close evaluation of co-occurring conditions to determine which medications are appropriate and may pose serious adverse effects.

SUMMARY

Older adults can potentially present with a myriad of chronic conditions, and these conditions can determine what medications may or may not be prescribed. The determination of the appropriateness of drug therapy in an older adult can be paramount when it comes to achieving desired therapeutic outcomes. A thorough assessment should be performed prior to the initiation of therapy, and there should be ongoing monitoring of effect with the continuation of therapy. The potential risks versus benefits of the initiation of therapy must be weighed, and if risks ever exceed benefits, the discontinuation of therapy must be considered.

REFERENCES

Karlamangla, A., Tinetti, M., Guralnik, J., Studenski, S., Wetle, T., & Reuben, D. (2007). Comorbidity: The ultimate geriatric syndrome. *Journal of Gerontology Series A: Biological Sciences and Medical Sciences, 62*(3), 296–300. doi:10.1093/gerona/62.3.296

Moini, J. (2013). *Focus on pharmacology: Essentials for health professionals* (2nd ed.). Upper Saddle River, NJ: Prentice Hall.

Nobili, A., Garattini, S., & Mannucci, P. (2011). Multiple diseases and polypharmacy in the elderly: Challenges for the internist of the third millennium. *Journal of Comorbidity, 1*, 28–44. Retrieved from https://www.ncbi.nlm.nih.gov/pmc/articles/PMC5556419

Ruscin, J. M., & Linnebur, S. A. (2018). Aging and drugs. *The Merck manual consumer version*. Retrieved from http://www.merckmanuals.com/home/older-people%E2%80%99s-health-issues/aging-and-drugs/aging-and-drugs

Shah, B., & Hajjar, E. (2012). Polypharmacy, adverse drug reactions, and geriatric syndromes. *Clinics in Geriatric Medicine, 28*, 173–186. doi:10.1016/j.cger.2012.01.002

9 Available Drug Therapies Utilized in Geriatric Patients

Abimbola Farinde

OBJECTIVES

1. Evaluate the currently available drug therapies that are prescribed in geriatric patients
2. Assess the potential therapeutic effect and adverse effects that can arise from the specific drug classes
3. Discuss what to evaluate when determining appropriateness of initiating medications in geriatric patients

INTRODUCTION

In the geriatric population, a myriad of medications can be utilized to manage or treat a variety of disease states or existing conditions. The ability to effectively optimize drug therapy is an essential component of caring for an older adult. When it comes to prescribing medications in this population, the process can be viewed as a complex one that can include elements of determining the drug's indication, determining the type of drug, the dosage, frequency, formulation, and continuous monitoring for efficacy and toxicity.

When approaching geriatric medicine, there are basic principles that should be adhered to in order to achieve optimal therapeutic outcomes:

- Avoidance of unsafe medications
- The recognition of worsening condition with medications
- The use of evidence-based medicine to guide first-line therapies
- Drug therapy should be specific to the individual (Akhtar, 2018)

AVOIDING ADVERSE DRUG EFFECTS

A goal of initiating drug therapies in the geriatric population is to seek to avoid adverse drug effects that can become a consequence of inappropriate drug prescribing (Rochon, 2019). The drug therapies that are utilized in geriatric patients can encompass prescriptions, over-the-counter medications, and herbal preparations. As aging can be associated with a variety of physiological changes and multiple disease states such as diabetes, hypertension, arthritis, and high cholesterol to name a few, the responses to drug selections may be altered. This change must be factored when considering the use of drug classes such as nonsteroidal anti-inflammatory drugs, benzodiazepines, or opioids. Table 9.1 lists some of the commonly encountered drugs in older adults and the potential adverse effects that can be experienced.

TABLE 9.1 Commonly Used Drugs and Their Adverse Effects in Older Adults

Drugs	Adverse Effects
First-generation antihistamines	
Promethazine, hydroxyzine	
Low potent antipsychotics	
Chlorpromazine	Strong anticholinergic and sedative effect
Prochlorperazine	Extrapyramidal and orthostatic adverse events
Long-acting benzodiazepines	
Nitrazepam	Long half-life resulting in prolonged sedation, causing falls and fractures
Flunitrazepam	
Analgesics	
Pethidine	Causes convulsions and renal failure
Propoxyphene	
Combination of NSAID with warfarin	Increases GI bleeding
ACE inhibitor	Renal failure
SSRI	Increases GI bleeding
Diuretics	Reduces the effect of diuretics

ACE, angiotensin-converting enzyme; GI, gastrointestinal; NSAID, nonsteroidal anti-inflammatory drug; SSRI, selective serotonin reuptake inhibitor.

Antihistamines

Drugs that possess antihistaminergic properties have the potential to cause sedative and anticholinergic effects. The first-generation antihistamines have low receptor specificity and can interact with both peripheral and central histamine receptors. This action can lead to central nervous system effects that along with sedation include drowsiness, fatigue, cognitive decline, and a loss of coordination (Coggins, 2017). Additionally, the muscarinic receptor antagonist effects of the antihistamines can cause anticholinergic side effects that include urinary retention, dry mouth, blurry vision, or constipation (Coggins, 2017).

Benzodiazepines

Some benzodiazepines (e.g., diazepam) have active metabolites, which can remain in the system and cause problems for older patients. Geriatric patients with liver impairments can have problems with eliminating long-acting benzodiazepines, and this can produce side effects such as confusion or gait disturbances. The use of short-acting benzodiazepines (triazolam) is typically preferred for insomnia as they can produce less sedation or drowsiness. Prior to the initiation of benzodiazepines, nonpharmacological approaches such as sleep restriction and cognitive behavioral therapy should be applied and should have demonstrated failure (Markota, Rummans, Bostwick, & Lapid, 2016).

CHALLENGES SPECIFIC TO INITIATING DRUG THERAPIES IN GERIATRIC PATIENTS

A challenge with initiating drug therapies in geriatric patients can be the underrepresentation of this population in randomized clinical trials. It can be difficult to select beneficial treatments with the fewest risks. For any commonly used drug in the geriatric patient regardless of the history of use, it is always important to evaluate the potential for adverse effects and adjust therapy accordingly to the patient case. As a healthcare professional, it becomes a standard of practice to become cognizant of these effects and take them into consideration prior to the initiation of any therapeutic agent.

SUMMARY

The geriatric patient population represents a complex one, and in order to provide effective and optimal treatment, a clinician must be aware of the pharmacodynamic properties that make them distinct from their younger counterparts. Whereas pharmacokinetics focuses on the absorption, distribution, distribution, biotransformation, and excretion of drugs, pharmacodynamics focuses on how these drugs will react once they are inside the human body. Both of these factors must be considered when it comes to the selection and subsequent dosing of a drug in a geriatric patient. The aging process can also play an important role when it comes to drug selection. The diminished capacities of liver and kidney function decrease in gastrointestinal blood flow, motility, and gastric acid secretion can be observed in older adults; so this has the potential to impact the therapeutic outcomes of medications that are given to this population. Drug-related problems can occur in older adults, and consideration must be given for potential drug–drug interactions as well as drug–food interactions. Ultimately, the decision to initiate any given drug in a geriatric individual can entail a number of factors, but striving to achieve optimal therapeutic outcomes while minimizing the potential for adverse effects is a key component to treating this unique patient population.

REFERENCES

Akhtar, S. (2018). Pharmacological considerations in the elderly. *Current Opinion in Anesthesiology, 31*(1), 11–18. doi:10.1097/ACO.0000000000000544

Coggins, M. (2017). Antihistamine risks. *Aging Well, 6*(2), 6. Retrieved from http://www.todaysgeriatricmedicine.com/archive/0313p6.shtml

Markota, M. M., Rummans, T., Bostwick, J., & Lapid, M. (2016). Benzodiazepines use in older adults: Dangers, management, and alternative therapies. *Mayo Clinic Proceedings, 91*(1), 1632–1639. doi:10.1016/j.mayocp.2016.07.024

Rochon, P. (2019). Drug prescribing for older adults. In K. E. Schmader (Ed.), *UpToDate*. Retrieved from https://www.uptodate.com/contents/drug-prescribing-for-older-adults

III Guidelines for Dosing Geriatric Patients by Disorders/Body Systems

10 Guidelines for Dosing Geriatric Patients

Abimbola Farinde

OBJECTIVES
1. Discuss the complexities that might exist with dosing geriatric patients
2. Review glomerular filtration rate (GFR) and renal dosing
3. Analyze drugs or drug classes to avoid in those with chronic kidney disease (CKD)
4. Discuss clinician awareness of how psychological changes can impact medication selection and dosing in geriatric patients

INTRODUCTION
The geriatric population represents a unique group that can present with a myriad of conditions and disease states. According to the U.S. Census Bureau, it is reported that during the 20th century, the number of persons aged 65 or older jumped by a factor of 11. By 2050, as many as 1 in 5 Americans could be older adults (United States Census Bureau, 2011). In some cases, a geriatric patient can present with a combination of conditions all at once. Older adults are known to have a greater prevalence of chronic and multiple illnesses compared to other age groups as well as physiological changes (decreased volume of distribution, slow metabolism, and increased drug sensitivity) that can be associated with aging, which may present as several illnesses (Akhar & Ramani, 2015; Milton, 2008). With the degree of complexity that exists with this patient population, there comes the need for a comprehensive assessment whenever the decision is made to initiate most medications. Geriatric patients typically can present with a variety of diseases and conditions that require the administration of a variety of medications for proper management of symptoms and overall patient condition. Additionally, with the higher prevalence of chronic illnesses coupled with physiological changes associated with the aging process, all of these factors should be taken into consideration when selecting a specific dosage of a given medication for a geriatric patient (Tidy, 2014). However, these medications can at times be prescribed in inappropriate or even unsafe doses. Given that more than 90% of individuals who are 65 years of age or older use one medication per week, there is the potential for inappropriate medication prescribing to take place (Gurwitz, 2003). There are studies that have indicated that two-thirds of older patients can receive high doses of drugs that are renally cleared, but to a larger extent this may be due to a lack of awareness of the elements and management of CKD (Hanlon et al., 2009). The use of the GFR has been linked to renal drug elimination, which can prove to be useful in determining dosage adjustments (Olyaei & Bennet, 2009). Most drugs and their associated metabolites can be removed renally through glomerular filtration. In those patients

with CKD, there should be an emphasis on a thorough patient assessment to reduce the likelihood of adverse events that can be associated with the administration of certain medications (Lassiter, Bennett, & Olyaei, 2013). The cumulative incidence of adverse drug reactions that can be observed in patients with kidney disease is about three- to tenfold higher in comparison to those without kidney disease (Olyaei & Bennett, 2009).

DRUG CLASS CONSIDERATIONS

Given the potential adverse outcomes that can result from a number of medications that can be given to geriatric patients, it is important for clinicians to be mindful of the most common ones. There are specific drug classes that should be used with caution or completely avoided in patients with CKD due to the potential for toxicity. Table 10.1 lists classes of drugs that should be considered with caution or potentially avoided in geriatric patients due to possible negative effects that can result from therapy.

The ability to dose and prescribe medications in this special population can present specific challenges, and this must be taken into consideration by every prescriber when making the final decision to initiate therapy. Absolute care must be taken with drug dosages, given the pharmacokinetic/pharmacodynamic parameters that can come into play with this population. For example, an older adult can present with an increased volume of distribution, decreased drug clearance due to decline in renal function, or increasing age can lead to more sensitivity to specific drugs, which all must be taken into consideration (Rochon, 2019). The number of prescriptions can

TABLE 10.1 Agents to Be Avoided or Used With Caution in Patients With CKD

Class	Examples
Antibiotics	Aminoglycosides, vancomycin, sulfamethoxazole
Antifungals	Amphotericin B
Antivirals	Foscarnet, indinavir, cidofovir
Anticoagulants	Low molecular weight heparins, warfarin
Cardiac drugs	Digoxin, sotalol, ACE-I, ARB, DRIs
Opioids	Morphine, meperidine, propoxyphene
Psychotropics/anticonvulsants	Amisulpride, gabapentin, lithium, levetiracetam, topiramate, vigabatrin
Hypoglycemic drugs	Metformin, glyburide, insulin
Drugs for gout	Allopurinol, colchicine
Others	Methotrexate, penicillamine, nonsteroidal anti-inflammatory drugs

ACE-I, angiotensin-converting enzyme inhibitor; ARB, angiotensin II receptor blocker; CKD, chronic kidney disease; DRI, direct renin inhibitor.

Source: From Olyaei, A., & Bennet, W. (2009). Drug dosing and renal toxicity in the elderly patient. In American Society of Nephrology (Ed.), *Geriatric nephrology curriculum*. Washington, DC: Editor. Retrieved from https://www.asn-online.org/education/distancelearning/curricula/geriatrics/Chapter9.pdf

be significantly higher in patients with CKD, and in the geriatric population these newly identified adverse drug reactions can be viewed as morbidity related to the aging process (Olyaei & Bennet, 2009; Snowden, 2008). One of the most notable pharmacokinetic changes that can be observed with older age is the reduction in the excretory capacity of the kidney, but the rate of decline of drug metabolism can be less significant (Turnheim, 1998; Nygaard, Nalik, Ruths, & Kruger, 2004). In most cases, a prescriber will come across lists of agents that are to be avoided or used with extreme caution in older patients. Along with these, there are also efforts to identify the potential for adverse effects and to work to reduce the risk of initiating those medications that have the potential to cause harm. The practice of inappropriate drug prescribing in the geriatric population has become an observed occurrence, because they often take a large number of medications (Zhan et al., 2001). This practice increases the chances of adverse events but this can be minimized through the use of formularies, appropriate dosages, and use of guidelines specific to older patients (Milton, 2008). The guidelines that suggest the use of as few prescribers as possible are evidence based (Green, Hawley, & Rask, 2007). Some examples of recommendations include the presence of a regular medication review and the patient also agreeing with any changes that are made to the regimen. There should be a continuous effort to discontinue any medication regimen that is not indicated based on the patient's case. Prescribers should also initiate only new drug therapies that have clear indications or valid reasons for initiation in an older adult (Green et al., 2007). Periodically, a review of drug regimens and associated indications should be performed by prescribers as a means of continuing medications that are warranted or discontinuing medications that are not needed. A medication should always seek to match a diagnosis or therapeutic indication (Bushardt, Massey, Simpson, Ariail, & Simpson, 2008).

Additionally, if possible, there should be the avoidance of drugs that are known to cause harmful effects in elderly patients, and the reduction of the dosages of these medications should be made whenever considered appropriate (Green et al., 2007; Milton, 2008). When prescribing and dosing these medications, it is important to strive to limit the number of prescribers who are on the patient's case if at all possible. This strategy can minimize incidences of polypharmacy or overprescribing habits that can lead to irreversible outcomes. The national service framework designated for older adults recommends the performance of regular medication review, particularly in those taking four or more drugs, not only to assess dosage and indication but also the evaluation of appropriateness of use. While the dosing criteria should not seek to take the place of clinical judgment, they should be used as guidance for care in order to reduce dosing and duration of inappropriately prescribed medications to work toward improving patient outcomes (Weston & Weston, 2015).

EVALUATION OF MEDICATION SUBSETS

In the geriatric population, there is a subset of medications that can be associated with dosing errors as well as preventable adverse events that can occur during the prescribing stage (Gurwitz, 2003). Some of the medications have the potential to cause serious adverse events or can prove to be fatal if not prescribed appropriately. Examples of medication classes that can be associated with prescribing errors include cardiovascular medications (e.g., digoxin, angiotensin-converting enzyme inhibitors, diuretics) (Gurwitz, 2003). There are also nonopioid analgesics, hypoglycemics, anticholinergics, and anticoagulants (Gurwitz, 2003). With a rate of about 50.01 per 1,000 person-years for adverse drug events, it has been found that approximately 28% of these incidences can be prevented. The implementation of specific strategies that are designed to reduce or prevent the effects of adverse drug events in most settings, clinical or otherwise, has the ability to significantly shape the manner in which patient medications are dosed. As a rule of thumb, it is important to maintain an awareness that there are specific medications or classes of drug according to the Beers Criteria that should be avoided in individuals who are 65 years of age or older either due to being ineffective or, most notably, posing a high risk of adverse events in this population. Clinicians can be challenged when it comes to the complex needs of the geriatric population and matching these needs with those of the disease-specific clinical practice guidelines (Rochon, 2019). The presence of multiple medications requiring accurate dosing is required when managing older adults, with this being regarded as a standard of practice when addressing this population. For any clinician working with older patients, there must be awareness of the physiological differences that exist with this population in comparison to their younger counterparts. The differences that can exist with older adults should always be taken into consideration as it relates to dosing strategies and the risks compared to the benefits that can be associated with the selection of a specific drug when compared to another.

SUMMARY

The presentation of pharmacokinetic and pharmacodynamic changes that can occur in geriatric patients can make this population extremely susceptible to adverse drug events resulting from overprescribing or inappropriate prescribing of specific medications or medication classes. For any clinician engaged in the process of initiating drug therapy in older adults, a myriad of factors must be taken into consideration when making selection among the various therapeutic options that are available on the market. Given the vulnerability and potential for these drug effects to develop with geriatric patients, it is important for clinicians to incorporate the use of a stepwise approach to prescribing for older adults. This approach should include an ongoing and comprehensive review of a patient's current drug therapies, the removal of any and all drugs that are deemed to be unnecessary or do not have an existing diagnosis to support continuation, the use of nonmedicine interventions to treat mild to moderate conditions, and consideration being given to alternative agents that can be viewed to be safer. Last, the use of the lowest but effective dose that can be prescribed to provide optimal benefits to the patient is the desired goal of any clinician and all patient cases. Geriatric patients represent a unique group, and the dosing of any medication should be performed with the utmost care taking into consideration not only the benefits of initiation but negative effects that may be experienced. The intended goal of geriatric dosing is to treat the patient and prevent any harm that can be inflicted to deliver effective treatment. In order to achieve this outcome, there must be a clear understanding of the special circumstances that can be associated with this particular population (Comaty, 2015). The specific medication classes that have the ability to lead to adverse drug effects should be avoided in favor of the selection of more appropriate medication to manage diseases' states and achieve optimal therapeutic outcomes. The awareness that clinicians possess to appropriately dose geriatric patients can have an impact on the course of treatment and quality-of-life outcomes that can result. The approach of a case-by-case assessment of older adults will most likely aid a clinician in determining what will deliver optimal therapeutic outcomes.

DERMATOLOGY INTERPROFESSIONAL CASE STUDY
Megan Hebdon

Patient Presentation
Graham is a 72-year-old male who presents to the clinic with a rash on the left side of his face that started yesterday. Prior to the rash, he noted a tingling sensation to the tip of his nose and across his left cheek for several days. He reports more tingling and burning today, and the rash has increased in intensity. He has not tried anything for the rash.

History
Graham has been a widower for the past 2 years. He is active socially, and currently in a monogamous relationship with a male partner. His spouse was a female. He rides on a recumbent bicycle daily, enjoys meat but also eats fruits and vegetables, has three to four alcoholic drinks per day, does not use tobacco or other substances, and he is up to date on his vaccines. He had testing for sexually transmitted infections (STIs) when he became intimate with his current partner, and the testing was negative. He has one child and no other living relatives. His past medical history is significant for hypertension, hyperlipidemia, erectile dysfunction, and seasonal allergies. He had a hernia repair in his early 30s; otherwise, he had no surgeries.

Medications
Losartan 20 mg for hypertension, rosuvastatin 20 mg for hyperlipidemia, sildenafil 10 mg for erectile dysfunction, and Claritin 10 mg for seasonal allergies.

Physical Exam
You note an erythematous, vesicular rash to the left side of his face that does not cross the midline. There is no crusting or drainage from the lesions. His vision is 20/20 with corrective lenses, and the fundoscopic exam is unremarkable. He rates his pain at 8/10.

Diagnostic Testing
None obtained at the appointment today, but creatinine clearance was 96 mL/min 3 months ago.

Plan of Care
Graham is diagnosed with herpes zoster and is started on a regimen of valacyclovir 1,000 mg three times daily for 7 days. You call his pharmacist to check the price. The ease of dosing and improved neuralgia outcomes make this a preferred choice over acyclovir, but the cost could be prohibitive for him. You share the treatment options with him, and he opts to take valacyclovir. No dose adjustments are made due to adequate creatinine clearance levels. He is encouraged to provide good skin care and to watch for signs and symptoms of infection including increased redness, honey crusting, increased pain, warmth, and swelling to the area.

His pain will be initially managed with tramadol 50 every 8 hours for a maximum of 5 days and then de-escalated to acetaminophen 500 mg every 6 hours. A discussion about pregabalin and gabapentin is broached for subacute and postherpetic neuralgia, but this will be determined when he follows up. You plan short-term follow-up in 1 week to address any acute issues and a second follow-up at 1 month to assess for persistent neuralgia. Any pain that persists beyond 4 months will be treated based on patient symptoms and treatment preferences.

Interprofessional Collaboration

Graham is referred to an ophthalmologist for a same-day evaluation to complete a thorough fundoscopic exam and as a precaution for any ophthalmic complications. They may consider topical or oral corticosteroid therapy in addition to the antiviral therapy. You also discuss a herpes zoster vaccination with him but plan to wait 3 years to refer him to his pharmacist for the vaccination. You make a note in the medical record to address this at that time.

Case Study References

Albrecht, M. A. (2018). Treatment of herpes zoster in the immunocompetent host. In M. S. Hirsch & J. Mitty (Eds.), *UpToDate*. Retrieved from https://www.uptodate.com/contents/treatment-of-herpes-zoster-in-the-immunocompetent-host

Albrecht, M. A. & Levin, M. J. (2019a). Epidemiology, clinical manifestations, and diagnosis of herpes zoster. In M. S. Hirsch & J. Mitty (Eds.), *UpToDate*. Retrieved from https://www.uptodate.com/contents/epidemiology-clinical-manifestations-and-diagnosis-of-herpes-zoster

Albrecht, M. A., & Levin, M. J. (2019b). Vaccination for the prevention of shingles (herpes zoster). In M. S. Hirsch & J. Mitty (Eds.), *UpToDate*. Retrieved from https://www.uptodate.com/contents/vaccination-for-the-prevention-of-shingles-herpes-zoster

Ortega, E. (2019). Postherpetic neuralgia. In J. M. Shefner & A. F. Eichler (Eds.), *UpToDate*. Retrieved from https://www.uptodate.com/contents/postherpetic-neuralgia

Vrcek, I., Choudhury, E., & Durairaj, V. (2017). Herpes zoster ophthalmicus: A review for the internist. *The American Journal of Medicine, 130*(1), 21–26. doi:10.1016/j.amjmed.2016.08.039

REFERENCES

Akhar, S., & Ramani, R. (2015). Geriatric pharmacology. *Anesthesiology Clinics, 33*(3), 457–469. doi:10.1016/j.anclin.2015.05.004

Bushardt, R. L., Massey, E. B., Simpson, T. W., Ariail, J. C., & Simpson, K. N. (2008). Polypharmacy: Misleading, but manageable. *Clinical Interventions in Aging, 3*(2), 383–389. doi:10.2147/cia.s2468

Comaty, J. (2015). Geriatric pharmacotherapy. *The Tablet*. Retrieved from http://www.apadivisions.org/division-55/publications/tablet/2015/12/geriatric-medicine.aspx

Green, J. L., Hawley, J. N., & Rask, K. J. (2007). Is the number of prescribing physicians an independent risk factor for adverse drug events in an elderly outpatient population? *American Journal of Geriatric Pharmacotherapy, 5*, 31–39. doi:10.1016/j.amjopharm.2007.03.004

Gurwitz, J. H. (2003). Incidence and preventability of adverse drug events among older persons in the ambulatory setting. *Journal of American Medical Association, 289*, 1107–1116. doi:10.1001/jama.289.9.1107

Hanlon, J. T., Aspinall, S. L., Semla, T. P., Weisbord, S. D., Fried, L. F., Good, C. B., . . . Handler, S. M. (2009). Consensus guidelines for oral dosing of primarily renally cleared medications in older adults. *Journal of American Geriatric Society, 57*(2), 335–340. doi:10.1111/j.1532-5415.2008.02098.x

Lassiter, J., Bennett, W. M., & Olyaei, A. J. (2013). Drug dosing in elderly patients with chronic kidney disease. *Clinics in Geriatric Medicine, 29*(3), 657–705. doi:10.1016/j.cger.2013.05.008

Milton, J. (2008). Prescribing for older people. *The British Journal of Medicine, 336*, 606–609. doi:10.1136/bmj.39503.424653.80

Nygaard, H. A., Nalik, M., Ruths, S., & Kruger, K. (2004). Clinically important renal impairment in various groups. *Scandinavian Journal of Primary Health Care, 22*(3), 152–156. doi:10.1080/02813430410006468-1

Olyaei, A., & Bennet, W. (2009). Drug dosing and renal toxicity in the elderly patient. In American Society of Nephrology (Ed.), *Geriatric nephrology curriculum*. Washington, DC: Editor. Retrieved from https://www.asn-online.org/education/distancelearning/curricula/geriatrics/Chapter9.pdf

Rochon, P. (2017). Drug prescribing for older adults. In K. E. Schmader (Ed.), *UpToDate*. Retrieved from https://www.uptodate.com/contents/drug-prescribing-for-older-adults

Snowden, A. (2008). Medication management in older adults: A critique of concordance. *British Journal of Nursing, 17*, 114–119.

Tidy, C. (2014). Prescribing for the older patient. Retrieved from https://patient.info/doctor/prescribing-for-the-older-patient

Turnheim, K. (1998). Drug dosage in the elderly. Is it rational? *Drugs & Aging, 13*(5), 357–379. doi:10.2165/00002512-199813050-00003

United States Census Bureau. (2011). Sixty-five plus in the United States. Retrieved from https://www.census.gov/population/socdemo/statbriefs/agebrief.html

Weston, C., & Weston, J. (2015). Applying the Beers and STOPP criteria to care of the critically ill older adult. *Critical Care Nursing Quarterly, 38*(3), 231–236. doi:10.1097/CNQ.0000000000000077

Zhan, C., Sangl, J., Bierman, A. S., Miller, M. R., Friedman, B., & Wickizer, S. W. (2001). Potentially inappropriate medication use in community-dwelling elderly. Finding from the 1996 medical expenditure panel survey. *Journal of the American Medical Association, 286*, 2823–2829. doi:10.1001/jama.286.22.2823

11
Auditory Disorders

Abimbola Farinde

OBJECTIVES

1. Evaluate the development of hearing loss and resultant outcome in an older adult
2. Discuss the outcomes that can be observed in an older adult experiencing hearing loss
3. Review methods for prevention or minimization of hearing loss in older adults
4. Discuss the available options for management and treatment approach of hearing loss

INTRODUCTION

It is well established that older adults can experience physiological and physical changes with the progression of age. Along with this process, there is an increased likelihood of experiencing hearing impairment during one point or another. Hearing loss is reported to impact about one-third of adults 61 to 70 years of age and over 80% who are older than 85 years (Walling & Dickson, 2012). The percentage of higher loss appears to be greater in males compared to females and can contribute to dysfunction in the performance of activities of daily living. The presence of hearing loss or hearing impairment is a problem that can impact one or more parts of the ear and has the potential to interrupt the manner in which sounds travel through the hearing system up to the brain. "Hearing loss" is defined as a gradual reduction in the ability to perceive sounds, whether this is a partial or complete impairment that is temporary or permanent (Harvard Health Publications, 2018). When any type of sound enters the ear, it comes into contact with the eardrum, which causes a vibration to occur. Within the ear, the sounds are then transformed into nerve impulses, which make their way to the brain (Figure 11.1). The ability to hear and interpret sound is imperative for an older adult's day-to-day functioning and quality of life.

The development of hearing loss is recognized as a natural consequence of the aging process (Monahan & Sieminski, n.d.). It is noted that hearing loss can result from disorders or damage to the ear or the brain. It has the capacity to impact every part of the human ear, with the most notable damage occurring with the inner ear. Some of the most notable causes of hearing loss in adults can include disease of the middle ear in the form of a bacterial infection, persistent loud noise causing damage to the cells of the ear, an abnormal growth of one or more of the bones in the middle ear (otosclerosis), Meniere's disease, trauma, exposure to loud noise, sudden sensorineural hearing loss, or specific drugs (e.g., chemotherapeutic agents, antimalarial agents, and ototoxic medications). There are more than 100 causes of hearing loss; so

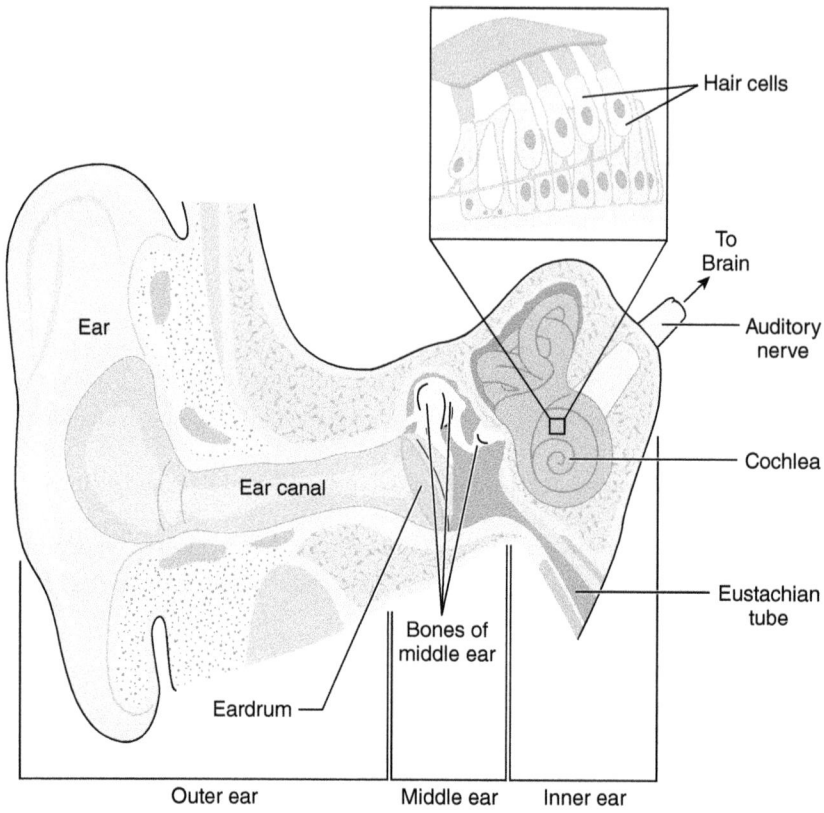

FIGURE 11.1 Hearing process.

it is ultimately the role of the clinician to determine what may be the primary cause of the condition.

BACKGROUND ON HEARING DEFICITS

It is reported that 25% of individuals over the age of 60 have some degree of hearing loss, with this increasing to 50% in those over the age of 70 (California Ear Institute, n.d.). The ability to understand and follow speech can become compromised in older adults when compared with their younger counterparts. This deficit can become increasingly observable in noisy environments where older adults struggle to compensate for the loss (Martin & Jerger, 2005). The various issues that can arise with listening difficulties in older adults can be attributed to their presbycusic high-frequency hearing losses. Hearing loss can be divided into three specific categories: conductive, sensorineural, and central. The type of hearing loss that is experienced will ultimately determine the treatment approach that is taken. In some instances, the hearing loss can be idiopathic. The presence of a conductive hearing loss can stem from the presence of cerumen buildup, which does not fall out with normal washing. For older adults who present with conductive hearing loss, they often state that their own voices can sound loud while other voices that they hear can be muffled. Furthermore, there is also the additional symptom of having a ringing in the ears.

For many sufferers of this type of hearing loss, there is the potential for this to be corrected with medication or surgical interventions. In the event that these interventions are not successful, there is also the implementation of hearing aids to assist with the amplification of the sounds that they hear on a daily basis (California Ear Institute, n.d.). The sensorineural hearing loss can stem from continuous and prolonged exposure to loud noises and diseases that lead to ear infections and can damage the hair cells of the cochlea. For older adults who experience sensorineural hearing loss, it may impact only a portion of their sound spectrum, and they may have deteriorating hearing in higher frequencies than the lower frequencies. The use of digital hearing aids can prove to be advantageous for this particular type of hearing loss due to the fact that there is an amplification of the section of the sound spectrum that has worsened or has been lost while enabling the filtration of background noise. Central hearing loss is considered to be a rare form compared to sensorineural or conductive types of hearing but when it develops, it can occur with inconsistent auditory behavior in which individuals can experience reactions that are out of their character to sounds in their environment even though there may not be the presence of any loud noises. Patients may perceive themselves to be deaf even though they have reactions to sounds that can arise from their environment (Hain, 2017). Given that the majority of hearing loss can be experienced in later years, which can be associated with previous trauma or events, it is important that efforts are taken to minimize hearing loss with prevention being the key measure. The prevention of hearing loss and other auditory issues should encompass the avoidance of situations that can damage hearing or, at least, attempts should be made to protect the ear as much as possible from negative exposures.

The loss of hearing in older adults can cause significant issues related to communication as well as unnecessarily induced stress due to the inability to react in situations (Dewane, 2010). It can cause struggles with everyday living, with adults reporting that it can impact not only how they do not react to others but also the day-to day-stressors that they can encounter. There can be associated negative elements of hearing loss that can become a recognized part of an individual's personality. The presentation of physical manifestation such as tension and psychological changes can dramatically alter the personality. Hearing loss can produce moments of crises in an individual's life as well as depression or adjustment disorder. The mental health aspect of hearing loss is one that is not always recognized but should be considered a part of the assessment process for any clinician. It has the potential to cause confinement within an individual and cause issues related to thinking, concentrating, paying attention, or boredom (Dewane, 2010). The direct impact that hearing loss can have on mental illness is a key element that a clinician should be aware of and take the necessary steps to address, given the substantial impact it can have on quality of life. For any clinician, the ability to understand how hearing loss can affect the individual can help with addressing the problem (Cunningham & Tucci, 2017).

MANAGEMENT OF HEARING LOSS IN OLDER ADULTS

The presentation of idiopathic sudden sensorineural hearing loss can be within 72 hours and restricted to one side (Rauch, 2008). It is reported that about 90% of older individuals can present with age-related sensorineural hearing loss, which can be progressive in nature (Walling & Dickson, 2012). Typically, sensorineural hearing loss can entail problems related to the conversion of mechanical vibrations (Walling & Dickson, 2012). It is important to perform an MRI in order to determine the underlying cause of the condition. One of the most commonly recognized treatment interventions for this condition is the use of steroids, but this may not prove to be effective in all patients and an in-depth assessment should be performed.

Conductive hearing loss is most commonly associated with age-related hearing loss resulting from the accumulation of ear wax. This can contribute to the worsening of hearing loss in about 30% of older individuals. The removal of the ear wax through various techniques such as curetting or solutions containing hydrogen peroxide has demonstrated significant benefit as well as the use of warm water irrigation (Memel et al., 2002). Weber and Rinne tests are utilized to distinguish conductive from sensorineural hearing loss through the comparison of air and bone conduction (Walling & Dickson, 2012). The use of laboratory as well as imaging tests should be specific to the individual depending on the presentation of the hearing loss, and this can ultimately assist with determining the type of hearing loss that is being experienced by the older adult. Once the type of impairment is identified, strategies can be developed to optimize management/treatment.

The management of hearing loss requires an analysis of the cause, contributing factors, or co-occurring conditions that led to the loss and the identification of strategies to optimize hearing. The implementation of effective therapeutic interventions can help to improve an older individual's quality of life, which can include social and emotional performance, communication, and cognitive function (Walling & Dickson, 2012). While the benefits of treatment recommendations are observable, the potential for nonadherence to these can be common. The perception that an older individual has about improvement of hearing and the use of assistive listening devices are also contributing factors to adherence (Mulrow et al., 1990; Walling & Dickson, 2012). Overall, the treatment approaches that are applied to hearing loss should be individualized in order to optimize therapeutic interventions. Other potential factors that can affect management can include barriers such as cost, social norms, or negative societal perceptions that can be associated with the use of hearing aids, which is why treatment must be patient centered and focus on the desires of the patient (Pacal & Yueh, 2012).

SUMMARY

The ability to avoid potential risk factors and excessive exposure to noise that can be destructive to hearing is critical to preventing age-related hearing loss. Upon development of hearing loss, proper management requires a patient-specific approach and also adherence on the part of the older adult in order to optimize treatment and achieve a good quality of life. Over time, it is important not only for the clinician to assess for the development of hearing loss or other impairments but also for the individual to be mindful of the signs and symptoms that would lead to this presentation.

AUDITORY DISORDERS INTERPROFESSIONAL CASE STUDY
Megan Hebdon

Patient Presentation

Mr. H, a 72-year-old male, presents to the clinic with a chief complaint of hearing loss and pressure in his right ear. He denies dizziness and headache. He has also noted upper respiratory symptoms such as runny nose, congestion, and itchy eyes. He reports occasionally having seasonal allergies in the spring, but they generally resolve without treatment. He feels his symptoms are much worse this year. He is wondering whether it is due to his recent move to the area. He is 72 years old, and he is an avid golfer. He has been having trouble hearing his friends out on the golf course. He worked as a lawyer prior to his retirement and has not engaged in any leisure activities with a large amount of noise exposure. In addition to golf, he enjoys reading and going to dinner with friends.

History

Mr. H is married, reports being monogamous, and has two children and three grandchildren living nearby. He is currently being treated for osteoarthritis in his knees, hypertension, and hyperlipidemia. Otherwise, he has no other chronic health conditions. He had an appendectomy when he was 23, but he denies any other surgeries. He exercises daily either with walking on the golf course or swimming at the local recreation center. He enjoys meat, but he tries to eat a "balanced diet." He smokes an occasional cigar with friends and drinks socially on the weekends. He still drives and uses corrective lenses for nearsightedness. He is up to date on his vaccines.

Medications

Mr. H reports no medication allergies. He is currently taking diclofenac gel for his knees twice daily, lisinopril 20 mg daily, and pravastatin 20 mg daily.

Physical Exam

Vital signs are Pulse: 72 beats per minute; Respirations: 18 breaths per minute; Blood Pressure: 180/82 mmHg; Temperature: 98.2 degrees F. He is pleasant, cooperative, and in no acute distress. He has mild erythema to his conjunctiva bilaterally and clear nasal discharge with pale and boggy turbinates. His right external auditory canal is occluded with cerumen and his left ear canal is clear with a pearly gray tympanic membrane with intact cone of light. His oral mucous membranes are pink and moist, and there is cobblestoning to his posterior pharynx. His cardiovascular and pulmonary exam is unremarkable. He has a steady gait with coordinated movement and equal strength to upper and lower extremities. Cranial nerves II–XII are intact, minus a failed whisper test to the right ear. Negative Rinne test on the right and asymmetric Weber test, being louder on the right, are obtained.

Diagnostic Testing

You consider ordering a hearing screening if hearing has not improved with irrigation of his right ear canal.

Plan of Care

You diagnose Mr. H with cerumen impaction and hearing loss. The plan of care will start with irrigation of his right ear. After several large pieces of dark, yellow wax are removed from his ear with irrigation, the right ear canal and tympanic membrane are reinspected. His ear canal is moist with a small amount of wax remaining. His tympanic membrane is visible with mild erythema and intact cone of light. He reports feeling instant pressure relief after the irrigation, and he responds to the whisper test on both sides. You recheck the Rinne and Weber tests, and they are both within normal limits. You provide education on the use of either mineral oil once a month or Debrox over the counter to help with cerumen impaction in the future.

For his allergic rhinitis symptoms, you discuss treatment options including a short-term second-generation antihistamine, an intranasal corticosteroid, an intranasal antihistamine, or nonpharmacologic saline nasal irrigation. You discuss the risks and benefits including minimal risk of cognitive side effects with the oral antihistamine, nosebleeds with the intranasal medications, and increased infection risk with nasal irrigation if poor cleaning practices are used. He would like to try an intranasal antihistamine, so you prescribe olopatadine 0.6%, two sprays in each nostril twice daily. You counsel Mr. H on follow-up for his annual exam including vision and labs such as complete blood count (CBC), comprehensive metabolic panel (CMP), a lipid panel, and an annual flu shot. He verbalizes understanding.

Interprofessional Collaboration

Mr. H's condition resolved with a simple in-office procedure. If he returns reporting hearing loss that is not associated with a cerumen impaction, then the next step would be a referral to audiology for a hearing screening. Hearing loss can either be sensorineural or conductive. In this case, Mr. H was experiencing conductive hearing loss related to the cerumen, but other factors contributing to conductive hearing loss include otitis externa, foreign body, perforation of the tympanic membrane, acute otitis media, serous otitis, and otosclerosis. Contributing factors related to sensorineural hearing loss that the nurse practitioner should consider in the future include meningitis, viral infections such as measles, mumps, or rubella, ototoxic medications such as aminoglycoside agents, loop diuretics, or large doses of aspirin, trauma causing damage to the cochlea and auditory nerve, acoustic neuroma, and Meniere's disease.

Case Study References

American Geriatrics Society Beers Criteria Update Expert Panel. (2019). American Geriatrics Society 2019 updated AGS Beers Criteria for potentially inappropriate medication use in older adults. *Journal of the American Geriatric Society, 67*(4), 674-694. doi:10.1111/jgs.15767

Armstrong, C. (2009). Diagnosis and management of cerumen impaction. *American Family Physician, 80*(9), 1011–1013. Retrieved from https://www.aafp.org/afp/2009/1101/p1011.html

Baptist, A. P., & Nyenhuis, S. (2016). Rhinitis in the elderly. *Immunology & Allergy Clinics of North America, 36*(2), 343–357. doi:10.1016/j.iac.2015.12.010

Coggins, M. D. (2013). Antihistamine risks. *Aging Well, 6*(2), 6.

Seidman, M. D., Gurgel, R. K., Lin, S. Y., Schwartz, S. R., Baroody, F. M., Bonner, J. R., . . . Nnacheta, L. C. (2015). Clinical practice guideline: Allergic rhinitis. *Otolaryngology: Head & Neck Surgery, 152*(Suppl 1), S1–S43.

Turton, L., & Batty, S. (2016). Recommended procedure: Rinne and Weber tuning fork tests. Bathgate, Scotland: British Society of Audiology. Retrieved from https://www.thebsa.org.uk/wp-content/uploads/1987/04/Recommended-Procedure-Tuning-Forks-2016.pdf

Weber, P.C. (2019). Evaluation of hearing loss in adults. *UpToDate*. Retrieved from https://www.uptodate.com/contents/evaluation-of-hearing-loss-in-adults

REFERENCES

California Ear Institute. (n.d.). Common causes of hearing impairment in seniors. Retrieved from http://www.californiaearinstitute.com/hearing-device-center-common-causes-hearing-impairment-seniors.php

Cunningham, L., & Tucci, D. (2017). Hearing loos in adults. *New England Journal of Medicine, 377*, 2465–2473. doi:10.1056/nejmra1616601

Dewane, C. (2010). Hearing loss in older adults — Its effect on mental health. *Social Work Today, 10*(4), 18

Hain, T. (2017). Central hearing loss. Otoneurology Education Index. Retrieved from http://www.tchain.com/otoneurology/disorders/hearing/cent_hearing.html

Harvard Health Publications. (2018). Hearing loss in adults. Retrieved from https://www.drugs.com/health-guide/hearing-loss-in-adults.html

Martin, J., & Jerger, J. (2005). Some effects of aging on central auditory processing. *Journal of Rehabilitation Research & Development, 42*(4), 25–44. doi:10.1682/jrrd.2004.12.0164

Memel,D., Langley, C,, Watkins, C., Laue, B., Birchall, M, Bachmann, M. (2002). Effectiveness of ear syringing in general practice: a randomised controlled trial and patients' experiences. *British Journal of Geneeral Practice, 52*(484), 906–911.

Monahan, R., & Sieminski, L. (n.d.). Hearing loss—Undiagnosed and undertreated. *Today's Geriatric Medicine, 7*(3), 14. Retrieved from https://www.todaysgeriatricmedicine.com/archive/052714p14.shtml

Mulrow, C., Aguilar, C., Endicott, J. E., Tuley, M. R., Velez, R., Charlip, W. S., . . . DeNino, L. A. (1990). Quality-of-life changes and hearing impairment: A randomized trial. *Annals of Internal Medicine, 113*(3), 188–194. doi:10.7326/0003-4819-113-3-188

Pacal, J. T., & Yueh, B. (2012). Hearing deficits in the older patient: I didn't notice anything. *Journal of the American Medical Association, 307*(11), 1185–1194. doi:10.1001/jama.2012.305

Rauch, S. D. (2008). Idiopathic sudden sensorineural hearing loss. *New England Journal of Medicine, 359*(8), 833–840. doi:10.1056/nejmcp0802129

Walling, A., & Dickson, G. (2012). Hearing loss in older adults. *American Family Physician, 85*(12), 1150–1156. Retrieved from https://www.aafp.org/afp/2012/0615/p1150.html

12 Neurologic Disorders

Abimbola Farinde

OBJECTIVES

1. Discuss common types of neurologic disorders that occur in older adults
2. Discuss the pathological hallmarks of Parkinson's disease and Alzheimer's disease
3. Review the mainstay of management of common neurologic disorders, Parkinson's disease, and Alzheimer's disease

INTRODUCTION

It is widely recognized that as humans age, the brain and central nervous system also undergo a certain type of aging process. Neurologic disorders are frequent in older adults, affecting between 5% and 55% of people who are 55 years of age and older. The development of neurologic disorders can be associated with a high prevalence of adverse health outcomes that can include but are not limited to disability, institutionalization, hospitalization, and mortality (Broe et al., 1978; Callixte et al., 2015). Commonly identified neurologic disorders that affect older adults include strokes, neuropathy, Alzheimer's disease, and Parkinson's disease which one or more individuals.

STROKE

Stroke is recognized as the fourth leading cause of death, with the mortality rate being slightly higher in women compared to men. More than 80% of cardiovascular accidents (e.g., atherothrombotic, lacunar, cardioembolic) can occur in those above the age of 70 with the mean age of about 72 years and hemorrhagic stroke (intracerebral) with a mean age of about 79 years. The most commonly identified risk factors for stroke can include hypertension, diabetes, smoking, cardiac arrhythmias, and lipid abnormalities. It is unclear if managing the risk factors after the presentation of an initial stroke can reduce poststroke mortality or not (De Jong, 2003). The treatment of stroke can entail the administration of alteplase or tissue plasminogen activator (TPA). It is important that no aspirin or anticoagulation is administered for at least 24 hours after TPA administration. Afterward, aspirin or anticoagulation therapy can be initiated depending on the patient and circumstances.

PARKINSON'S DISEASE

Parkinson's disease is recognized as the second most common neurodegenerative disorder as well as a movement disorder (Heyn & Davis, 2017). The development of Parkinson's disease can be associated with a reduction of dopamine due to the destruction of pigmented neuronal cells in the substantia nigra in the basal ganglia. When levels of dopamine in the communication level that exists between the substantia nigra and corpus striatum can become increasingly inefficient, with time the movement of an affected individual becomes influenced. Men are 50% more likely to develop the disease, with the reason for this occurrence still yet to be understood, but the typical presentation of Parkinson's disease can be exhibited in those who are 60 years of age and older. The primary symptoms of Parkinson's disease include tremors, vertigo, rigidity, and bradykinesia while the secondary symptoms include anxiety, depression, and anxiety. While the etiology and epidemiology of neurologic disorders in older adults are not well-known in developing countries, progress has been made with the identification and management of these conditions in many developed countries. One of the more commonly known and recognized conditions is Parkinson's disease, which is a chronic and progressive movement disorder that can affect those over 65 years of age, with 1% being seniors.

Parkinson's Disease Management

To date, there is no cure for Parkinson's disease, but efforts are made to manage the symptoms of the disease. Commonly utilized pharmacologic therapeutic approaches can include anti-parkinsonian medications, anticholinergics, antiviral therapy, dopamine agonists, monoamine oxidase inhibitors (MAOIs), catechol-O-methyl-transferase (COMT) inhibitors, antidepressants, and antihistamines. Surgical management can be reserved as a last resort in some cases with the use of thalamotomy and pallidotomy, neural transplantation, and deep brain stimulation. All of these therapeutic approaches can be employed to slow the progressive nature of Parkinson's disease.

ALZHEIMER'S DISEASE

Alzheimer's disease is a commonly occurring form of dementia in the older population accounting for about 60% to 80% of dementia cases. It is recognized as the sixth leading cause of death in the United States (Alzheimer's Association, n.d.). Alzheimer's disease is commonly associated with memory loss and cognitive abilities can be observed, but as previously indicated, Alzheimer's disease is not always a normal part of the aging process. There are genetic risk factors that have been noted to be associated with Alzheimer's disease. At least half of these early-onset patients have inherited gene mutations that can be associated with Alzheimer's disease, with the most commonly studied being the apoE gene, which has three forms (alleles): apoE2, apoE3, and apoE4. Given that the most significant risk factor is increasing age, it is understandable that it can be viewed as a part of aging, but it is not to be considered a disease of old age. It has been reported that about 200,000 individuals who are younger than 65 years have early-onset Alzheimer's disease. Similar to most other dementias, Alzheimer's disease is considered to be a progressive neurodegenerative disorder that becomes worse over time. During the beginning phase of this disorder, an older adult may experience mild memory loss, but as the disease progresses to the later phase, an individual can lose the ability to carry on conversations as well as appropriately respond to stimuli from the environment (Alzheimer's Association, n.d.).

Alzheimer's Disease Management

The mainstay of management of Alzheimer's disease can consist of medication and nonmedication-based treatment interventions. For any individual who is diagnosed with Alzheimer's disease, including older adults, cholinesterase inhibitors and partial glutamate antagonists can be prescribed. Cholinesterase inhibitors can work by reversibly and noncompetitively inhibiting centrally active acetylcholinesterase, an enzyme that is responsible for the hydrolysis of acetylcholine. This is believed to lead to increased concentrations of acetylcholine that is available for synaptic transmission into the central nervous system. Regardless of the neurologic disorder that is diagnosed in an older adult, the mission is to strive to formulate an appropriate therapeutic intervention that can help to maintain his or her quality of life for years to come. There is currently no cure for many of the existing neurologic disorders; so the goal is to seek to slow progression and damage that can be caused over time. In an older adult, the maintenance of quality of life is the desired outcome with the initiation of therapy to manage a neurologic condition, and this requires an assessment of the risks versus benefits.

SUMMARY

The development of a neurologic disorder can be a common occurrence in older adults, and proper management is of the utmost importance in order to maintain quality of life. While the therapeutic approach may not be curative, the goal can be to slow down disease progression and achieve symptom control. Older adults represent a unique patient population that can be predisposed to the development of neurologic disorders, and clinicians should perform a thorough evaluation of potential conditions in order to arrive at optimal outcomes for care. While the progressive nature of neurologic disorders can bring significant life stressors to an older adult, the ability to achieve proper management and control of these systems can aid with achieving a close to normal quality of life.

NEUROLOGIC INTERPROFESSIONAL CASE STUDY

Megan Hebdon

Patient Presentation

Roberto is a 67-year-old male patient who presents to the clinic reporting a tremor to his left arm. He has noted these symptoms over the past 6 months but initially disregarded them. He is coming in today for evaluation, because he has been having difficulty buttoning his shirts and has noted changes in his handwriting. He currently works part time in a community health clinic as an optometrist to keep him busy postretirement. He reports that his office staff have difficulty reading his handwriting. The only other symptoms he reports are increased fatigue and feeling less engaged in activities he usually enjoys.

History

His family history is not significant for neurologic issues. He has one older brother who was diagnosed with prostate cancer. His parents died in their 90s and were relatively healthy. He grew up on a farm, and his parents worked until the last few years of their lives. He currently works part time as an optometrist. He is heterosexual, divorced with two grown children, and he has had multiple sexual partners in the past year. He reports drinking a beer with his dinner 2 to 3 nights a week, eats a varied diet with fruits and vegetables, is an avid cycler, and denies tobacco or illicit drug use. His only surgery was a right knee anterior cruciate ligament (ACL) repair in his 40s. He is currently being treated for hypertension, and he has mildly elevated cholesterol, which is managed with diet. He also has symptoms related to benign prostatic hyperplasia (BPH), but prefers to manage symptoms without medication. He has no history of psychiatric illness or treatment.

Medications
Lisinopril 20 mg once daily.

Physical Exam
Vital signs are Blood pressure: 132/78 mmHg; Pulse: 66 beats per minute; Respirations: 18 breaths per minute; Oxygen saturation: 98%.

He is alert and oriented, pleasant, and well-spoken. Ears, nose, throat, cardiovascular, pulmonary, and gastrointestinal exams are unremarkable. Cranial nerves II–XII are intact. The Romberg test is negative, and his heel–toe walking reveals no balance or gait abnormalities. When he walks across the room, however, a resting tremor is noted in his left arm. Stereognosis and finger-to-nose test are within normal limits. With rapid alternating movements, a tremor is noted to the left hand and lower arm. You ask him to pick up coins with his left and right hands. He has greater difficulty with his left hand. You do a Mini-Mental State Exam, and that is within normal limits. You also test him for anxiety and depression using SIG E CAPS (sleep, interest, guilt, energy, concentration, and appetite, psychomotor, and suicidal ideation), the Geriatric Depression Scale (GDS), and the Generalized Anxiety Disorder 7-item (GAD-7) scale. He screens negative for suicidal or homicidal ideation and reports anhedonia, fatigue, reduced concentration, and appetite loss with SIG E CAPS. He screens positive for depression with the GDS, but has a subthreshold score for anxiety symptoms with the GAD-7.

Diagnostic Testing
You decide to do some baseline lab tests with the following: complete blood count (CBC), comprehensive metabolic panel (CMP), vitamin D, thyroid-stimulating hormone (TSH)/T4, and testosterone. All of the tests are within normal limits, except for a vitamin D level of 25 ng/ml, which is slightly low.

Plan of Care
You discuss the potential diagnoses of essential tremor or Parkinson's disease. Due to the unilateral onset, character of the tremor, and accompanying symptoms of fatigue and mild depression, you identify Parkinson's disease as most likely. You discuss the diagnosis being based on a good history and physical exam and by ruling out other potential causes. Patient education is provided regarding both conditions although Parkinson's disease is emphasized. Due to the newness of information and unconfirmed diagnosis, you focus on the patient's questions and concerns. Based on his younger age, you describe pharmacologic options such as ropinirole and pramipexole due to the lower risk of dyskinesias, although first-line therapy is levodopa/carbidopa in older age. You plan short-term follow-up to continue the conversation with the patient and allow him time to process the information. You discuss the importance of a neurology referral and a neuropsychiatric

exam to confirm the diagnosis. In addition, you suggest occupational therapy for the tremor.

The patient has a generally active and healthy lifestyle, so you address behavioral strategies to promote well-being. With the patient, you review the importance of good sleep, optimizing nutrition, and maintaining physical activity. He desires to remain active, so you address the importance of balancing safety with well-being. Together, you come up with the following strategies: continue his cycling on the road with a daily warm-up near home to assess his level of symptoms, and swimming and tai chi to supplement his cycling.

You discuss the positive depression screen with him and discuss potential options for treatment including short-term follow-up to reevaluate, initiation of a selective serotonin reuptake inhibitor if needed, and a referral for counseling. The lifestyle changes for his tremor will also help with depressive symptoms. He states that with all of the new information, he would like to plan on reevaluating his symptoms at his next appointment.

Finally, you ask him to buy a vitamin D (cholecalciferol) supplement of 600 to 800 international units daily, because this may help with his fatigue. You plan to recheck his vitamin D levels in 3 months.

Interprofessional Collaboration

As described earlier, you suggest a neurology referral and neuropsychiatric exam for confirmation of the diagnosis. You suggest short-term follow-up in a week to give the patient time to review the information you have provided and to identify questions or concerns. You also suggest an occupational therapy referral to help with the tremor. There may be future need for physical therapy, speech therapy, and referral to psychology to address motor symptoms, dysarthria, and mood, respectively. You also consider the importance of a palliative care approach focusing on pain and symptom management and quality of life. End-of-life decision-making is an importance piece of the treatment plan, but you plan to introduce this step by step as the patient comes to terms with the new diagnosis and the impact it will have on his life. You encourage the patient to reach out to family and friends for the support he needs as he makes decisions throughout the course of his illness. You also provide him with online resources and local support group information.

Case Study References

Chou, K. L. (2019). Clinical manifestations of Parkinson disease. In H. I. Hurtig (Ed.), *UpToDate*. Retrieved from https://www.uptodate.com/contents/clinical-manifestations-of-parkinson-disease

Deik, A., & Tarsy, D. (2019). Essential tremor: Treatment and prognosis. In H. I. Hurtig (Ed.), *UpToDate*. Retrieved from https://www.uptodate.com/contents/essential-tremor-treatment-and-prognosis

Friedman, M. B., Furst, L., Gellis, Z. D., & Williams, K. (2012). Identifying and treating anxiety disorders. *Aging Well, 5*(3), 14. Retrieved from https://www.todaysgeriatricmedicine.com/archive/050712p14.shtml

Jankovic, J. (2012). Distinguishing essential tremor from Parkinson's disease. *Practical Neurology*, 36–38. Retrieved from https://practicalneurology.com/articles/2012-nov-dec/distinguishing-essential-tremor-from-parkinsons-disease

National Initiative for the Care of the Elderly. (n.d.). Depression: Assessment and treatment for older adults. Retrieved from http://www.nicenet.ca/tools-depression-assessment-and-treatment-for-older-adults

Tello, M. (2018). Vitamin D: What's the "right" level? *Harvard Health Blog*. Retrieved from https://www.health.harvard.edu/blog/vitamin-d-whats-right-level-2016121910893

REFERENCES

Alzheimer's Association. (n.d.). What is Alzheimer's disease? Retrieved from https://alz.org/alzheimers_disease_what_is_alzheimers.asp

Broe, G., Akhtar, A., Andrews, G., Caird, F., Gilmore, A., & McLennan, W. (1978). Neurological disorders in the elderly at home. *Journal of Neurology, Neurosurgery & Psychiatry, 39*(4), 362–366. doi:10.1136/jnnp.39.4.362

Callixte, K.-T., Clet, T., Jacques, D., Faustin, Y., François, D., & Maturin, T.-T. (2015). The pattern of neurological diseases in elderly people in outpatient consultations in Sub-Saharan Africa. *Biomedical Central Research Notes, 8*, 159. doi:10.1186/s13104-015-1116-x

De Jong, G. (2003). Stroke parkinsonism and parkinson's disease. *Journal of Clinical Epidemiology, 56*, 262–268. doi:10.1016/s0895-4356(02)00572-3

Heyn, S., & Davis, C. (2017). Parkinson's disease. *MedicineNet*. Retrieved from https://www.medicinenet.com/parkinsons_disease/article.htm#what_are_the_early_and_later_signs_and_symptoms_of_parkinsons_disease

13 Hematologic Disorders

Abimbola Farinde

OBJECTIVES
1. Discuss the common hematologic disorders that can be identified in older adults
2. Review age-related assessment findings present in an older adult with a hematologic disorder

INTRODUCTION
Hematologic disorders are not specific to geriatric patients, but in this population special consideration must be given for reduced physiological reserves and concomitant illnesses (Balucci, Ershler, & de Gaetano, 2008; Walsh, 1981). Similar to neurological disorders such as Alzheimer's disease, the presentation of hematologic disorders in the geriatric population should not be always associated with advancing age, but a consideration can be given in some cases. In the United States, it is reported that approximately 10% of the older population are anemic and, if left untreated, this can present serious risks to individuals. The prevalence rate of anemia is reported to be higher in women than men aged less than 75 years, but at the age of 75 years, males tend to surpass females by 5% (Guralnik, Ershler, Schrier, & Picozzi, 2005). The condition can be associated with substantial functional impairment and at times even mortality (Guralnik et al., 2005). According to Ezekowitz, McAlister, and Armstrong (2003), there is an observed increase in mortality in elderly patients with congestive heart failure as compared to the nonanemic cohorts. As the incidence of blood disorder increases with age, so does the potential burden that can be placed on the healthcare system if not addressed.

ANEMIA AND VITAMIN DEFICIENCIES
The development of anemia in combination with other existing illnesses can indicate the need for immediate and direct therapeutic interventions. The most commonly observed anemia in older adults that can develop with age can include iron deficiency anemia and anemia of chronic disease (ACD; Makipour, Kanapuru, & Ershler, 2008). Older adults are unlikely to present with iron deficiency anemia unless there are problems associated with absorption in the intestines, or presence of blood in the stool (Cleveland Clinic, n.d.). If there is blood in the stool, a comprehensive test must be performed in order to determine the source of the bleeding incident. With ACD, there is an adequate amount of iron present in the body, but the bone marrow is unable to incorporate this into the red blood cells. ACD can be associated with cancer, collagen disease, and chronic infection to name a

few (Cleveland Clinic, n.d.). One-third of anemia can be due to vitamin B12 deficiency, folate deficiency, gastrointestinal bleeding, and myelodysplastic syndrome. Vitamin B12 deficiency is also referred to as "pernicious anemia," and oral or injectable formulation of vitamin B12 is administered to correct this issue (Cleveland Clinic, n.d.). According to the World Health Organization (WHO), the criteria for anemia constitute a hemoglobin of less than 12 g/dl (120 g/L) in women and less than 13 g/dL (130 g/L) in men (Smith, 2000). A hemoglobin level that is below the normal limit can be used as a marker to detect anemia, and it can be described as "microcytic" (red cells are smaller than normal size), "normocytic" (red cells are of normal size), or "macrocytic" (red cells are larger than normal size). The presenting symptoms of anemia can include weakness, shortness of breath, high heart rate, and headaches (Kernisan, 2018). The more quickly the anemia appears, it can be determined that the more severe the symptoms will be. The decision to treat anemia in a geriatric adult can at times be difficult due to co-occurring physical and mental disorders, which may impact the optimal management of the anemia (Walsh, 1981). A clinician must be cognizant of these coexisting conditions and how they will impact the course of treatment prior to initiation. The course of action that is ultimately taken in a geriatric patient will be highly dependent on the status of the existing conditions and the risks versus benefits of treatment. The presence of iron deficiency anemia in a geriatric patient is regarded as the second most common form of anemia that can result from blood loss from the gastrointestinal tract, inadequate intake and absorption of iron, or can be drug induced. In order to effectively diagnose the presence of iron deficiency anemia, the ferritin level should be analyzed. If the level is found to be less than 15 ng/ml or 15 mcg/L, a determination can be made for the presence of iron deficiency (American Society of Hematology, n.d.). Once the confirmation of iron deficiency anemia has been made in a geriatric patient, the steps toward management can begin. If the patient does not respond to iron therapy, a bone marrow biopsy might be necessary to measure iron stores directly.

Some of the more common follow-up tests can include performing a check on the signs of microscopic blood loss, review and check of the ferritin level, vitamin B12, and folate levels. One of the more important parameters to check for includes kidney performance and reticulocyte count, which serves as a marker for whether the bone marrow is attempting to produce more red blood cells in an effort to compensate for the presence of the anemia (Kernisan, 2018).

When addressing anemia in older adults, a thorough assessment of the areas of the body that can include nail beds, hair placement, and skin, to name a few, should be performed. The specific details of what should be observed with each area are provided in Table 13.1. When treating anemia in older adults, it is important to identify the underlying cause and from there steps can be taken to correct the problem, which can either be done quickly or may take time in some cases.

SUMMARY

The presence of a hematologic disorder in an older adult can potentially turn into a more serious matter if immediate action is not taken to address the issue. A hematologic issue in an older adult should not be ruled out as a minor finding not requiring intensive workup. The development of anemia or vitamin deficiencies can present as a common finding in older adults, and a trained clinician should focus on performing an initial thorough assessment and proceed with making adjustment with follow-up if deemed necessary.

TABLE 13.1 Age-Related Assessment Findings for the Hematologic System

Assessment Area	Hematologic System Findings	Older Adults' Changes and Significance
Nail beds (check for capillary refill)	Pallor, cyanosis, and decreased capillary refill are often noted in hematologic disorders.	• Nails are typically thickened and discolored. • Need to use another body area, such as the lips, to access capillary refill.
Hair distribution	Thin or absent hair on trunk and extremities may indicate poor oxygenation and blood supply to area.	• Older adults are losing body hair, but often in an even pattern distribution that has occurred slowly over time. • Lack of hair only on lower legs and toes may indicate poor circulation.
Skin moisture and color	Skin dryness, pallor, and jaundice may occur with anemia, leukemia, etc.	• Dry skin is a normal aspect of aging and thus becomes an unreliable indicator of skin moisture. • Pigment loss and skin changes along with some yellowing occur with aging. • Pallor that is not associated with anemia may be noted in older adults, because they tend not to go outdoors and get exposed to sunlight.

HEMATOLOGY INTERPROFESSIONAL CASE STUDY
Megan Hebdon

Patient Presentation

George, a 68-year-old homeless patient arrives at the clinic for a general checkup. He has been staying at the nearby homeless shelter that is associated with the clinic. He has had no routine healthcare for the past 10 years. He reports living in three different cities for the past 10 years and being a "pretty healthy guy." However, in the midst of the conversation, he starts to describe the following symptoms: pain and tingling in his fingers and toes like they are "on fire," swelling of his tongue, and noting more difficulty with doing crossword puzzles (a favorite pastime when he can find them). He states that when he last saw a provider, he was told that his blood pressure was high. This was during an ED visit for a tooth abscess.

History

He has been homeless for the past 20 years. He used to work as a welder but then had a worksite injury that resulted in job loss, chronic back pain, and depression. He self-treated with alcohol, became abusive to his wife, lost his house, and currently has no contact with his family. He has been a heavy drinker on and off for the past 20 years although he is 3 months sober due to an agreement with the current shelter. He is attending Alcoholics Anonymous (AA) meetings, and he is hoping to get his life back on track for his retirement. He has started a temporary job at Good Will. He has not had recent labs and does not recall which immunizations he has received. He denies current sexual activity and past or present intravenous (IV) drug use, but he has been in jail at several points over the past 20 years. He denies current or past tobacco use.

Medications

None

Physical Exam

Vital signs are Blood pressure: 174/100 mmHg; Pulse: 92 beats per minute; Respirations: 22 breaths per minute; Temperature: 97.4 degrees F; Oxygen saturation: 96%; Height: 70 inches; Weight: 156 pounds.

He is alert, oriented, and cooperative and reports no acute distress. Physical exam is unremarkable except for inflamed gums; multiple missing teeth; existing teeth with evidence of dental caries; widened gait; difficulty moving from chair to exam table; telangiectasia around nose and cheeks; and Patient Health Questionnaire-9 (PHQ-9): 15, Generalized Anxiety Disorder 7-item (GAD-7): 6, and Mood Disorder Questionnaire: negative for bipolar disorder. He denies suicidal or homicidal ideation, hallucinations, or delusions. The Mini-Mental State Exam (MMSE) is appropriate, and he exhibits the full spectrum of emotions; but he has poor eye contact.

Diagnostic Testing

His lab tests include complete blood count (CBC), comprehensive metabolic panel (CMP), lipid panel, vitamin B12, homocysteine, folic acid, methylmalonic acid (MMA), thyroid-stimulating hormone (TSH)/T4, B vitamins, vitamin D, A1C, HIV, and acute viral hepatitis panel.

His labs come back consistent with a megaloblastic anemia, low vitamin B12, low folic acid, and elevated MMA and homocysteine. His A1C is in the prediabetes range. He has elevated lipids with a cardiac risk index of 10%, his HIV and viral hepatitis tests are negative, his vitamin D is low, and he has elevated liver enzymes.

Plan of Care

He is diagnosed with vitamin B12 deficiency, folic acid deficiency, hypertension, prediabetes, hyperlipidemia, and vitamin D deficiency. He is started on B12 injections, folic acid supplementation, exercise and diet for the prediabetes, lisinopril/hydrochlorothiazide (HCTZ) 20/12.5 for the hypertension, fluoxetine 10 mg for depression with a goal of titrating to 20 mg, and pravastatin 20 mg for the hyperlipidemia. He is counseled on safe medication use, increasing fruits and vegetables in his diet within the limits of his current situation, and continuing his daily walking. He is encouraged to eat meat, when he has access, to increase absorption of B vitamins. Due to his history of alcohol use and risk for suicide with antidepressant, 2-week follow-up is planned. Screening for suicidal ideation and labs to recheck liver enzymes with the potential for further workup will be planned at the next visit. His blood pressure and other health needs will also be reevaluated.

Interprofessional Collaboration

In addition to his multiple chronic health conditions, this patient has extensive social needs. He is referred to the public health department for immunizations, food assistance, and for assistance with Medicare. He is also referred to a free dental clinic in the area. The in-office social worker plans a follow-up visit to ensure he receives the resources he needs for stable housing, healthcare, food resources, and employment. You request that he follows up in 1 month to see how he is tolerating the medication. He will eventually be transitioned to oral B12, but the injections ensure frequent contact. Once Medicare is in place, he can be referred to an internal medicine provider for ongoing management. He is also referred to the community services board for counseling services to support him in his recovery as well as his depression.

Case Study References

Hirschfeld, R. M. A., Cass, A. R., Holt, D. C. L., & Carlson, C. A. (2005). Screening for bipolar disorder in patients treated for depression in a family medicine clinic. *Journal of the American Board of Family Medicine, 18,* 233–239. doi:10.3122/jabfm.18.4.233

Institute of Medicine Committee on Health Care for Homeless People. (1988). *Homelessness, health, and human needs.* Washington, DC: National Academies Press.

Johnson, B. A. (2018, July 15). Pharmacotherapy for alcohol use disorder. In R. Saitz & R. Hermann (Eds.), *UpToDate.* Waltham, MA: Wolters Kluwer.

Jordan, P., Shedden-Mora, M. C., & Lowe, B. (2017). Psychometric analysis of the Generalized Anxiety Disorder scale (GAD-7) in primary care using modern item response theory. *PLoS One, 12*(8), e0182162. doi:10.1371/journal.pone.0182162

Kroenke, K., Spitzer, R., & Williams, W. (2001). The PHQ-9: Validity of a brief depression severity measure. *Journal of General Internal Medicine, 16,* 606–616. doi:10.1046/j.1525-1497.2001.016009606.x

Means, R. T., Jr., & Fairfield, K. M. (2019a, September 27). Clinical manifestations and diagnosis of vitamin B12 and folate deficiency. In W. C. Mentzer, J. S. Tirnauer, L. Kunins (Eds.), *UpToDate.* Retrieved from https://www.uptodate.com/contents/clinical-manifestations-and-diagnosis-of-vitamin-b12-and-folate-deficiency

Means, R. T., Jr., & Fairfield, K. M. (2019b, September 27). Treatment of vitamin B12 and folate deficiencies. In W. C. Mentzer, J. S. Tirnauer, & L. Kunins (Eds.), *UpToDate.* Retrieved from https://www.uptodate.com/contents/treatment-of-vitamin-b12-and-folate-deficiencies

Mueller, S., Seitz, H. K., & Rausch, V. (2014). Non-invasive diagnosis of alcoholic liver disease. *World Journal of Gastroenterology, 20*(40), 14526–14641. doi:10.3748/wjg.v20.i40.14626

Whelton, P. K., Carey, R. M., Aronow, W. S., Casey, D. E., Jr., Collins, K. J., Himmelfarb, C. D., . . . Wright, J. T., Jr. (2018). 2017 ACC/AHA/AAPA/ABC/ACPM/AGS/APhA/ASH/ASPC/NMA/PCNA guideline for the prevention, detection, evaluation, and management of high blood pressure in adults: A report of the American College of Cardiology/American Heart Association Task Force on Clinical Practice Guidelines. *Hypertension, 71,* e13–e115. doi:10.1161/HYP.0000000000000065

REFERENCES

American Society of Hematology. (n.d.). Anemia and older adults. Retrieved from http://www.hematology.org/Patients/Anemia/Adults.aspx

Balucci, L., Ershler, W., & de Gaetano, G. (Eds.). (2008). *Blood disorders in the elderly* (pp. i–xi). Cambridge, MA: Cambridge University Press. Retrieved from http://assets.cambridge.org/97805218/75738/frontmatter/9780521875738_frontmatter.pdf

Cleveland Clinic. (n.d.). Aging and anemia. Retrieved from https://my.clevelandclinic.org/health/articles/8964-aging--anemia

Ezekowitz, J., McAlister, F., & Armstrong, P. (2003). Anemia is common in heart failure and associated with poor outcomes: Insights from a cohort of 12,065 patients with new-onset heart failure. *Circulation, 107,* 223–225. doi:10.1161/01.cir.0000052622.51963.fc

Guralnik, J., Ershler, W., Schrier, S., & Picozzi, V. (2005). Anemia in the elderly: A public health crisis in hematology. *American Society of Hematology Education Book, 1,* 528–532. doi:10.1182/asheducation-2005.1.528

Kernisan, L. (2018). Anemia in the older adult: 10 common causes and what to ask. *Better Health While Aging.* Retrieved from https://betterhealthwhileaging.net/anemia-in-aging

Makipour, S., Kanapuru, B., & Ershler, W. (2008). Unexplained anemia in the elderly. *Seminars in Hematology, 45*(4), 250–254. doi:10.1053/j.seminhematol.2008.06.003

Smith, D. (2000). Anemia in the elderly. *American Family Physician, 62*(7), 1565–1572. Retrieved from https://www.aafp.org/afp/2000/1001/p1565.html

Walsh, J. (1981). Hematologic disorder in the elderly. *Western Journal of Medicine, 135*(6), 446–454. Retrieved from https://www.ncbi.nlm.nih.gov/pmc/articles/PMC1273318

14 Nutritional Issues

Abimbola Farinde

OBJECTIVES

1. Discuss the common nutritional issues that can arise in older adults
2. Evaluate the dietary needs and expectations for older adults
3. Review the changes that can occur with older adults that elicit nutritional deficiencies
4. Examine potential strategies for improving nutritional deficiencies in older adults

INTRODUCTION

The growing number of baby boomers and the increase in life expectancy have led to an associated increase in the number of older adults in America who can present with nutrition-related chronic disorders (Johnson et al., 2008). Based on data obtained on acute hospitalizations in older adults, it was suggested that approximately 71% are malnourished or experience a nutritional risk. These nutrition-related deficiencies can stem from poverty, an impaired appetite or sense of taste and smell, underlying conditions (e.g., depression or chronic illness), or the influence of medications (Bates, 2017). The presence of malnutrition can pose a serious mortality risk (Wallace, Schwartz, LaCroix, & Pearlman, 1995). With the aging process, older adults can present with some nutritional deficiencies that can impact their quality of life. Many older adults do not achieve adequate nutritional intake to support their needs and can be at risk for malnutrition (Nieuwenhuizen, Weenen, Rigby, & Hetherington, 2009).

THE AGING PROCESS

Notable improvements in nutrition can bring about benefits to older people and help to improve the healthy aging process of this population (Baugreet, Hamil, Kerry, & McCarthy, 2017). The aging process is associated with decreased organ system and potential disruption of homeostasis (Ritchie & Yukawa, 2019). These presenting deficiencies can result from the dietary changes that can occur with the aging process as well as other co-occurring factors (Institute of Medicine Food Forum, 2010). The nutritional demands of older adults can be attributed to various factors that include but are not limited to health problems, organ system issues, level of physical activity, energy use, and caloric requirements; for this reason, nutrition is regarded as an important aspect of health among older individuals (Amarya, Singh, & Sabharwal, 2015; Ritchie & Yukawam, 2019). The dietary needs of older adults tend to change based on several reasons, some of which can include reduction of metabolism, and their energy requirements can also lessen. The potential issues that can occur can lead to increased susceptibility to malnutrition. The prevalence of malnutrition is increasing with this population and can be associated with a reduction in functional status, reduction in bone mass, immune dysfunction, anemia, cognitive decline, and inability to heal from wounds (Amarya et al., 2015).

Additionally, the ability for older adults to take in and use a variety of nutrients can become less efficient; so the nutritional intake that is required can increase. Also, the presence of chronic disease states and medication can also have a significant impact on nutritional requirements for older adults. The ability to maintain a diet that contains appropriate nutritional content is important for older adults to maintain consistent health and functioning. For any older adult, having a consistent nutritional intake has the potential to improve overall health and functioning (Institute of Medicine Food Forum, 2010). While it is recognized that older adults may require a greater nutritional demand, the requirements are not always well-defined (World Health Organization [WHO], n.d.). According to the WHO, there has been an immediate need for the development of guidelines that are focused on addressing the nutritional demands of the increasing elderly population. A number of diseases that inflict older adults can result from dietary factors, which can then be increased by the aging process. The presence of poor nutrition is not always associated with aging, but older adults tend to be at a greater risk for malnutrition as a result of social, environmental, dietary, and psychological risk factors (Dimaria-Ghalili & Amella, n.d.).

A notable change that can occur with older adults is with their digestive system, which can impact gastric acid production and minimize the absorption of iron and essential vitamins such as vitamin B12 (Amarya et al., 2015). There is also the observance of a reduction in saliva and a subsequent reduction in constipation. Once the digestive system of an older adults becomes compromised, time is of the essence when it comes to restoration of these deficiencies and the reinstatement of proper functioning. The signs of nutritional deficiencies in older adults may not always be easy to identify as they can be mistaken as a normal aspect of the aging process, but this may not always be the case. The lack of adequate nutrition can contribute to deteriorated presentation of an older individual; so this must be carefully evaluated before consideration is given for a therapeutic approach.

Older adults can present with a myriad of chronic and progressively debilitating conditions, which can have a significant impact on nutritional status, daily activities of living, and quality of life. Some of these conditions can be degenerative in nature such as cardiovascular and cerebrovascular diseases (e.g., diabetes, cancer, stroke, osteoporosis), and this can be affected by dietary intake. Deficiencies in macronutrients are commonly identified in older adults due to reduced food intake and lack of diversity with the foods that are ultimately consumed. The ability to effectively make changes in the diet of an older adult can have a profound effect on overall health and longevity. In order to promote nutritional status, the general recommendation for a sedentary male is to consume 2,000 calories and for women who are 51 years of age and older, it is 1,600 calories. The consumption of fruits and vegetables is recognized as a cornerstone for improvement of nutritional status, and older adults can consume three to four servings (2 cups) of fruit and four to five servings (2.5 cups) of vegetables per day. Fruits and vegetables contain fibers, which are very beneficial to the diets of older adults who may have low fiber intake, and also have the capacity to serve as prevention against long-term diseases (Cooper, 2004).

There are a variety of methods that can be employed to identify the presence of a nutritional deficiency in an older adult. The presence of malnutrition can potentially stem from an underlying health condition that has been diagnosed or has yet to be identified. While many people may tend to focus their dietary intake around weight loss or disease prevention, the nutrition that surrounds older adults can start a substantially different approach. This is required in order to have a clear picture of the problem, and the assessment of each provides a window into a possible approach that can be taken (Bates, 2017). There is the use of biochemical indices of nutritional status that can be assessed by the measurement of blood, urine, or surface tissues for the presence of trace elements, which can provide more tangible estimates. When taking a dietary intake assessment of an older adult, it is crucial to have a reliable food intake record and then to change this to nutrient intake by means of a table that provides the nutrient contents of foods (Bates, 2017). There are a myriad of ways that food intake records can be obtained, which can include a 24-hour review of a patient's diet from the previous day to assess trends and patterns for possible changes. This can be a formatted or unformatted process that can utilize measures from all over an individual's home such as cups, teaspoons, or tablespoons to quantify portions of food that is being consumed. Second, there can also be the use of a log of food intake that can be assessed over a given period of time or even the inclusion of a device that measures the weight of all the food intakes.

The food intake and presence of adequate nutritional content can have a substantial role in the health status and well-being of older adults (Baugreet et al., 2017). The amount of energy that is lost in relation to intake can be far exceeded; so it is not surprising that older adults may experience weight loss, malnutrition, and other negative effects that can have a subsequent impact on activities of daily living. According to Robinson, Cooper, and Aihie Sayer (2012), the intake of food in older adults 70 years of age and older can decrease as much as 25%. Even in the most severe cases, a caloric intake of about 1,000 kcal per day has been identified in free-living older adults (Baugreet et al., 2017; Morley & Thomas, 2007). There are a number of factors that can contribute to diminished caloric and ultimately nutritional deficiencies in older adults. Some of these barriers can include reduced mobility, limited access to food choices, or a decreased appetite for the consumption of food due to an underlying medical condition. With decreased or minimal intake of essential proteins and micronutrient sources, older adults can lack capacity to thrive. Table 14.1 includes potential risk factors, both physiological and social factors, that can be associated with dietary intake and that can ultimately contribute to nutritional deficiencies in older adults.

TABLE 14.1 Risk Factors Contributing to the Development of Nutritional Deficiency in Older Adults

Cause of Nutritional Deficiency	Consequence
Physical and physiological	
Changes in body composition	Reduced metabolic rate and loss of muscle mass
Altered nutrient requirements	Insufficient energy and nutrient intake
Decreased physical activity	Progressive loss of body weight and reduced appetite
Sensory impairment	
Decreased sense of taste and smell	Reduced appetite
Loss of vision and hearing	Decreased ability to purchase and prepare food
Dental problems	Difficulty in chewing and poor-quality diet

(continued)

TABLE 14.1 Risk Factors Contributing to the Development of Nutritional Deficiency in Older Adults (*continued*)

Cause of Nutritional Deficiency	Consequence
Age-related issues	
Dementia	Decreased ability for self-care and increased morbidity
Sarcopenia	Decreased functional ability, assistance needed with ADLs, and increased frailty
Social determinants	
Financial restraints and poverty	Poor diet and limited access to food
Social isolation, reduced mobility, and lack of transport	Inappropriate food choices
Widowhood and bereavement	Food aversion
Decreased independence	Decreased food intake and inability to self-feed

ADLs, activities of daily living.

Notes: Cumulative effect → progressive undernutrition

Source: From Baugreet, S., Hamill, R., Kerry, J., & McCarthy, S. (2017). Mitigating nutrition and health deficiencies in older adults: A role for food innovation. *Journal of Food Science, 82*(4), 848–855. doi:10.1111/1750-3841

STRATEGIES TO IMPROVE NUTRITIONAL DEFICIENCIES IN OLDER ADULTS

It is vital that a thorough nutritional screening is performed in older adults (Posthauer, Collins, Dorner, & Sloan, 2013). There are screening tests in place to assess for nutritional deficiencies or undernutrition in older adults such as the Simplified Nutritional deficiencies or malnutrition can result from underlying health conditions, poor lifestyle choices, or other contributing factors. Some of the more notable factors can include loss of appetite, reduction in the sense of taste and/or smell, difficulty chewing, the loss of physical strength or mobility, and financial insecurity (Hollis & Henry, 2007). The prevalence of and impact of malnutrition in older adults can be an issue that can be underestimated when it comes to severity and management. Table 14.2 illustrates the prevalence of undernutrition that can exist in elderly individuals based on the population type.

Prior to addressing a nutritional deficiency, a clinician should be able to detect its presence, which may not always be easy to identify. However, there are specific features that can be identified such as muscle wasting, susceptibility to recurrence of infections, or low body weight. In many cases, the use of the body mass index (BMI) can serve as another index to gauge if an older adult is currently in a malnourished state. Proper screening to determine if an older adult is in a malnourished state can be done with periodic health checkup, and this is particularly important in recognized risk groups. According to the National Institute for Health and Care Excellence (NICE) guidelines, the recommendation is to have the culmination of scores for BMI,

TABLE 14.2 Estimates of Prevalence of Undernutrition in Elderly People

Prevalence	Type of population
Over 10%	Noninstitutional elderly people
10%–50%	Hospitalized for acute illness
10%–70%	Long-term care units or nursing homes

Source: From Best Practice Advocacy Centre New Zealand. (2011). Strategies to improve nutrition in elderly people. Retrieved from https://bpac.org.nz/BPJ/2011/May/elderly.aspx

unintentional weight loss (over 3 to 6 months), and the presence of an illness or lack of food intake for more than 5 days (NICE, 2017).

The advent of nutritional support can extend beyond providing older adults with supplementation in the form of oral supplements or enteral feeding. Before enteral feeding is initiated, a clinician should strive to build up an individual's nutritional intake that can be obtained from regular food and drinks. The beginning approach would be to increase the number of times that an individual eats and the energy density that is a part of the food and drink intake (NICE, 2017). In addition, if there is an identified loss of appetite, strategies can include: promoting the intake of three small meals per day with snacks in between each meal that contain high levels of protein and are full of energy; meal times can be made more enjoyable with less interruptions during these times; and meals can be made more appealing through size and appearance. If there is an identified problem with chewing that compromises nutritional status, there can be the promotion of adequate dental and mouth care to address the issue or the intake of softer foods that may not require as much chewing on the part of the older individual. The potential for swallowing difficulties can pose an additional challenge for older adults, and this may require an immediate modification of the consistency of foods that are eaten.

APPROACHES FOR FOOD SUGGESTIONS FOR MALNOURISHED OLDER ADULTS

For older adults, the promotion of a healthy eating style and the incorporation of eating guidelines can serve as the cornerstone for improved nutrition and health. The adoption of simplistic dietary approaches can include eating three small meals each day with snacks in between, the incorporation of two foods with each of the three meals each day, or having a nutritional drink such as soups or fruit drinks. An emphasis should also be placed on the distinction between light meals, main meals, and desserts. The intake of solid foods should be attempted in an older adult and if success is not achieved, there can be movement toward the use of oral nutritional supplementation. For those individuals who experience significant nutritional deficiencies, oral supplementation can provide the combination of essential macronutrients and micronutrients. A systematic review of 62 trials demonstrated the emergence of minimal weight gain based on the use of nutritional supplements for those who were undernourished (Milne, Potter, Vivanti, & Avenell, 2009). Furthermore, there is the reduction in associated complications when compared to previous reviews. The commonality that is associated with the reviews is that oral nutritional supplements are an acceptable means to increase energy and nutritional intake (Milne et al., 2009). While oral nutritional supplements have observed benefits, potential drawbacks can include adverse effects that can be experienced by older adults, associated costs, and diminished or lack of appropriate compliance.

Another viable therapeutic approach that can be used with malnourished older adults is parenteral nutrition, which provides immediate and direct nutrition into the venous system. This can be provided through the use of a central line. The use of parenteral nutrition has the ability to bypass parts of the digestive system that can minimize the delivery of nutritional content. If not immediately assessed and administered, the presence of malnutrition can be associated with significant complications and premature deaths among older adults (Dimaria-Ghalili & Amelia, n.d.). Prior to the administration of parenteral nutrition, an assessment must be performed to determine if an individual meets the criteria for initiation. Examples of indications for nutrition support can include an inadequate or unsafe use of oral or enteral nutrition intake or the presence of a leaking gastrointestinal tract (NICE, n.d.). The introduction of parenteral nutrition should be provided through a progressive process in an older adult like any other individual with close, ongoing monitoring with about no more than 50% of the estimated nutritional needs for the initial 24 to 48 hours (NICE, n.d.). For any older adult, the administration of parenteral nutrition can be removed once there is appropriate tolerance of oral or enteral nutrition. Additionally, it must be demonstrated that the nutritional status of an individual is adequate. The introduction of parenteral nutrition for any older adult must be patient specific, and withdrawal should be performed through a stepwise approach.

SUMMARY

For a clinician who is concerned about the nutritional status of an older adult who may present with issues related to malnutrition, it is important that there must be a step-by-step approach that is taken to ensure that the total nutritional intake that is provided takes into account energy, protein, fluid, electrolyte, mineral, micronutrients, and fiber requirements to name a few. The improvement of an older adult's nutritional status is the key to increased longevity during the course of the aging process.

The presence of nutritional deficits in an older adult can prove to be detrimental to health if this is not immediately addressed. The ability to properly assess an adult's energy expenditure and caloric intake requirement, evaluate co-occurring health problems that may be attributing to the condition, and adjust dietary intake based on these parameters is vitally important to the survival of the individual.

The nutritional needs of older adults can be based on a number of factors, including health problems, organ-related issues, level of activity, energy expenditure, or food selection to name a few. A clinician providing treatment to this particular type of patient must take all of these factors into consideration and select a therapeutic approach that is viewed to produce desirable outcomes.

NUTRITION INTERPROFESSIONAL CASE STUDY

Megan Hebdon

Patient Presentation

Maria is an 88-year-old Italian American female who presents to the clinic with her husband and daughter. They have brought her into the clinic because she has lost 10 pounds in the past 2 months. She has been on a soft diet because she has been waiting for a bridge implant. She is currently living at an assisted living facility with her husband, and she refuses to eat in the dining room. She is uncomfortable with the fact that she is on a soft versus a regular diet. She also reports that she has little to no appetite, because she does not like the texture of her food. She has not had an evaluation by a dietitian.

History

Maria has six daughters, but only five are living. She is married and monogamous but reports not being sexually active right now. Her father died due to a heart attack, and five of her six brothers died due to complications from heart attack or stroke. She lives in an assisted living facility because her husband could no longer take care of her at home. She has persistently declined over the past 4 years due to two hip fractures, depressive symptoms, and irritable bowel syndrome (IBS) with fecal incontinence that started after her last hospitalization. She has had two hip replacements, a total hysterectomy, and a minor heart attack. She is currently being treated for peripheral neuropathy, depression, essential tremor, hypertension, and hyperlipidemia. She is receiving biofeedback for the fecal incontinence, and this has significantly improved.

Medications

Gabapentin 300 mg twice daily, escitalopram 10 mg daily, propranolol 40 mg twice daily, lisinopril 20 mg, and cholestyramine 4 grams twice daily.
    She is allergic to sulfa drugs and statins.

Physical Exam

Vital signs are Blood presure: 100/52 mmHg; Pulse: 58 beats per minute; Respirations: 20 breaths per minute; Oxygen saturation: 96%; height: 57 inches; weight: 122 lbs (10-pound weight loss since the last visit).
    Maria is cooperative with the exam. Her skin is pale and has decreased turgor. Her physical exam is unremarkable besides gray, thinning hair, evidence of cachexia with temporal wasting, loose clothing, and missing her right first and second molars and her left second and third molars.

Diagnostic Testing

Comprehensive metabolic panel (CMP; specifically focused on albumin), complete blood count (CBC) with peripheral smear, iron, total iron-binding capacity (TIBC), B12, folic acid, thyroid-stimulating hormone (TSH)/T4, C-reactive protein (CRP), and vitamin D.

Plan of Care

While waiting for lab results, you discuss strategies to address Maria's appetite and overall health with her husband and daughter. First, you strategize about how to make mealtimes more comfortable including having a set time, eating in her room with family until she is more comfortable eating with other residents, and focusing on soft foods she does enjoy. You also discuss strategies to make her food more nutrient dense including adding extra butter and cream to the foods she eats, eating small, frequent meals, supplementing with protein shakes, taking a daily multivitamin, ensuring her food has enough seasoning, and eating what she prefers. You are concerned about her current blood pressure level and pulse. You discuss reducing her propranolol to 20 mg twice daily. Additionally, you are concerned about bowel obstruction with the cholestyramine; so you discuss tapering off that and adding a psyllium fiber supplement as a bulking agent for her diarrhea. Finally, you address medication options for appetite stimulation such as megestrol (risk of thrombus formation), dronabinol (central nervous system side effects), and mirtazapine (could also be adjunctive for depression). They state they will consider the options and follow up if they want to give one a trial. You plan a 1-week follow-up for reevaluation.

Interprofessional Collaboration

Appetite changes, weight loss, and nutritional imbalances can contribute significantly to frailty in older adults; so Maria needs an interprofessional team for adequate support. You suggest a dietitian referral, which the family readily accepts. You also write a note to the assisted living facility with recommendations to help with Maria's nutritional needs, including a prescription for a protein-based snack or shake twice daily. You also discuss the importance of social engagement with mealtime; so you encourage Maria's husband and daughter to coordinate family member presence during major meals. Finally, you recognize that sometimes appetite decline and weight loss occur as a patient nears the end of life. You recommend that Maria and her family have frank discussions regarding her health-related goals so that her wishes will be reflected with each decision regarding her care.

Case Study References

Braunstein, E. M. (2018). Evaluation of anemia. *Merck manual professional version*. Kenilworth, NJ: Merck & Co. Retrieved from https://www.merckmanuals.com/professional/hematology-and-oncology/approach-to-the-patient-with-anemia/evaluation-of-anemia

Pilgrim, A., & Sayer, A. A. (2015). An overview of appetite decline in older people. *Nursing in Older People, 27*(5), 29–35. doi:10.7748/nop.27.5.29.e697

Ritchie, C., & Yukawa, M. (2019). Geriatric nutrition: Nutritional issues in older adults. In K. E. Schmader, D. Seres, & J. Givens (Eds.), *UpToDate*. Retrieved from https://www.uptodate.com/contents/geriatric-nutrition-nutritional-issues-in-older-adults

Youdin, A. (2018). Nutrition in clinical medicine. *Merck manual professional version*. Kenilworth, NJ: Merck & Co. Retrieved from https://www.merckmanuals.com/professional/nutritional-disorders/nutrition-general-considerations/nutrition-in-clinical-medicine

REFERENCES

Amarya, S., Singh, K., & Sabharwal, M. (2015). Changes during aging and their association with malnutrition. *Journal of Clinical Gerontology and Geriatrics, 6*(3), 78–84. doi:10.1016/j.jcgg.2015.05.003

Bates, C. (2017). Common nutrient deficiencies in older adults. In C. Watkins Bale, & C. Seel Ritchie (Eds.), *Handbook of clinical nutrition and aging* (pp. 103–125). Totowa, NJ: Humana Press. doi:10.1007/978-1-59259-391-0_6

Baugreet, S., Hamill, R., Kerry, J., & McCarthy, S. (2017). Mitigating nutrition and health deficiencies in older adults: A role for food innovation. *Journal of Food Science, 82*, 848–855. doi:10.1111/1750-3841.13674

Best Practice Advocacy Centre New Zealand. (2011). Strategies to improve nutrition in elderly people. Retrieved from https://bpac.org.nz/BPJ/2011/May/elderly.aspx

Cooper, D. A. (2004). Carotenoids in health and disease: Recent scientific evaluations, research recommendations and the consumer. *Journal of Nutrition, 134*(1 Suppl.), 221S–224S. doi:10.1093/jn/134.1.221s

DiMaria-Ghalili, R. A., & Amella, E. J. (n.d.). Assessing nutrition in older adults. Retrieved from https://consultgeri.org/try-this/general-assessment/issue-9

Hollis, J. H., & Henry, C. J. (2007). Dietary variety and its effect on food intake of elderly adults. *Journal of Human Nutrition and Dietetics, 20*(4), 345–351. doi:10.1111/j.1365-277x.2007.00796.x

Institute of Medicine Food Forum. (2010). *Providing healthy and safe foods as we age: Workshop summary*. Washington, DC: National Academies Press. Retrieved from https://www.ncbi.nlm.nih.gov/books/NBK51837

Johnson, M. A., Park, S., Penn, D., McClelland, J. W., Brown, K., & Adler, A. (2008). Nutrition education issues for older adults. *The Forum for Family and Consumer Issues, 13*(3). Retrieved from https://www.theforumjournal.org/2008/01/03/nutrition-education-issues-for-older-adults

Milne, A. C., Potter, J., Vivanti, A., & Avenell, A. (2009). Protein and energy supplementation in elderly people at risk from malnutrition. *Cochrane Database of Systematic Reviews*, (2), CD003288. doi:10.1002/14651858.CD003288.pub3

Morley, J, E., & Thomas, D. R. (Eds.). (2007). *Geriatric nutrition*. London, UK: CRC Press.

National Institute for Health and Care Excellence. (n.d.). Parenteral nutrition. NICE pathways. Retrieved from https://pathways.nice.org.uk/pathways/nutrition-support-in-adults/parenteral-nutrition

National Institute for Health and Care Excellence. (2017). Nutritional support for adults: Oral nutrition support, enteral tube feeding and parenteral nutrition. Retrieved from https://www.nice.org.uk/Guidance/CG32

Nieuwenhuizen, W., Weenen, H., Rigby, P., & Hetherington, M. (2009). Older adults and patients in need of nutritional support: Review of current treatment options and factors influencing nutritional intake. *Clinical Nutrition, 29*(2), 160–169. doi:10.1016/j.clnu.2009.09.003

Posthauer, M. E., Collins, N., Dorner, B., & Sloan, C. (2013). Nutritional strategies for frail older adults. *Advances in Skin & Wound Care, 26*(3), 128–140. doi:10.1097/01.asw.0000427920.74379.8c

Ritchie, C., & Yukawa, M. (2019). Geriatric nutrition: Nutritional issues in older adults. In K. E. Schmader, & D. Seres (Eds.), *UpToDate*. Retrieved from https://www.uptodate.com/contents/geriatric-nutrition-nutritional-issues-in-older-adults

Robinson, S., Cooper, C., & Aihie Sayer, A. (2012). Nutrition and sarcopenia: A review of the evidence and implications for preventive strategies. *Journal of Aging Research, 2012*, 1–6. doi:10.1155/2012/510801

Wallace, J., Schwartz, R., LaCroix, A., & Pearlman, R. (1995). Involuntary weight loss in older adults: Incidence and clinical significance. *Journal of the American Geriatric Society, 43*(4), 329–337. doi:10.1111/j.1532-5415.1995.tb05803.x

World Health Organization. (n.d.). Nutrition for older persons. Retrieved from http://www.who.int/nutrition/topics/ageing/en/index1.html

15 Endocrine Disorders

Megan Hebdon

OBJECTIVES
1. Provide an overview of aging changes in the endocrine system
2. Identify endocrine diseases that frequently impact the aging population
3. Outline pharmacologic considerations for endocrine disease treatment in geriatric patients
4. Describe pharmacologic and nonpharmacologic management of endocrine diseases in the geriatric population

INTRODUCTION
There are multiple changes to the endocrine system that occur with aging. Management of endocrine diseases in the geriatric population can often be complex due to comorbid conditions and polypharmacy. Nurse practitioners in primary care must balance managing symptoms, preventing worsening of illness or the incidence of other related illnesses, goals of care, and life expectancy.

The diagnoses that are addressed in this chapter include type 2 diabetes mellitus, thyroid disease, parathyroid disease, and osteoporosis.

TYPE 2 DIABETES MELLITUS
The incidence of type 2 diabetes mellitus increases with age (Munshi, 2019). For the purposes of this discussion, diagnosis and treatment are focused on type 2 diabetes mellitus rather than type 1 although principles of insulin management are also applicable to type 1 diabetes. Adults over the age of 65 have the same risk of developing microvascular complications, but with later development of disease the complications are of shorter duration (Munshi, 2019). They are at higher risk of macrovascular complications, polypharmacy, functional issues, and cognitive decline that may be associated with diabetes and its treatment (Munshi, 2019).

Screening and Diagnosis
Diabetes is generally diagnosed using a fasting blood glucose or A1C. Other methods include an oral glucose tolerance test or a random plasma glucose test in individuals with classic symptoms of hyperglycemia and/or hyperglycemic crisis (American Diabetes Association [ADA], 2018; Munshi, 2019). Screening for older adults should occur based on the level of risk and life expectancy. Risk factors for type 2 diabetes include:

- Family history
- Obesity

- Sedentary lifestyle
- Race/ethnicity
- History of gestational diabetes or delivery of a large baby
- History of hypertension (HTN) or cardiovascular disease (CVD)
- Dyslipidemia
- Polycystic ovary syndrome (PCOS) or acanthosis nigricans
- Peripheral vascular disease (ADA, 2018; Munshi, 2019)

All older adults with prediabetes may be screened annually, and women with a history of gestational diabetes should be screened every 3 years. If initial testing is normal, then follow-up screening should occur every 3 years (ADA, 2018; Munshi, 2019). Additionally, autoantibody testing can be considered with diabetes screening if an individual has a first-degree relative with type 1 diabetes (Munshi, 2019). The risk of type 1 diabetes mellitus is lower in older adults; so nurse practitioners must balance the presentation and risk with the decision to test. The decision to screen and treat should always return to quality of life, potential for disease-related health outcomes, and optimal functioning.

When diagnosing a patient with type 2 diabetes mellitus, providers should conduct a careful health history including personal and family risk factors for diabetes. A thorough physical exam should also be conducted to evaluate microvascular and macrovascular complications. Microvascular complications include:

- Nephropathy
- Retinopathy
- Neuropathy (ADA, 2018; Munshi, 2019)

Diabetes is diagnosed based on the lab result findings indicated in Table 15.1.

TABLE 15.1 Diagnostic Criteria for Diabetes Mellitus

Test	Level	Other Notes
Fasting plasma glucose	≥126 mg/dL (7.0 mmol/L)	Fasting defined as no caloric intake for at least 8 hours
Oral glucose tolerance test	2-hour plasma glucose ≥200 mg/dL (11.1 mmol/L)	Performed as described by WHO
A1C	≥6.5% (48 mmol/mol)	Performed in a lab that is NGSP certified and standardized to the DCCT assay
Random plasma glucose	≥200 mg/dL (11.1 mmol/L)	In patients with classic signs of hyperglycemia or in a hyperglycemic crisis

DCCT, Diabetes Control and Complications Trial; WHO, World Health Organization.

Source: Data from American Diabetes Association. (2018). 15. Diabetes advocacy: Standards of medical care in diabetes—2018. *Diabetes Care, 41*(Suppl. 1), S152–S153. doi:10.2337/dc18-s015; Munshi, M. (2019). Treatment of type 2 diabetes mellitus in the older patient. In D. M. Nathan, K. E. Schmader, & J. E. Mulder (Eds.), *UpToDate*. Retrieved from https://www.uptodate.com/contents/treatment-of-type-2-diabetes-mellitus-in-the-older-patient

A1C measurement may not be accurate in older adults due to anemia, chronic kidney disease, recent transfusions, recent illness or hospitalization, and liver disease. These issues are all encountered with greater frequency in aging patients (Munshi, 2019).

Treatment of Hyperglycemia

Management of hyperglycemia in older adults is based on health, risk of hypoglycemia, and life expectancy (Munshi, 2019). Some guiding principles include the following:

- For individuals with life expectancy of greater than 10 years, an A1C goal of <7.5% (58.5 mmol/mol) may be appropriate—fasting and premeal targets of 140 to 150 mg/dL will help achieve this goal.
- A goal of A1C ≤8% is higher in frail older adults with comorbid conditions, functional limitations, and life expectancy <10 years.
- For the very old, A1C goals should focus on quality of life, avoidance of hypoglycemia and severe hyperglycemia (>350 mg/dL). An average glucose of 200 mg/dL or A1C of 8.5% may be appropriate (ADA, 2018; Munshi, 2019)

Hyperglycemia may contribute to visual and cognitive impairments and increase the risk of dehydration and infections, but hypoglycemia increases the risk of falls. Providers face the inherent tension between preventing macrovascular/microvascular complications and hyperglycemia symptoms and safety issues related to hypoglycemia (ADA, 2018; Munshi, 2019). An additional goal of treatment is cardiovascular risk reduction by emphasizing smoking cessation, managing HTN and dyslipidemia, aspirin therapy, and exercise.

Behavioral Changes

Emphasis on lifestyle changes with diet, exercise, weight reduction, and behavioral change will help improve glycemic control and reduce complications (ADA, 2018; Munshi, 2019). Exercise or physical activity goals should be tailored to the individual patients, and coordination with physical therapy and occupational therapy may help those with functional or physical limitations. Medical nutrition therapy should be tailored to the needs of patients due to aging issues such as changes in taste, dentition alterations, functional barriers, and comorbidities that affect nutrition. Referring patients for dietary counseling with a dietitian and/or certified diabetes educator can help balance these factors with dietary goals (ADA, 2018; Munshi, 2019).

Medications

Older patients may require pharmacologic therapy along with lifestyle changes to manage hyperglycemia (see Table 15.2). For adults who do not have renal impairment or unstable, acute heart failure, metformin may be used as initial therapy (ADA, 2018; Munshi, 2019). A short-acting sulfonylurea such as glipizide or glimepiride may be considered as second-line therapy, but clinicians should be aware of the hypoglycemia risks associated with this drug class. In general, thiazolidinediones should be avoided in older adults due to weight gain, increased risk of heart failure, and osteoporotic fracture. If patients are not achieving the goal of blood glucose control, then a second agent may be added (ADA, 2018; Munshi, 2019). Consideration of cost, comorbid conditions, hypoglycemia risk, and avoiding weight gain can help with the decision-making process. If patients fail to achieve glycemic goals with two agents, then initiating or intensifying insulin therapy should be considered. Sulfonylureas should be discontinued in this situation. An alternative for three-agent therapy is two oral agents and a GLP-1 receptor agonist (ADA, 2018; Munshi, 2019).

TABLE 15.2 Diabetic Medications

Class (Drugs)	Initial Dose	Advantages	Disadvantages
Biguanides (Metformin)	500 mg BID	1%–1.5% A1C reduction Weight neutral Reduces CVD events Tx of prediabetes Lack of hypoglycemia as monotherapy	Diarrhea/abdominal sx B12 deficiency Lactic acidosis (rare) Watch renal function
Sulfonylureas (glyburide, glipizide, glimepiride)	Glyburide: 2.5 mg daily Glipizide: 5 mg daily Glimepiride: 1 mg daily	1%–1.5% A1C reduction Good efficacy initially Inexpensive	Hypoglycemia (less with glimepiride) Weight gain Reduced efficacy over time Start low in older adults D/C with complex insulin regimens
Thiazolidinediones (pioglitazone, rosiglitazone)	Pioglitazone: 15 mg daily Rosiglitazone: 4 mg daily	1%–1.5% A1C reduction Lack of hypoglycemia Improves HDL levels Reduced triglycerides (pioglitazone) May reduce CVD (pioglitazone)	Weight gain Fluid retention (CHF) Increased fracture risk Increased LDL (rosiglitazone) Increased risk of bladder cancer (pioglitazone)

DPP-4 inhibitors (alogliptin, linagliptin, saxagliptin, sitagliptin)	Alogliptin: 25 mg daily Linagliptin: 5 mg daily Saxagliptin: 2.5–5 mg daily Sitagliptin: 100 mg daily	0.5%–1% A1C reduction Lack of hypoglycemia with monotherapy Weight neutral Well tolerated	Dosage modification with renal impairment CYP3A4 interactions (saxagliptin, linagliptin) Associated with pancreatitis Worsen heart failure (saxagliptin) Cause severe joint pain
SGLT2 inhibitors (canagliflozin, dapagliflozin, empagliflozin)	Canagliflozin: 100 mg daily Dapagliflozin: 5 mg daily Empagliflozin: 10 mg daily	0.5%–1% A1C reduction Lack of hypoglycemia as monotherapy Weight loss Decrease BP	Fungal infections/UTI/frequency Hypotension Increase LDL Cannot use for decreased eGFR Fractures/decreased BMD Increased bladder cancer risk (canagliflozin) Association with ketoacidosis
GLP-1 agonists (albiglutide, dulaglutide, exenatide, exenatide ER, liraglutide)	Albiglutide: 30 mg SC weekly Dulaglutide: 0.75 mg SC weekly Exenatide: 5 mcg SC BID Exenatide ER: 2 mg SC once weekly Liraglutide: 0.6 mg SC once daily x 1wk, then 1.2 mg SC once daily	1%–1.5% A1C reduction Lack of hypoglycemia as monotherapy Weight loss Reduces postprandial glucose levels Emerging as a good choice for patients needing more than 1–2 meds, combination with basal insulin	Headache Nausea (transient)/diarrhea Renal dose adjustment Avoid in severe renal impairment (exenatide) Associated with pancreatitis Associated with thyroid cell cancer in rodents Associated with renal insufficiency Injectable

(continued)

TABLE 15.2 Diabetic Medications *(continued)*

Class (Drugs)	Initial Dose	Advantages	Disadvantages
Alpha-glucosidase inhibitor (acarbose, miglitol)	Acarbose: 25 mg TID Miglitol: 25 mg TID	0.5%–1% Lack of hypoglycemia as monotherapy Weight neutral Reduces postprandial glucose values Not absorbed Reduces CVD events (acarbose) Tx of prediabetes (acarbose)	Modest effect on A1C Flatulence/Diarrhea Frequent dosing
SGLT2 inhibitors (canagliflozin, dapagliflozin, empagliflozin)	Canagliflozin: 100 mg daily Dapagliflozin: 5 mg daily Empagliflozin: 10 mg daily	0.5%–1% A1C reduction Lack of hypoglycemia as monotherapy Weight loss Decrease BP	Fungal infections/UTI/frequency Hypotension Increase LDL Cannot use for decreased eGFR Fractures/decreased BMD Increased bladder cancer risk (canagliflozin) Association with ketoacidosis

GLP-1 agonists (albiglutide, dulaglutide, exenatide, exenatide ER, liraglutide)	Albiglutide: 30 mg SC weekly Dulaglutide: 0.75 mg SC weekly Exenatide: 5 mcg SC BID Exenatide ER: 2 mg SC once weekly Liraglutide: 0.6 mg SC once daily × 1 wk, then 1.2 mg SC once daily	1%–1.5% A1C reduction Lack of hypoglycemia as monotherapy Weight loss Reduces postprandial glucose levels Emerging as a good choice for patients needing more than 1–2 meds, combination with basal insulin	Headache Nausea (transient)/diarrhea Renal dose adjustment Avoid in severe renal impairment (exenatide) Associated with pancreatitis Associated with thyroid cell cancer in rodents Associated with renal insufficiency Injectable
Alpha-glucosidase inhibitor (acarbose, miglitol)	Acarbose: 25 mg TID Miglitol: 25 mg TID	0.5%–1% Lack of hypoglycemia as monotherapy Weight neutral Reduces postprandial glucose values Not absorbed Reduces CVD events (acarbose) Tx of prediabetes (acarbose)	Modest effect on A1C Flatulence/Diarrhea Frequent dosing

BID, two times per day; BMD, bone mineral density; BP, blood pressure; CHF, congestive heart failure; CVD, cardiovascular disease; D/C, discontinue; eGFR, estimated glomerular filtration rate; HDL, high-density lipoprotein; LDL, low-density lipoprotein; SC, subcutaneous; sx, symptoms; TID, three times per day; Tx, treatment; UTI, urinary tract infection.

Source: Data from American Diabetes Association. (2018). 15. Diabetes advocacy: Standards of medical care in diabetes—2018. *Diabetes Care, 41*(Suppl. 1), S152–S153. doi:10.2337/dc18-s015; Pharmacist's Letter. (2015). *Drugs for type 2 diabetes.* Retrieved from http://pharmacistsletter. therapeuticresearch.com/pl/ArticleDD.aspx?nidchk=1&cs=&s=PL&pt=2&segment=4407&dd=280601; Munshi, M. (2019). Treatment of type 2 diabetes mellitus in the older patient. In D. M. Nathan, K. E. Schmader, & J. E. Mulder (Eds.), *UpToDate.* Retrieved from https://www.uptodate.com/contents/treatment-of-type-2-diabetes-mellitus-in-the-older-patient

TABLE 15.3 Insulin Overview

Insulin Category	Examples
Rapid-acting analogs	Lispro, aspart, inhaled insulin
Short-acting analogs	Human regular
Intermediate-acting analogs	Human NPH
Basal insulin analogs	Glargine, detemir
Premixed insulin products	NPH/Regular 70/30 70/30 aspart mix 75/25 lispro mix 50/50 lispro mix

Source: Data from American Diabetes Association. (2018). 15. Diabetes advocacy: Standards of medical care in diabetes—2018. *Diabetes Care, 41*(Suppl. 1), S152–S153. doi:10.2337/dc18-s015; Munshi, M. (2019). Treatment of type 2 diabetes mellitus in the older patient. In D. M. Nathan, K. E. Schmader, & J. E. Mulder (Eds.), *UpToDate*. Retrieved from https://www.uptodate.com/contents/treatment-of-type-2-diabetes-mellitus-in-the-older-patient

Insulin therapy is becoming easier to administer, but physical or cognitive limitations should be considered before initiating therapy. Family members or a pharmacist may be able to prepare a week's worth of fixed dose insulin syringes for patients who are not physically or cognitively able to do the task themselves (Munshi, 2019). Starting with a bedtime intermediate-acting or long-acting insulin at a base dose of 10 units or 0.2 units per kg is appropriate. Dose adjustments may be made on a weekly basis to achieve glycemic goals (see Table 15.3).

If the provider and patient decide that insulin therapy will be the emphasis of treatment, then a basal/bolus insulin approach may be used. The basal to bolus ratio should be 50/50 (Moses, 2019). If bolus insulin is initiated, then sulfonylureas, DPP-4 inhibitors, meglitinides, and GLP-1 receptor agonists should be discontinued. The bolus dose should start with 0.1 units/kg before the largest meal with a corresponding reduction of basal insulin by 0.1 units/kg (Moses, 2019). There are multiple approaches for dosing including the following:

- Based on postprandial glucose levels
- Dosed to cover carbohydrate load
- Dosed with correction for elevated glucose levels (Moses, 2019)

Providers should remember that less complicated regimens are optimal for those with functional and cognitive limitations. In addition, less insulin is needed in individuals with chronic renal failure due to impaired insulin metabolism (Munshi, 2019).

Treatment Response

Nurse practitioners should be aware of the risks related to polypharmacy in older patients and ensure accurate medication lists, provide good follow-up, and be careful about overtreatment or complicated regimens. To assess response to therapy, A1C measurement should occur twice a year for individuals who are well controlled or quarterly in patients with therapy changes or who fail to achieve glycemic goals (ADA, 2018).

THYROID DISEASE

Both hypothyroidism and hyperthyroidism are encountered in older adults, and they can contribute to significant distress if misdiagnosed or untreated. Older adults are susceptible to thyroid conditions due to aging changes, and studies have noted increased thyroid-stimulating hormone (TSH) levels in older age. The primary care nurse practitioner needs to be cognizant of thyroid disease in older adults and recognize that symptoms might be attenuated by comorbid conditions or medications (American Thyroid Association [ATA], n.d.; Papaleontiou & Haymart, 2012).

Hyperthyroidism

Hyperthyroidism in older adults may be related to Graves disease, multinodular goiter, or toxic nodular adenomas (Papaleontiou & Haymart, 2012). Elderly patients may present with classic symptoms such as tremors, anxiety, palpitations, weight loss, and heat intolerance. However, one-third of patients will present with less dramatic symptoms (Papaleontiou & Haymart, 2012). Weight loss, apathy, and tachycardia tend to be the most common symptoms (Ross, 2019a). Older adults may also have subclinical hyperthyroidism, which occurs more commonly in women than men. It is important to recognize hyperthyroidism in aging patients because the complications of this disease (atrial fibrillation, cardiovascular mortality, and osteoporosis) can be significant (Papaleontiou & Haymart, 2012; Ross, 2019a).

Diagnosis

Initial testing for hyperthyroidism is a serum TSH although providers should note that low TSH may be present in acutely ill patients in the hospital (Papaleontiou & Haymart, 2012). In most cases, nurse practitioners in primary care would refer patients to an endocrinologist for further evaluation, especially if the patient does not have Graves disease. There may be cases where further workup in primary care should occur with referral for radioactive iodine uptake to identify disease nodules or other disease etiology (Papaleontiou & Haymart, 2012; Ross, 2019a).

Treatment

Treatment of hyperthyroidism should address symptoms of tachycardia through beta-blockade. Additionally, treatment should address the root cause through iodine ablation, antithyroid medications, or thyroidectomy (Papaleontiou & Haymart, 2012). Ablation is a modality often used in older adults due to safety and efficacy. The main issue with this approach is the slow reversal of hyperthyroidism and the need to manage cardiac sequelae until thyrotoxicosis is reversed. Subsequently, most patients develop hypothyroidism and require thyroid hormone therapy (Papaleontiou & Haymart, 2012). If antithyroid medication is used to treat hyperthyroidism, methimazole is the preferred agent. Older adults are at greater risk for recurrence and for medication side effects with both methimazole and propylthiouracil. Surgical treatment is generally the last resort due to increased morbidity. This approach may be used for large goiters or malignancy (Papaleontiou & Haymart, 2012; Ross, 2019a). Subclinical hyperthyroidism may be treated in older adults if the TSH is <0.1 mIU/L or considered if the TSH is 0.1 to 0.5 mIU/L (Papaleontiou & Haymart, 2012).

Hypothyroidism

Hypothyroidism incidence increases with age, especially due to increased risk of Hashimoto's thyroiditis (Papaleontiou & Haymart, 2012). Sometimes a diagnosis of hypothyroidism is missed in older adults because cold intolerance, constipation, fatigue, weakness, and dry skin may be attributed to aging, medications, or comorbid conditions (ATA, n.d.; Papaleontiou & Haymart, 2012; Ross, 2019b). Depressive symptoms related to hypothyroidism are relatively common in older adults, and the most common symptoms in older adults are fatigue and weakness. Identifying and treating hypothyroidism is of the utmost importance due to increased risk of cognitive impairment, cardiovascular side effects, and myxedema coma (this has a high mortality rate); see Papaleontiou and Haymart (2012).

Diagnosis and Treatment

Just as in hyperthyroidism, initial screening is completed with a serum TSH. An elevated TSH is an indicator of hypothyroidism and may be further evaluated with free T4 levels (thyroxine). With corresponding low T4 levels, this is a good indication of hypothyroidism. Primary hypothyroidism should be treated unless it is transient due to a subacute condition or reversible etiology (Papaleontiou & Haymart, 2012; Ross, 2019b).

The standard clinical treatment for hypothyroidism is synthetic thyroxine (T4) or levothyroxine. Older adults often require lower levothyroxine doses; so initiation at 12.5 to 25 mcg or 25 to 50 mcg versus 1.6 mcg/kg/day may be appropriate (Papaleontiou & Haymart, 2012; Ross, 2019b). Dosage increases can occur every 6 weeks as needed, and lower titration increments (12.5–25 mcg) may be preferable. Treatment targets should be a normal TSH level, symptom control, reduction in goiter (if present), and avoiding overtreatment (Papaleontiou & Haymart, 2012; Ross, 2019b).

Treatment of subclinical hypothyroidism (high TSH and normal free T4) is controversial due to research demonstrating no net benefit with treatment. Other researchers recommend levothyroxine with consistently elevated TSH and symptoms associated with low thyroid function, family history of thyroid disease, or severe hyperlipidemia that is attributable to thyroid dysfunction (Papaleontiou & Haymart, 2012; Ross, 2019b).

PARATHYROID DISEASE

Parathyroid disease in older adults is relatively common, and it is an important disease for primary care nurse practitioners to identify due to the complications of calcium imbalances, such as fracture or renal stones (Fuleihan, 2019; Goltzman, 2019). While management may not occur solely in the primary care setting, an understanding of the conditions and treatment will help nurse practitioners identify treatment response and appropriately manage comorbidities. A brief overview of hypoparathyroidism and hyperparathyroidism is presented in the following.

Hypoparathyroidism

Acquired hypoparathyroidism generally occurs due to surgery or an autoimmune response. In adults, head and neck surgeries are the most common cause of parathyroid dysfunction (Goltzman, 2019). Decreased secretion of parathyroid hormone results in decreased calcium secretion; so the symptoms range from mild to severe manifestations of hypocalcemia including:

- Tetany
- Fatigue
- Irritability
- Anxiety/depression
- Seizures
- Heart failure
- QT prolongation
- Arrhythmias (Goltzman, 2019)

Chronic hypocalcemia related to hypoparathyroidism may result in basal ganglia calcifications, increased bone mineral density (BMD), cataracts, dental issues, and skin manifestations (Fuleihan, 2019).

Diagnosis

Hypoparathyroidism can be identified through laboratory testing. The findings indicate hypocalcemia and low or inappropriately normal parathyroid hormone. Serum phosphorus levels are usually elevated, serum 25-hydroxyvitamin D is usually normal, and magnesium and creatinine are normal. Individuals may have increased urine calcium due to high urinary calcium excretion (Goltzman, 2019). In older patients who are more prone to nutritional deficiencies, nurse practitioners should be aware of calcium corrections based on albumin levels.

Treatment

After a diagnosis of hyperparathyroidism is established, a 24-hour urine should be collected prior to initiating treatment due to the risk of kidney stones with restored calcium levels in this population. Treatment of this condition may range from supplementation with oral calcium and vitamin D in mild cases to intravenous calcium plus oral calcitriol supplementation in acute, severe cases. Restoration of low normal calcium levels (8.0–8.5 mg/dL or 2.0–2.1 mmol/L) and prevention of kidney stones should be the treatment goal. Correction of low vitamin D and magnesium levels should also be addressed (Goltzman, 2019).

Hyperparathyroidism

Patients with hyperparathyroidism are often asymptomatic, even with elevated calcium levels. The classic manifestation of hyperparathyroidism includes kidney stones, abdominal pains, bone disease, and mental instability (Fuleihan, 2019). Other nonspecific symptoms include fatigue, thirst, increased urination, weakness, decreased appetite, depression, cognitive impairment, and neuromuscular dysfunction. Patients with hyperparathyroidism may experience cardiovascular complications including elevated blood pressure, arrhythmias, ventricular hypertrophy, and vascular/valvular calcification (Fuleihan, 2019).

Diagnosis

Diagnosis is made based on laboratory findings including normal to elevated calcium levels, elevated parathyroid hormone levels, low phosphorus levels, vitamin D imbalances, and normal to low magnesium levels. Patients may also have metabolic acidosis and normochromic/normocytic anemia. Nurse practitioners need to be aware of the manifestations and workup for this condition due to cardiovascular mortality risk (Fuleihan, 2019).

Treatment

Parathyroidectomy is the definitive treatment for hyperparathyroidism, but this may be prohibitive in older adults with frailty or multimorbidity (Marcoci, Bollerslev, Khan, & Shoback, 2014; Morris, Zelada, Wu, Hahn, & Yeh, 2010). Low vitamin D levels should be corrected and normal calcium supplementation may occur (Marcoci et al., 2014). Cinacalcet may be used as a nonsurgical approach, but it does not appear to affect parathyroid hormone levels or bone density. Alendronate does improve BMD but does not alter serum calcium levels. Combination therapy may be used, but there is no strong evidence for this approach (Fuleihan, 2019; Marcoci et al., 2014).

OSTEOPOROSIS

Osteoporosis is a significant clinical issue in the aging population due to increased incidence in aging along with coincidental risk of falls and fracture (Jeremiah, Unwin, Greenawald, & Casiano, 2015). It occurs when the balance of bone resorption and deposition is disrupted. With excessive resorption, bone density decreases, bones weaken (osteopenia), and eventually become brittle (osteoporosis; International Osteoporosis Foundation, n.d.). Osteoporosis occurs more commonly in women, but it is also a consideration in men (Jeremiah et al., 2015).

Screening and Diagnosis

Nurse practitioners should be prepared to diagnose and treat osteoporosis to reduce the risk of mortality, disability, and increased healthcare costs in aging patients. Risk factors for osteoporosis include:

- Excessive alcohol intake
- Gonadal hormone deficiency
- Immobility and sedentary lifestyle
- Age
- Low body weight
- Low calcium and vitamin D intake
- Personal history of fracture or family history of osteoporotic fracture
- Smoking
- White or Asian race (Jeremiah et al., 2015)

Screening for osteoporosis may occur with an annual health exam in those who meet criteria, or it may be assessed if a patient has a low-velocity or fragility fracture. If a patient has multiple risk factors, the Fracture Risk Assessment Tool (FRAX) provides an overview of 10-year risk. Those with normal BMD should be rescreened every 4 years, and repeat BMD testing should not exceed every 2 years (Jeremiah et al., 2014; Rosen & Drezner, 2019). See Box 15.1 for screening recommendations.

Diagnosis of osteoporosis is made based on BMD findings from dual energy x-ray absorptiometry (DEXA) scan. Diagnostic criteria have been established by the World

BOX 15.1 Osteoporosis Screening Recommendations

> Recommendation for screening with BMD testing in men and women.
> Women 65 years and older should be screened for osteoporosis.
> Postmenopausal women younger than 65 should be screened for osteoporosis using a risk assessment tool. If 10-year fracture risk equals or exceeds the risk of a 65-year-old White woman with no risk factors, then BMD testing is a reasonable approach.
> There is insufficient evidence to balance benefits and harms for routine osteoporosis screening in men. Providers should consider individual clinical risk factors and determine screening on an individual basis.

BMD, bone mineral density.

Source: Data from Jeremiah, M. P., Unwin, B. K., Greenawald, M. H., & Casiano, V. E. (2015). Diagnosis and management of osteoporosis. *American Family Physician, 92*(4), 261–268. Retrieved from https://www.aafp.org/afp/2015/0815/p261.html; U.S. Preventive Services Task Force. (2018). *Osteoporosis to prevent fractures: Screening.* Retrieved from https://www.uspreventiveservicestaskforce.org/Page/Document/RecommendationStatementFinal/osteoporosis-screening1

TABLE 15.4 Diagnostic Criteria for Osteoporosis and Osteopenia in Women and Men Older Than 50 Years

Diagnostic Category	Bone Mineral Density
Normal bone density	Bone density within 1.0 SD below young adult mean (T-score ≥−1.0)
Osteopenia or decreased bone density	Bone density between 1.0 and 2.5 SDs below young adult mean (T-score <−1.0 and >−2.5)
Osteoporosis	Bone density ≥2.5 SDs below young adult mean (T-score ≤−2.5)
Severe or established osteoporosis	Bone density ≥2.5 SDs below young adult mean and presence of one or more fractures related to osteoporosis

SD, standard deviation.

Source: Data from Jeremiah, M. P., Unwin, B. K., Greenawald, M. H., & Casiano, V. E. (2015). Diagnosis and management of osteoporosis. *American Family Physician, 92*(4), 261–268. Retrieved from https://www.aafp.org/afp/2015/0815/p261.html; National Institutes of Health Osteoporosis and RelatedBone DiseasesNational Resource Center. (2018). *Bone mass measurement: What the numbers mean*. Retrieved from https://www.bones.nih.gov/health-info/bone/bone-health/bone-mass-measure

Health Organization in women and men older than 50 years (Jeremiah et al., 2015; National Institutes of Health, 2018). See Table 15.4 for a summary of these criteria.

In children and premenopausal women, the z-score should be used, and a score of −2.0 or less is below the expected range. In men younger than 50 years old, bone density cannot be used alone to diagnose osteoporosis (Jeremiah et al., 2015).

Treatment

Treatment of osteopenia or osteoporosis in men and postmenopausal women should occur according to the following criteria:

- Personal history of hip or vertebral fracture
- T-score of −2.5 or less
- Combination of osteopenia (T-score between −1 and −2.5) and 10-year probability of hip fracture of at least 3% or any major fracture of at least 20% (based on the FRAX)

All patients should be educated on nonpharmacologic treatment measures including weight-bearing exercise, physical therapy when needed, vitamin D supplementation if appropriate, smoking cessation, alcohol reduction, limiting caffeine, and diet high in protein, calcium, vitamin D, vegetables, and fruits (Jeremiah et al., 2015; Rosen & Drezner, 2019).

Pharmacologic treatment includes:

- Bisphosphonates (alendronate, ibandronate, risedronate, and zoledronic acid). Some serious considerations in this class include risk of femoral shaft fractures, osteonecrosis of the jaw, and esophageal ulceration or perforations. Other side effects include upper gastrointestinal (GI) discomfort, bleeding, and muscular and joint pain. Elderly patients may be at higher risk of the following contraindications: esophageal abnormalities, inability to stand or sit for at least 30 minutes, chronic kidney disease (estimated glomerular filtration rate [eGFR] <30 mL/min),

and increased risk of aspiration or dysphagia. Drug discontinuation should be considered after 5 years in patients who are at low risk.
- Raloxifene: This is indicated only for vertebral fractures. Serious side effects include thromboembolic events like pulmonary emboli. Due to these side effects, raloxifene may be inappropriate in older adults at higher risk for venous thromboembolism.
- Teriparatide: This is for the treatment of high-risk patients. Common side effects with this medication include pain, nausea, transient orthostasis, hypercalcemia, and hyperuricemia. There is a risk of angioedema and anaphylaxis.
- Denosumab: This is also a treatment for high-risk patients. Older women with poor dental hygiene or cancer are at risk of osteonecrosis of the jaw. It may cause muscular and joint pain. This is contraindicated in individuals with hypocalcemia (Jeremiah et al., 2015).

Oral bisphosphonates are generally inexpensive and effective; so they are an excellent first-line option. Ibandronate is only indicated for vertebral fracture; so it may not be optimal for all patients. If patients remain at high risk for fracture after 5 years of bisphosphonate treatment, providers should consider continuing treatment or switching to an agent like denosumab (Jeremiah et al., 2015; Rosen & Drezner, 2019). Drug holidays for stable patients after 3 to 5 years are indicated only for bisphosphonates (North American Menopause Society, 2017).

SUMMARY

Primary care nurse practitioners are often the first stop for patients who may be experiencing symptoms related to endocrine disease. Nurse practitioners may also make ongoing treatment and referral decisions regarding type 2 diabetes, thyroid and parathyroid disease, and osteoporosis. It is essential to understand the recommended pharmacologic therapies, lifestyle management, and long-term outcomes associated with these endocrine disorders.

ENDOCRINE INTERPROFESSIONAL CASE STUDY
Megan Hebdon

Patient Presentation

Mrs. Reyes is an 82 year-old Filipino woman who presents to your clinic reporting burning in her fingers and toes. She is accompanied by her daughter. They are both bilingual with English and Filipino. She has noted these symptoms for a long time (over 10 years), but reports that they are affecting her ability to cook and clean. She rarely comes in for appointments, because she is "too busy" and "what will be will be." She has been taking metformin for 5 years for her diabetes. She reports no changes in taste or smell, no tongue enlargement, and mild fatigue. Her HTN is stable; last A1c was 7.2. Her review of systems reveals no additional concerns.

History

She has had five live births and two miscarriages. She went through menopause at 54, and she was diagnosed with breast cancer at 65 (treated with docetaxel, doxorubicin, and cyclophosphamide). Her family history is unknown. She had a lumpectomy on the right; otherwise she had no surgeries. She denies alcohol, tobacco, and drug use. Her husband is deceased; she lives alone but has family nearby, and she is active in her church community. She eats mostly Filipino food, which she cooks, and walks every day with her daughter.

Medications

Metformin 1,000 mg twice daily, losartan 10 mg daily, and aspirin 81 mg daily. No known allergies to medications or other substances.

Physical Exam

Vital signs are Pulse: 64 beats per minute; Blood pressure: 128/72 mmHg; Respirations: 18 breaths per minute; Temperature: 97.2 degrees F; Oxygen saturation: 98%.

She is alert, oriented, pleasant, and cooperative. Her physical exam is unremarkable besides the following findings: steady gait, equal strength in bilateral upper and lower extremities, and full range of motion (ROM) to upper and lower extremities bilaterally. Timed up and go test was 24 seconds. Cranial nerves II–XII intact, intact deep tendon reflexes (DTRs), and negative Romberg. Foot exam with skin intact, no pain to palpation, arches intact bilaterally, and callouses noted to the plantar forefoot. Monofilament test with diminished sensation to R great toe and third toe and L great toe, third, and fifth toes. Patient unable to pick up pennies off of the desk with pincer grasp. She has a normal affect, full spectrum of emotions, and intact judgment and insight.

Diagnostic Testing

Complete blood count (CBC) shows mild microcytic anemia, comprehensive metabolic panel (CMP) with fasting glucose 102, and stage I chronic kidney disease (CKD), A1C 7.0, B12 within normal limits (WNL), TSH/T4 WNL, homocysteine WNL, folic acid WNL, and vitamin D mildly deficient.

Plan of Care

You diagnose the patient with peripheral neuropathy, although the origin is uncertain. The patient has a prior history of breast cancer and was treated with a taxane that can induce peripheral neuropathy. She also has a history of diabetes although this is well controlled. Due to her age, her A1C goal could even be increased to closer to 8.0. This is something you discuss with the patient and her daughter. They do not note any issues with hypoglycemia, dizziness, and do not think her fatigue is due to her blood glucose. You also discuss the importance of daily foot inspection and foot care, avoiding extreme temperatures, using good footwear, and following up for foot inspections by a provider every 3 to 6 months. The patient is less concerned with the pain, so is not interested in a prescription medication for this. You discuss potential topical treatments such as menthol or capsaicin cream.

Interprofessional Collaboration

Due to the infrequency of patient visits, the medical records from the patient's oncologists have never been obtained. You discuss having the patient complete paperwork so that her oncology records can be sent to the clinic. You discuss the benefits of occupational therapy in developing strategies to work around the limitations that the neuropathy imposes. She currently has no gait abnormalities although her timed up and go test was greater than 12 seconds. You discuss the benefits of physical therapy for fall prevention. The patient is in relatively good health at this time, but you discuss the importance of advanced directives with the patient and her daughter due to the patient's age and intact memory and judgment. They are both given a copy of Five Wishes to review at home with the rest of the family.

Case Study References

Aging with Dignity. (n.d.). *Five wishes*. Retrieved from https://fivewishes.org/shop/order/product/five-wishes

American Diabetes Association. (2018). 15. Diabetes advocacy: Standards of medical care in diabetes—2018. *Diabetes Care, 41*(Suppl. 1), S152–S153. doi:10.2337/dc18-s015

Centers for Disease Control and Prevention. (2017). *Assessment: Timed up and go (TUG)*. Retrieved from https://www.cdc.gov/steadi/pdf/TUG_Test-print.pdf

Feldman, E. L., & McCulloch, D. K. (2018, November 27). Treatment of diabetic neuropathy. In J. M. Shefner, D. M. Nathan, & A. F. Eichler (Eds.), *UpToDate*. Retrieved from https://www.uptodate.com/contents/treatment-of-diabetic-neuropathy

Health Resources and Services Administration. (2005). Diabetic foot screen for loss of protective sensation. Retrieved from https://www.hrsa.gov/sites/default/files/hansensdisease/pdfs/leapfilament.pdf

Hordon, L. D. (2018, January 12). Diabetic neuropathic arthropathy. In P. L. Romain, D. M. Nathan, & S. M. Helfgott (Eds.), *UpToDate*. Retrieved from https://www.uptodate.com/contents/diabetic-neuropathic-arthropathy

Loprinzi, C. L. (2019, August 23). Prevention and treatment of chemotherapy-induced peripheral neuropathy. In D. M. F. Savarese, R. E. Drews, & R. M. Goldberg (Eds.), *UpToDate*. Retrieved from https://www.uptodate.com/contents/prevention-and-treatment-of-chemotherapy-induced-peripheral-neuropathy/print

REFERENCES

American Diabetes Association. (2018). 15. Diabetes advocacy: Standards of medical care in diabetes—2018. *Diabetes Care, 41*(Suppl. 1), S152–S153. doi:10.2337/dc18-s015

American Thyroid Association. (n.d.). *Older patients and thyroid disease*. Retrieved from https://www.thyroid.org/thyroid-disease-older-patient

Fuleihan, G. E.-H., & Silverberg, S. J. (2019). Primary hyperparathyroidism: Clinical manifestations. In C. J. Rosen & J. E. Mulder (Eds.), *UpToDate*. Retrieved from https://www.uptodate.com/contents/primary-hyperparathyroidism-clinical-manifestations/print

Goltzman, D. (2019). Hypoparathyroidism. In C. J. Rosen, J. I. Wolfsdorf, & J. E. Mulder (Eds.), *UpToDate*. Retrieved from https://www.uptodate.com/contents/hypoparathyroidism/print

International Osteoporosis Foundation. (n.d.). *Pathophysiology: Biological causes of osteoporosis*. Retrieved from https://www.iofbonehealth.org/pathophysiology-biological-causes-osteoporosis

Jeremiah, M. P., Unwin, B. K., Greenawald, M. H., & Casiano, V. E. (2015). Diagnosis and management of osteoporosis. *American Family Physician, 92*(4), 261–268. Retrieved from https://www.aafp.org/afp/2015/0815/p261.html

Marcoci, C., Bollerslev, J., Khan, A. A., & Shoback, D. M. (2014). Medical management of primary hyperparathyroidism: Proceedings of the fourth international workshop on the management of hyperparathyroidism. *The Journal of Clinical Endocrinology & Metabolism, 99*(10), 3607–3618. doi:10.1210/jc.2014-1417

Morris, L. F., Zelada, J., Wu, B., Hahn, T. J., & Yeh, M. W. (2010). Parathyroid surgery in the elderly. *The Oncologist, 15*(12), 1273–1284. doi:10.1634/theoncologist.2010-0158

Moses, S. (2019). Insulin dosing in type 2 diabetes. *Family Practice Notebook*. Retrieved from http://www.fpnotebook.com/Endo/Pharm/InslnDsngInTypDbts1.htm

Munshi, M. (2019). Treatment of type 2 diabetes mellitus in the older patient. In D. M. Nathan, K. E. Schmader, & J. E. Mulder (Eds.), *UpToDate*. Retrieved from https://www.uptodate.com/contents/treatment-of-type-2-diabetes-mellitus-in-the-older-patient

National Institutes of Health Osteoporosis and Related Bone Diseases National Resource Center. (2018). *Bone mass measurement: What the numbers mean*. Retrieved from https://www.bones.nih.gov/health-info/bone/bone-health/bone-mass-measure

North American Menopause Society. (2017). Confusion about long-term treatment of osteoporosis clarified. *ScienceDaily*. Retrieved from https://www.sciencedaily.com/releases/2017/10/171011091800.htm

Papaleontiou, M., & Haymart, M. R. (2012). Approach to and treatment of thyroid disorders in the elderly. *Medical Clinics of North America, 96*(2), 297–310. doi:10.1016/j.mcna.2012.01.013

Pharmacist's Letter. (2015). *Drugs for type 2 diabetes*. Retrieved from https://pharmacist.therapeuticresearch.com/Content/Segments/PRL/2015/Jun/Drugs-for-Type-2-Diabetes-8509

Rosen, H. N., & Drezner, M. K. (2019). Overview of the management of osteoporosis in postmenopausal women. In C. J. Rosen, K. E. Schmader, & J. E. Mulder (Eds.), *UpToDate*. Retrieved from https://www.uptodate.com/contents/overview-of-the-management-of-osteoporosis-in-postmenopausal-women

Ross, D. S. (2019a). Overview of the clinical manifestations of hyperthyroidism in adults. In D. S. Cooper & J. E. Mulder (Eds.), *UpToDate*. Retrieved from https://www.uptodate.com/contents/overview-of-the-clinical-manifestations-of-hyperthyroidism-in-adults

Ross, D. (2019b). Treatment of primary hypothyroidism in adults. In D. S. Cooper & J. E. Mulder (Eds.), *UpToDate*. Retrieved from https://www.uptodate.com/contents/treatment-of-primary-hypothyroidism-in-adults

U.S. Preventive Services Task Force. (2018). *Osteoporosis to prevent fractures: Screening*. Retrieved from https://www.uspreventiveservicestaskforce.org/Page/Document/RecommendationStatementFinal/osteoporosis-screening1

16 Hyperlipidemia

Megan Hebdon

OBJECTIVES

1. Describe lipid disorders in older adults and the association with cardiovascular disease
2. Identify patient risk factors and risk stratification for cardiovascular disease prevention
3. Discuss outline treatment goals and considerations for lipid disorder management and cardiovascular disease prevention in older adults

INTRODUCTION

Dyslipidemia is characterized by abnormal levels of low-density lipoprotein cholesterol (LDL-C), high-density lipoprotein cholesterol (HDL-C), triglycerides, or lipoprotein(a) (Lp[a]); see Rosenson and Durrington (2018). High levels of LDL-C with corresponding low levels of HDL-C are a major risk factor for heart attack, stroke, renal disease, dementia, and peripheral arterial disease. Clinically significant hypertriglyceridemia may put patients at risk for pancreatic disease and may also increase cardiovascular disease risk. Management of lipid disorders is often a priority in primary care for patients of any age but comes with key considerations in older adults. The major concerns related to treatment of lipid disorders include individual risk factors, comorbid conditions, and quality of life. In this chapter, a background of lipid disorders is reviewed, an overview of evidence-based guidelines is outlined, and application of guidelines is addressed in the geriatric population.

LIPID DISORDER BACKGROUND

Lipids are insoluble particles circulating in plasma that are carried by lipoproteins. They are used for energy, lipid deposition, hormone production, and the formation of bile acid. Lipoproteins have been classified according to size and concentration (Rosenson, 2019); see Table 16.1. Total serum cholesterol and lipoprotein carriers are related to atherosclerotic cardiovascular disease (ASCVD). The combination of LDL-C and very low density lipoprotein cholesterol (VLDL-C) is non-HDL-C; this is considered more atherogenic than LDL-C alone. Additionally, apolipoprotein B (apoB), the main protein in low-density lipoprotein (LDL) and VLDL, indicates atherogenicity more strongly than LDL-C alone (Grundy et al., 2018).

TABLE 16.1 Lipoprotein Classification

Lipoprotein	Description
Chylomicrons	Large particles carrying dietary fats, atherogenicity uncertain
VLDL	Carry cholesterol and endogenous triglycerides, atherogenic
LDL	Carry cholesterol esters, dominant atherogenic cholesterol
HDL	Carry cholesterol esters, not atherogenic

HDL, high-density lipoprotein; LDL, low-density lipoprotein; VLDL, very low density lipoprotein.

Sources: Data from Grundy, S. M., Stone, N. J., Bailey, A. L., Beam, C., Birtcher, K. K., Blumental, R. S., . . . Yeboah, J. (2018). 2018 AHA/ACC/AACVPR/AAPA/ABC/ACPM/ADA/AGS/APHA/ASPC/NLA/PCNA guideline on the management of blood cholesterol: A report of the American College of Cardiology/American Heart Association Task Force on Clinical Practice Guidelines. *Circulation, 139*, e1082–e1143. doi:10.1161/cir.0000000000000625; Rosenson, R. S. (2019). Lipoprotein classification, metabolism, and role in atherosclerosis. In M. W. Freeman & G. M. Saperia (Eds.), *UpToDate*. Retrieved from https://www.uptodate.com/contents/lipoprotein-classification-metabolism-and-role-in-atherosclerosis

ATHEROSCLEROTIC CARDIOVASCULAR DISEASE RISK AND LIPID DISORDERS

Over the past 10 years, there has been a move to treat lipid disorders based on the level of atherosclerotic cardiovascular disease (ASCVD) risk (Grundy et al., 2018; Jellinger et al., 2017). Box 16.1 provides an overview of risk-enhancing factors for ASCVD.

The following are definitions for specific lipid disorders:

- Lipid disorders: disorders of lipoprotein metabolism, lipodystrophies, and some lipid storage disorders; used to describe disorders with abnormal total, high-density lipoprotein (HDL), and LDL cholesterol, along with triglycerides
- Lipoprotein disorder: disorders of lipoproteins that carry cholesterol and triglyceride
- Dyslipidemia: elevated total or LDL cholesterol levels, or low HDL cholesterol levels; increases risk for atherosclerosis and cardiovascular disease.
- Hyperlipidemia: umbrella term for elevated lipids (fats, cholesterol, and triglycerides)
- Mixed hyperlipidemia: elevated LDL and triglyceride levels
- Hypertriglyceridemia: elevated triglycerides (Uphold, 2013)

SCREENING AND DIAGNOSIS OF LIPID DISORDERS

Due to the emphasis on prevention of ASCVD, periodic screening is recommended to help diagnose and treat lipid disorders and prevent heart attack, stroke, and peripheral arterial disease. Relevant screening criteria for older adults include the following:

- Screen for familial hypercholesterolemia (FH): indicated by family history of premature ASCVD and elevated cholesterol levels consistent with FH.

Hyperlipidemia

BOX 16.1 Factors Contributing to Enhanced Risk for ASCVD

Major Risk Factors

- Older age
- Primary hypercholesterolemia (non-HDL-C 190–219 mg/dL; LDL-C 160–189 mg/dL)
- Metabolic syndrome:
  - Abdominal obesity
  - Elevated triglycerides (>175 mg/dL)
  - Elevated blood pressure
  - Elevated blood glucose
  - Decreased HDL-C levels (<40 mg/dL in men and <50 mg/dL in women)
  - Total of three of the preceding syndromes being diagnostic
- Diabetes mellitus, hypertension, and chronic kidney disease
- Psoriasis, rheumatoid arthritis, AIDS, and other chronic inflammatory conditions
- Cigarette smoking
- Family history of premature ASCVD (men younger than 55 and women younger than 65) or hyperlipidemia
- Specific issues in women: PCOS, premature menopause, and pregnancy-related issues such as preeclampsia
- Having a high-risk ethnic background, such as being from South Asia
- Dyslipidemic triad: hypertriglyceridemia, low HDL-C, and excess of small dense LDL-C
- Other lipid/biomarker factors:
  - Persistently elevated triglycerides (>175 mg/dL)
  - Increased lipoprotein(a), clotting factors, and inflammation markers (CRP, Lp-PLA$_2$), homocysteine levels, uric acid, and triglyceride-rich remnants
  - Apo E4 isoform
  - Ankle–brachial index <0.9

ASCVD, atherosclerotic cardiovascular disease; CRP, C-reactive protein; HDL-C, high-density lipoprotein cholesterol; LDL-C, low-density lipoprotein cholesterol; Lp-PLA, lipoprotein-associated phospholipase A; PCOS, polycystic ovary syndrome.

Sources: Data from Grundy, S. M., Stone, N. J., Bailey, A. L., Beam, C., Birtcher, K. K., Blumental, R. S., . . . Yeboah, J. (2018). 2018 AHA/ACC/AACVPR/AAPA/ABC/ACPM/ADA/AGS/APHA/ASPC/NLA/PCNA guideline on the management of blood cholesterol: A report of the American College of Cardiology/American Heart Association Task Force on Clinical Practice Guidelines. *Circulation, 139*, e1082–e1143. doi:10.1161/cir.0000000000000625; Jellinger, P. S., Handelsman, Y., Rosenblit, P. D., Bloomgarden, Z. T., Fonseca, V. A., Garber, A. J., . . . Davidson, M. (2017). American Association of Clinical Endocrinologists and American College of Endocrinology guidelines for management of dyslipidemia and prevention of cardiovascular disease. *Endocrine Practice, 23*(Suppl. 2), 1–87. doi:10.4158/ep171764.appgl

- Screen individuals with diabetes mellitus annually.
- Screen adults 55 to 65 years every 1 to 2 years, more frequently if multiple risk factors are present.
- Screen adults 65 years and older annually.
- In adults 75 years and older, consider frailty, comorbid disease, goals of care, and cardiac risk; may continue to screen if the patient has long life expectancy and current quality of life.

In addition to screening with fasting lipid levels, some patients may benefit from receiving apoB screening, such as those with hypertriglyceridemia (triglyceride >200 mg/dL). This additional test may be cost-prohibitive and less accurate. Additionally, evaluating Lp(a) may be beneficial for patients with family history of premature ASCVD or personal history of ASCVD that is not explained by major risk factors (Grundy et al., 2018). However, the predictive utility in women is minimal (Grundy et al., 2018).

When conducting screening for lipid disorders, consider secondary sources of lipid abnormalities. For total cholesterol and LDL-C elevations, hypothyroidism, nephrosis, dysgammaglobulinemia in systemic lupus erythematosus (SLE) and multiple myeloma (MM), progestin or anabolic steroid treatment, cholestatic diseases of the liver, and protease inhibitors for HIV infection may be factors in increased levels (Jellinger et al., 2017). Chronic renal failure, type 2 diabetes mellitus, obesity, excessive alcohol intake, hypothyroidism, thiazide diuretics, beta-blockers, corticosteroids, oral estrogens, oral contraceptives, pregnancy, and protease inhibitors may contribute to increased triglyceride and VLDL-C levels (Jellinger et al., 2017).

Risk stratification of patients should occur to guide the decision to treat and treatment goals. The American Heart Association and the American College of Cardiology recommend using risk estimator tools, such as the ASCVD Risk Estimator tool, the Pooled Cohort Equation (PCE), the Framingham General CVD Risk Profile, and the Reynolds Risk Score (Lloyd-Jones et al., 2019). These should be used only with patients with no known ASCVD or FH (Lloyd-Jones et al., 2019). They also recommend assessing adults for ASCVD risk every 4 to 6 years. Patients can be categorized into four categories of risk, from low to high. High risk includes individuals with existing ASCVD, followed by individuals with LDL-C levels ≥190 mg/dL. Adults 40 to 75 years of age with diabetes mellitus should be started on a moderate-intensity statin, and further risk stratification may be conducted. The last category is individuals 40 to 75 years of age with a high 10-year risk as estimated by a risk assessment tool (Grundy et al., 2018). When determining the level of risk, conversations should be carried out with patients regarding maximizing lifestyle change, presence of risk-enhancing issues, and potential for adverse drug events related to statin therapy (Grundy et al., 2018). Grundy et al. (2018) describe the following risk-enhancing factors, which have similarities to the risks addressed by the American College of Endocrinology (ACE)/American Association of Clinical Endocrinologists (AACE) guidelines and are also outlined in Box 16.1:

- Family history of early ASCVD (males <55 years, females <65 years)
- Primary hypercholesterolemia
- Metabolic syndrome
- Chronic kidney disease
- Inflammatory conditions: psoriasis, rheumatoid arthritis (RA), and HIV/AIDS
- Premature menopause and/or preeclampsia
- High-risk race/ethnicities
- Lipid biomarkers
  - Persistently elevated triglycerides (≥175 mg/dL)
  - Elevated C-reactive protein (CRP)
  - Elevated Lp(a)
  - Elevated apoB
  - ABI <0.9

Treatment to Address ASCVD Risk

Treatment to reduce ASCVD risk includes lifestyle interventions: whole grains, increased fruits and vegetables, lean meats, low-fat dairy, plant-based fats, and limited added sugar. Weight loss should be a goal for individuals who are overweight or obese. Exercise recommendations include moderate to vigorous physical activity for 40 minutes, 3 to 4 times per week (Grundy et al., 2018). Additional interventions may be required for individuals with metabolic syndrome and/or difficulty losing weight or maintaining weight loss.

Along with lifestyle changes, statins are the cornerstone of lipid-lowering therapies. Statins are divided into low, moderate, and high intensity (see Table 16.2). Monitoring for response to statin therapy should be focused on percentage reduction of LDL-C because this has a corresponding reduction in ASCVD risk (Grundy et al., 2018). Statin side effects are outlined in Table 16.3. Nonstatin therapies that also reduce LDL-C include ezetimibe, bile acid sequestrants, and PCSK9 inhibitors. The side-effect profile for ezetimibe is fairly clean; bile acid sequestrants are associated with significant gastrointestinal side effects and may cause severe hypertriglyceridemia; and PCSK9 inhibitors are well tolerated, but long-term safety has not been established. Niacin and fibrates may have minimal effect on lowering LDL-C levels.

Individuals with known ASCVD should be treated with high-intensity statins, if tolerated. If poor statin tolerance occurs, then moderate-intensity statins should be used. For individuals over 75 years of age, statin initiation should be balanced with the following considerations: lowering ASCVD risk, adverse drug reactions, patient frailty, and patient and family goals of care (Grundy et al., 2018). Individuals older than 75 who are tolerating statin therapy may choose to remain on statin therapy, with discussions about ongoing ASCVD risk reduction, balancing adverse drug reactions, patient health status, and goals of care.

TABLE 16.2 Statin Intensity Levels

	High Intensity	Moderate Intensity	Low Intensity
LDL-C Lowering	≥50%	30%–49%	<30%
Statins	Atorvastatin 40–80 mg Rosuvastatin 20–40 mg	Atorvastatin 10–20 mg Rosuvastatin 5–10 mg Simvastatin 20–40 mg	Simvastatin 10 mg
		Pravastatin 40–80 mg Lovastatin 40–80 mg Fluvastatin XL 80 mg Fluvastatin 40 mg twice daily Pitavastatin 1–4 mg	Pravastatin 10–20 mg Lovastatin 20 mg Fluvastatin 20–40 mg

Source: From Grundy, S. M., Stone, N. J., Bailey, A. L., Beam, C., Birtcher, K. K., Blumental, R. S., . . . Yeboah, J. (2018). 2018 AHA/ACC/AACVPR/AAPA/ABC/ACPM/ADA/AGS/APHA/ASPC/NLA/PCNA guideline on the management of blood cholesterol: A report of the American College of Cardiology/American Heart Association Task Force on Clinical Practice Guidelines. *Circulation, 139,* e1082–e1143. doi:10.1161/cir.0000000000000625

TABLE 16.3 Statin-Associated Side Effects

Statin-Associated Side Effects	Predisposing Factors
Myalgias, myositis/myopathies (CK > ULN), rhabdomyolysis (CK >10 × ULN, plus renal injury), statin-associated autoimmune myopathy (HMGCR antibodies, incomplete resolution)	Age, female sex, low BMI, high-risk medications (CYP3A4 and OATP1B1 inhibitors), comorbid conditions (HIV, renal and liver disease, thyroid disease, existing myopathy), Asian ancestry, excess alcohol intake, high levels of physical activity, and trauma
New-onset diabetes mellitus	Diabetes mellitus risk factors, metabolic syndrome, high-intensity statin therapy

BMI, body mass index; CK, creatine kinase; HMGCR, 3-hydroxy-3-methylglutaryl-coenzyme A reductase; ULN, upper limit of normal.

If treatment goals are not being achieved with maximal statin therapy in patients with ASCVD who are 75 years or younger or with very high risk ASCVD, then ezetimibe may be added to therapy. If this does not produce the desired results, then a PCSK9 inhibitor may be added. Individuals at very high risk include the following:

- Recent myocardial infarction (MI)
- History of MI
- History of ischemic stroke
- Symptomatic peripheral arterial disease
- Sixty-five years or older
- Familial hypercholesterolemia
- History of coronary bypass surgery or percutaneous coronary intervention
- Diabetes mellitus
- Hypertension
- Chronic kidney disease stage 3
- Current smoking
- Elevated LDL-C despite maximum statin therapy and ezetimibe
- History of heart failure

In older individuals up to age 75 with severe hypercholesterolemia (LDL-C ≥190 mg/dL), high-intensity statins are recommended. If there is less than 50% reduction in LDL-C, then ezetimibe may be added. If there is less than 50% reduction with combination statin and ezetimibe, then a bile acid sequestrant may be considered, as long as triglycerides are ≤300 mg/dL. Individuals with heterozygous FH and LDL-C ≥100 mg/dL taking statins and ezetimibe may also consider adding a PCSK9 inhibitor. Grundy et al. (2018) describe additional recommendations for lipid management according to the presence of diabetes (use of moderate- to high-intensity statin) and high 10-year risk after risk stratification.

For older individuals, ongoing conversations about statin therapy should occur. For individuals older than age 75, moderate-intensity statin may be considered for LDL-C levels 70 to 189. Additionally, statin therapy may be discontinued if patients have functional or cognitive decline, frailty, multiple chronic illnesses, or decreased life expectancy (Grundy et al., 2018). Response to LDL-C lowering therapies should be evaluated 4 to 12 weeks after initiating statin therapy or after making dose adjustment. Response can then be evaluated every 3 to 12 months based on need (Grundy et al., 2018).

Treatment of Hypertriglyceridemia

Elevated triglycerides may contribute to cardiac risk; so they should be evaluated as part of the ASCVD risk assessment. Lifestyle changes to address obesity and metabolic syndrome should be encouraged, and secondary factors (diabetes mellitus, hypothyroidism, liver and kidney disease, and nephrotic syndrome) should be addressed (Grundy et al., 2018). For individuals with moderate (175–499 mg/dL) to severe (≥500 mg/dL) hypertriglyceridemia, initiation or intensification of statins, lifestyle therapy, and modifying risk from secondary causes may help reduce ASCVD risk. With very elevated triglyceride levels (≥500 mg/dL to ≥1000 mg/dL), intensifying lifestyle through a very low-fat diet, avoidance of alcohol and refined sugars, consumption of omega-3 fatty acids, and fibrate therapy should be considered to prevent pancreatitis (Grundy et al., 2018). Fibrate therapy in combination with statin therapy carries increased risk for myopathies and rhabdomyolysis; so nurse practitioners need to weigh the benefits of therapy with the risks related to drug–drug interactions. In older individuals, the risks of not treating severe hypertriglyceridemia with fibrates should be balanced with the risks related to adverse drug events due to both side effects and drug interactions.

SUMMARY

The management and reduction of ASCVD risk is of primary importance in older adults due to the higher incidence of predisposing factors. For nurse practitioners caring for geriatric patients, there is tension between reducing the risk of heart attack, stroke, and peripheral arterial disease and the potential for side effects and decreased quality of life, especially in patients older than 75. Ongoing conversations related to screening, risk assessment, treatment, and therapy intensification should occur with the need to reduce adverse drug events, promote ongoing function, and honor patient and family desires for care.

HYPERLIPIDEMIA INTERPROFESSIONAL CASE STUDY

Katie R. Katz

Patient Presentation

Lawrence is an 80-year-old male patient whom you are seeing in your clinic for routine chronic disease management and medication refills. His only complaint is discomfort bilaterally in his knees. He medication list was reviewed and he reports taking medications as prescribed, but he has added over-the-counter ibuprofen for his knee pain. He does have a prescription for Voltaren Gel that he uses intermittently when the ibuprofen "isn't enough." He reports that his job always kept him very active while he was working and that when he retired, he went walking daily at the mall for exercise. Since his knees started bothering him a few months ago, he has stopped his regular walking and has put on 13 pounds since his last office visit. He denies feeling fatigued and having chest pain or shortness of breath at rest or with activity. He also denies changes in his bowels and bladder. He tries to eat healthy foods, but reports that he and his wife do not like cooking just for two people, so they eat out nearly every day. He denies neurological changes including changes with his memory. He denies heat/cold intolerance and changes to his appetite.

History

He reports that his mother had Alzheimer's, his father died in World War II, and that he believes his siblings take medicine for high blood pressure, arthritis, and low thyroid. He is a retired railroad worker. He is married and has three living children, who he reports are doing well. He has had a history of hypertension, prostate cancer, and basal cell carcinoma of the skin. He has never routinely used tobacco products. His surgical history includes inguinal hernia repair at age 40, prostatectomy at age 61, and various skin biopsies. He has never had a cardiovascular evaluation more thorough than an EKG, which was normal when last completed 4 years ago. He has Railroad Medicare. He reports that they have saved well for retirement and feel that they are living comfortably at this time. He is able to travel often to see his adult children and their families in nearby states as well as travel for pleasure.

Medications

His prescriptions include lisinopril/hydrochlorothiazide (HCTZ) 20 mg/12.5 mg daily and Viagra 50 mg prn. These have not changed in the past 3 years. He also has a prescription for Voltaren Gel but reports he does not use it often.

He reports allergies to sulfa drugs but does not know what type of reaction he has.

Physical Exam

On physical exam, he is calm and cooperative. He presents well-dressed and has a positive disposition. His gait is slow but steady. He makes good eye contact and converses with ease. His Mini-Mental State Exam (MMSE) was a 29/30. His lungs are clear throughout. His cardiac assessment reveals regular rate and rhythm, with no abnormal sounds. He does have weakened, 1+, dorsalis pedis pulses. His abdomen is soft, nontender, and nondistended with active bowel sounds. He has one irregularly shaped reddened area on his forehead. He has slightly limited range of motion in bilateral knees, but acute assessment tests are normal.

His vital signs are Blood pressure: 126/82 mmHg; Pulse: 84 beats per minute; Respirations: 16 breaths per minute; Oxygen saturation: 99%.

Diagnostic Testing

He came in to the clinic last week to have fasting labs drawn prior to this visit. These labs include the routine labs done over the past years: complete blood count (CBC), comprehensive metabolic panel (CMP), lipids, vitamin D, and prostate-specific antigen (PSA). Results include the following:

- CBC: white blood cell (WBC) 5.8, red blood cell (RBC) 5.13, hemoglobin 15.5, hematocrit 46.7, mean corpuscular volume 91.0, mean corpuscular hemoglobin 30.2, mean corpuscular hemoglobin concentration 33.2, red cell distribution width 13.0, platelets 181, and mean platelet volume 11.2

- CMP: glucose 101, BUN 9, creatinine 1.08, glomerular filtration rate (GFR) 84, sodium 143, potassium 4.8, chloride 109, carbon dioxide 26, calcium 9.5, total protein 6.6, albumin 4.5, globulin 2.1, albumin/globulin ratio 2.1, bilirubin total 0.8, alkaline phosphatase 86, aspartate aminotransferase (AST) 35, and alanine aminotransferase (ALT) 45
- Lipids: total cholesterol 215, LDL 134, HDL 32, and triglycerides 153
- Vitamin D: 31
- PSA: 0.001

These labs are consistent with previous labs, with the exception of the mildly elevated glucose level and the cholesterol panel. The last lipid panel was a total cholesterol of 145, LDL 89, HDL 49, and triglycerides 133.

Plan of Care and Interprofessional Collaboration

Lawrence was aware that not walking daily and eating out more had caused his weight gain, but he is surprised to learn how much it has also changed his cardiovascular risks. With these noteworthy changes in lipids and weight gain, it is important to work with interprofessional teams to assess for appropriate interventions. First, a more thorough assessment of the knee is necessary and may include imaging of the knee, starting with a knee x-ray. If the x-ray findings support no structural changes beyond osteoarthritis, the patient should be referred to physical therapy to promote mobility, conditioning, and potentially improve pain levels. Increasing his physical activity will improve his cardiovascular risk assessment. Additionally, he should be referred to a registered dietitian and provided with information on how to cook healthy meals for two and how to make better decisions for the times that he does eat out. With an increase in physical activity and improved nutrition, he will also likely see an improvement in the elevated fasting glucose level. His fasting labs should be reassessed in 4 to 6 months with these lifestyle changes.

It may seem that Lawrence needs to consider treatment for his hyperlipidemia, but it is critical for the nurse practitioner to consider the patient holistically. His lipid panel has worsened, but this correlates to a decline in physical activity as well as a change in eating habits. Most of the large studies done on lipid management have not included older adults. Therefore, the Heart Risk Calculator, which is supported by the American College of Cardiology and the American Heart Association, provides calculations of 10-year risk of heart disease or stroke only for patients up to the age of 79. All medications and interventions carry a certain risk. That risk has to be weighed with the potential benefit. Statins are effective in preventing heart disease in appropriate populations, but they come with many side effects including myopathy or a slight increased risk in new-onset diabetes. Therapeutic lifestyle changes should always be considered prior to pharmacologic intervention. In the older adult, that consideration should weigh even heavier, due to the lack of evidence in the geriatric population.

In the newest 2018 Guidelines on the Management of Blood Cholesterol from the American College of Cardiology, there are new recommendations to measure a coronary artery calcium level for older patients with low burden risk factors who question whether they would benefit from statin therapy.

Case Study References

American College of Cardiology. (2014). ASCVD Risk Estimator plus. Retrieved from http://tools.acc.org/ascvd-risk-estimator-plus/#!/calculate/estimate

Banach, M., & Serban, M. C. (2016). Discussion around statin discontinuation in older adults and patients with wasting diseases. *Journal of Cachexia, Sarcopenia and Muscle, 7*(4), 396–399. doi:10.1002/jcsm.12109

Cifu, A. S., & Davis, A. M. (2017). Prevention, detection, evaluation, and management of high blood pressure in adults. *Journal of the American Medical Association, 318*(21), 2132–2134. doi:10.1001/jama.2017.18706

Curfman, G. (2017). Risks of statin therapy in older adults. *Journal of the American Medical Association Internal Medicine, 177*(7), 966. doi:10.1001/jamainternmed.2017.1457

Grundy, S. M., Stone, N. J., Bailey, A. L., Beam, C., Birtcher, K. K., Blumental, R. S., . . . Yeboah, J. (2018). *2018 guideline on the management of blood cholesterol.* Retrieved from https://www.acc.org/gmscholesterol

Gurwitz, J. H., Go, A. S., & Fortmann, S. P. (2016). Statins for primary prevention in older adults: Uncertainty and the need for more evidence. *Journal of the American Medical Association, 316*(19), 1971–1972. doi:10.1001/jama.2016.15212

Han, B. H., Sutin, D., Williamson, J. D., Davis, B. R., Piller, L. B., Pervin, H., . . . Blaum, C. S. (2017). Effect of statin treatment vs usual care on primary cardiovascular prevention among older adults: The ALLHAT-LLT randomized clinical trial [published online May 22, 2017]. *Journal of the American Medical Association Internal Medicine, 177*(7), 955. doi: 10.1001/jamainternmed.2017.1442

Last, A. R., Ference, J. D., & Falleroni, J. (2011). Pharmacologic treatment of hyperlipidemia. *American Family Physician, 84*(5): 551–558. Retrieved from https://www.aafp.org/afp/2011/0901/p551.html

Last, A. R., Ference, J. D., Menzel, E. R. (2017). Hyperlipidemia: Drugs for cardiovascular risk reduction in adults. *American Family Physician, 95*(2), 78–87. Retrieved from https://www.aafp.org/afp/2017/0115/p78.html

Sagon, C. (2016, November 15). New guidelines on who should take statins. Retrieved from https://www.aarp.org/health/drugs-supplements/info-2016/new-guidelines-on-who-should-take-statins-cs.html

U.S. Preventive Services Task Force. (2009). Using nontraditional risk factors in coronary heart disease risk assessment: U.S. Preventive Services Task Force recommendation statement. *Annals of Internal Medicine, 151*(7), 474–482. doi:10.7326/0003-4819-151-7-200910060-00008

U.S. Preventive Services Task Force. (2016). Final recommendation statement: Statin use for the primary prevention of cardiovascular disease in adults: Preventive medication. Retrieved from https://www.uspreventiveservicestaskforce.org/Page/Document/RecommendationStatementFinal/statin-use-in-adults-preventive-medication1

U.S. Preventive Services Task Force. (2017). Statin use for the primary prevention of cardiovascular disease in adults: Recommendation statement. *American Family Physician, 95*(2). Retrieved from https://www.aafp.org/afp/2017/0115/od1.html

Vaughan Tuohy, C., & Dodson, J. A. (2015). *Statins for primary prevention in older adults.* Retrieved from https://www.acc.org/latest-in-cardiology/articles/2015/03/10/07/46/statins-for-primary-prevention-in-older-adults

REFERENCES

Grundy, S. M., Stone, N. J., Bailey, A. L., Beam, C., Birtcher, K. K., Blumental, R. S., . . . Yeboah, J. (2018). 2018 AHA/ACC/AACVPR/AAPA/ABC/ACPM/ADA/AGS/APHA/ASPC/NLA/PCNA guideline on the management of blood cholesterol: A report of the American College of Cardiology/American Heart Association Task Force on Clinical Practice Guidelines. *Circulation, 139*, e1082–e1143. doi:10.1161/cir.0000000000000625

Jellinger, P. S., Handelsman, Y., Rosenblit, P. D., Bloomgarden, Z. T., Fonseca, V. A., Garber, A. J., . . . Davidson, M. (2017). American Association of Clinical Endocrinologists and American College of Endocrinology guidelines for management of dyslipidemia and prevention of cardiovascular disease. *Endocrine Practice, 23*(Suppl. 2), 1–87. doi:10.4158/ep171764.appgl

Lloyd-Jones, D. M., Braun, L. T., Ndumele, C. E., Smith, S.C., Sperling, L. S., Virani, S. S., & Blumenthal, R. S. (2019). Use of risk assessment tools to guide decision-making in the primary prevention of atherosclerotic cardiovascular disease: A special report from the American Heart Association and American College of Cardiology. *Journal of the American College of Cardiology, 73*(24), 3153–3167. doi:10.1016/j.jacc.2018.11.005

Rosenson, R. S. (2019). Lipoprotein classification, metabolism, and role in atherosclerosis. In M. W. Freeman & G. M. Saperia (Eds.), *UpToDate*. Retrieved from https://www.uptodate.com/contents/lipoprotein-classification-metabolism-and-role-in-atherosclerosis

Rosenson, R. S., & Durrington, P. (2018). Inherited disorders of LDL-cholesterol metabolism other than familial hypercholesterolemia. In W. Freeman, F. Cosentino, & G. M. Saperia (Eds.), *UpToDate*. Retrieved from https://www.uptodate.com/contents/inherited-disorders-of-ldl-cholesterol-metabolism-other-than-familial-hypercholesterolemia

Uphold, C. R. (2013). Metabolic and endocrine problems. In C. R. Uphold & M. V. Graham (Eds.), *Clinical guidelines in family practice* (5th ed., pp. 516–574). Gainesville, FL: Barmarrae Books.

17 Cardiovascular Disorders

Abimbola Farinde

OBJECTIVES

1. Discuss the development and prevalence of cardiovascular disease (CVD) in older adults
2. Evaluate coronary artery disease development in older adults
3. Discuss preventive measures for CVD in older adults
4. Review the long-term goals of management in older adults with CVD

INTRODUCTION

CVD is known to contribute to an increase in morbidity, mortality, disability, and healthcare costs with older adults in the United States. It is a leading cause of death and medical costs globally and is expected to remain this way for some time (Jones-Lloyd, 2016). All of the CVDs combined are expected to remain the leading causes of death in the United States. It has the potential to affect both men and women as they transition from one decade to the next in their lives. As individuals age, the blood vessels can become stiff, there is the migration of smooth muscle cells, and a notable decline in vasomotor function (Holliman, 2018). Heart disease is recognized as the leading cause of death in the United States. Heart failure, coronary artery disease, and atrial fibrillation are identified as primary reasons for hospital stays and healthcare visits. According to the Centers for Disease Control and Prevention, about 610,000 people die annually from heart disease, which equates to 1 in every 4 deaths. In terms of morbidity, it is estimated that 80 million Americans have some form of CVD and almost half of those individuals are 60 years of age or older (Yazdanyar & Newman, 2010). The yearly rates of the first cardiovascular event can increase from 3 per 1,000 men at 35 to 44 years of age to 74 per 1,000 men at 85 to 94 years of age. On the other hand for women, similar rates can be seen 10 years later in life (American Heart Association, 2013). There are a number of risk factors that can predispose an individual, including an older adult, to cardiovascular disorders, and these can include a number of medical conditions and lifestyle choices such as diabetes, being overweight or obese, sedentary lifestyle, and excessive consumption of alcohol. The age-related growth in CVD morbidity and mortality can be appreciated by factors related to population-based, disease-specific incidence, and the rates of CVD that include valvular heart disease, stroke, peripheral arterial disease, and coronary heart disease (CHD; Yazdanyar & Newman, 2010). The management of CVD can be complicated by the presence of comorbidities. As an adult ages, there is an increased prevalence of coronary risk factors, but there is also a benefit that can be gained from reduction in cardiovascular events with optimal and effective therapy.

BACKGROUND OF CORONARY HEART DISEASE

The heart possesses two sides. The right side of the heart pumps blood to the lungs to get oxygen and aid with the elimination of carbon dioxide. On the other hand, the left side of the heart works to pump oxygen-rich blood to the body. CHD is known to contribute to about half of all CVD-related deaths, and this incidence generally increases with advancing age regardless of race or gender. In the United States, it is estimated that about 15.4 million adults have CHD, with having a myocardial infarction. It is a condition that can be the result of atherosclerosis. At about the age of 70 years, the lifetime risk of CHD is comparable between men and women.

There are a number of risk factors that have been established for CVD based on specificity, temporality, and biologic plausibility (Eckel et al., 2014; Lewington, et al., 2007). There are significant risk factors that contribute to CHD, and these can include cigarette smoking, high cholesterol, hypertension, elevated apolipoprotein B to apolipoprotein A1 ratio, abdominal obesity, alcohol intake, and physical inactivity (Kannel & Levin, 2003). Some of the modifiable risk factors can include smoking, alcohol intake, physical inactivity, and hypertension. Many of these risk factors can cluster into what is known as "metabolic syndrome," which is characterized by abdominal obesity, insulin resistance, hyperglycemia, elevated blood pressure, elevated triglyceride levels, and having a lower high-density (high-density lipoprotein [HDL]) cholesterol level. The nonmodifiable risk factor age is regarded as the most powerful risk factor for the development of most CVDs, particularly stroke, heart failure, and atrial fibrillation. The development of CVD appears to double with at least each additional decade of a person's life, and there is an increased burden that can contribute to mortality (Jones-Lloyd, 2016). Other risk factors are gender (more women are dying from CVD annually), race (believed to be an independent risk factor for CVD, and some of the cardiovascular risk differences that are seen across race and ethnic groups can be attributed to difference in socioeconomic status), and family history (heritability of optimal cardiovascular health is less than 20%, thereby suggesting strong environmental and behavioral influence on this trait). Currently, there are more than 5 million Americans living with chronic heart failure, with equal distribution among men and women; so urgent identification and management is of the utmost importance (Jones-Lloyd, 2016).

In an older adult, the presence of the total serum cholesterol level and low-density lipoprotein (LDL) cholesterol can have a significant connection with the risk of CHD as well as peripheral arterial disease (Kleczk & Benjamin, 2018). It is vital for any clinician who is treating this patient population to be aware of these potential risk factors as screeners for CVD. On the other hand, cigarette smoking is considered to be one of the strongest risk factors for CVD events; so any older adult engaged in this practice must be mindful of the outcomes. It has been shown that smoking can confer a two- to threefold higher risk for all manifestations of CVD, and steps taken to cease smoking can dramatically reduce an individual's risk. The risk factors and cholesterol panel are markers that are used to assess the degree of damage or impact on cardiovascular health.

PREVENTION OF CARDIOVASCULAR HEART DISEASE

The ability to strive to prevent heart disease is one of the largest factors that lower the risk of death. There are three types of preventive measures that include primordial, primary, and secondary prevention. Each of these three preventative measures may share similar elements but are distinctive in the approach that is taken to minimize risk. The primordial prevention consists of working to minimize or prevent the occurrence of inflammation, atherosclerosis, or endothelial dysfunction by reducing one's weight, decreasing cholesterol, or lowering high blood pressure (Harvard C.H. Chan School of Public Health, 2018). When it comes to the application of primordial prevention, it is best to initiate it as soon as possible and work to potentially decrease the occurrence of heart disease. These preventive measures include the removal of inflammation, atherosclerosis, or presence of endothelial dysfunction by addressing identifiable risk factors of hypertension, hypercholesterolemia, or obesity. While primordial prevention has not been widely recognized as primary or secondary prevention, it is gaining attention to become the hallmark for the American Heart Association's stance of what defines optimal heart health and the methods that may be employed to attain this. The earlier that individuals can begin to incorporate primordial prevention into their lifestyles, even as early as their childhood, the chances of prevention against heart disease can increase.

The primary prevention is to provide an older adult who has a notable risk of heart disease as a result of an initial occurrence with a heart attack or stroke that requires immediate intervention. The intent of primary prevention is usually targeted toward older adults who have existing cardiovascular risk factors that can include high cholesterol and high blood pressure and working to minimize any potential progression of these factors that can predispose a person to more fatal outcomes (Harvard C.H. Chan School of Public Health, 2018). Some of the notable preventive measures include lifestyle modifications, both dietary and medication related to assist with offsetting the progression.

The adoption of secondary prevention generally begins after an older adult has experienced a heart attack or stroke or has undergone angioplasty or bypass surgery or the presence of an existing heart disease or condition. This type of prevention can entail taking medications such as aspirin and/or a lipid-lowering medication such as a statin, the cessation of smoking, or taking steps to lose weight if applicable, and incorporate a healthy eating habit. Secondary prevention does appear to include elements of primordial and primary prevention, and its goal is to work to achieve optimal outcomes. These steps are designed to prevent the recurrence of a heart attack, stroke, or even fatality. Unfortunately, a large number of individuals who experience an initial heart attack and are survivors of this can die as a result of a second heart attack or stroke; so prevention can be the key to saving a life.

For any older adult, one of the most important strategies that can be adopted for improved health is not begin or continue to use tobacco of any form. Once this habit begins, it can become increasingly difficult to stop it even though it is regarded as a significant contributor to heart disease. According to research, there is believed to be a link between cigarette smoking and cessation in terms of mortality based on a decades-long perspective study (Harvard C.H. Chan School of Public Health, 2018). It was identified that with over 100,000 women, 64% of the deaths were with existing smokers and 28% of the deaths were among former smokers (given their past history of cigarette smoking). As a result, it has been noted that much of the associated risk of smoking as well as the all-cause mortality can be diminished if the habit is stopped.

Furthermore, the ability to maintain a healthy weight can lower the risk of heart disease as well as other ailments that may be found in an older adult. The inclusion of exercise and other physical activities has the potential to help maintain a good body weight and prevent heart disease and lower high blood pressure. Exercise and physical activity have a benefit on the body while having a lifestyle that is sedentary can have the opposite effect.

SUMMARY

CVD can be viewed as a significant and life-threatening issue for older adults. Clinicians should be aware of not only treatment options but also preventive measures that can be implemented to eliminate risk if at all possible. The implementation of primary and/or secondary preventive measures can mean the difference between risk development and quality-of-life adjustments or death if not immediately identified and therapeutic measures are implemented.

CARDIOVASCULAR INTERPROFESSIONAL CASE STUDY
Wendy R. Downey

Patient Presentation
You are working in an internal medicine office when James McNeely, a 79-year-old African American male, presents with elevated blood pressure, shortness of breath (SOB), and chest pain 8/10 without nausea and vomiting. He states that he has been feeling tired for the past 3 weeks and began having chest discomfort last night after dinner. He decided to make an appointment once he was unable to rest due to the pain and SOB. He has been transported by his wife.

On arrival to the clinic, you do a stat ECG, which shows atrial fibrillation. He is started on 2 LPM oxygen via nasal cannula and emergency transport is contacted. On arrival to the ED, a second ECG, troponin I, and chest x-ray were obtained per protocol. The stat ECG continues to show atrial fibrillation. He is placed on 2 LPM of oxygen via nasal cannula and given morphine 5 mg IV. The chest x-ray shows an enlarged cardiac silhouette without evidence of pneumothorax or consolidation. The troponin I is elevated at 0.45. The ED provider admits him to the cardiac telemetry progressive care unit (PCU).

History
Mr. McNeely lives at home with his wife of 54 years and has one son who also lives in the community. He enjoys spending time with his large extended family, most of whom live locally and attend the same church. He is retired from a physically demanding job as an electrician at the local auto manufacturing plant, where he worked his entire adult life. He draws a pension that "gets us by" and is now insured through Medicare. Since his heart attack, he and his wife take occasional walks in the evening after supper, but this is his only form of activity.

Three weeks ago, Mr. McNeely was hospitalized for acute or chronic diastolic heart failure with an ejection fraction of 35% to 40%, likely the result of an anterior ST elevation myocardial infarction (STEMI) 2 years ago. He has a past medical history of primary hypertension, hyperlipidemia, atrial fibrillation, type 2 diabetes, chronic kidney disease stage II, peripheral neuropathy (bilateral feet), obstructive sleep apnea, osteoarthritis, and benign prostate hyperplasia. His surgical history includes percutaneous coronary angioplasty (PTCA) with two stents, cardioversion, cholecystectomy, and cataract removal.

Medications
Metoprolol 25 mg BID, HCTZ 50 mg BID, Lasix 40 mg QD, diltiazem 120 mg QD, atorvastatin 80 mg QD, metformin 1 g BID, glipizide 5 mg BID, gabapentin 100 mg TID, finasteride 5 mg QD, aspirin 81 mg QD, nitroglycerin spray, and ibuprofen 600 mg PRN.

Physical Exam

Outpatient: vital signs are Blood presure: 196/102 mmHg; Pulse: 146 beats per minute; Respirations: 18 breaths per minute; Temperature: 98.7 degrees F; Oxygen saturation: 97% on 2 liters per minute on O2 via nasal cannula. On examination, all systems are within normal range (WNL) except the following: respiratory assessment reveals rales in bilateral lower lobes with an occasional cough, dyspnea, and orthopnea. He becomes slightly panicked when lying supine, which he describes as the primary symptom that motivated him to seek care. Cardiovascular assessment shows irregular heart rhythm, prolonged capillary refill >3 seconds, and 2+ pitting edema of bilateral lower extremities. His skin is pale, and he appears thin for his height with general muscular atrophy.

Inpatient: Similar findings are noted by the ED physician and the hospitalist.

Diagnostic Testing

Inpatient: complete blood count (CBC), comprehensive metabolic panel (CMP), brain natriuretic peptide (BNP), serial troponin levels at 3 hours and 6 hours, and an echocardiogram. Results show: Hgb 10.3; hematocrit (HCT) 31.4; glomerular filtration rate (GFR) 48; BUN 40; creatinine 3.2; GFR 44; glucose 182; BNP 40,895. The echo reveals an ejection fraction of 30% with moderate mitral and tricuspid valve regurgitation. There is a mild pleural effusion. These results indicate systolic on diastolic heart failure, worsening kidney function with anemia, hyperglycemia, and normal electrolytes.

Plan of Care

Inpatient: Cardiology is consulted due to the patient's extensive cardiac history. Additional orders include bumetanide, diltiazem, hydralazine, fluid restriction, strict I&Os, daily weights, daily am ECG, low sodium/diabetic diet, and glucose monitoring before meals and at bedtime with a low-dose sliding scale of insulin. Daily labs include CBC, basic metabolic panel (BMP), and BNP.

Outpatient: When the patient is discharged, he is instructed to have a follow-up exam with you. You discuss goals of care with the patient, including preventing a return to the hospital. You reconcile his home medications with his hospital discharge plan; you reinforce a low sodium and glucose diet; and you review his blood glucose record with him. He continues to have elevated blood glucose levels. You order an A1C and discuss the potential for transitioning to basal insulin, such as glargine, and having him go off glipizide. He states he would like to think about it and will follow up with you in 1 week. Finally, his pain is addressed due to the change from ibuprofen to acetaminophen. You recommend other strategies for pain: heat/cold therapy for the arthritis, a transcutaneous electrical nerve stimulation (TENS) unit, and deep breathing exercises.

Interprofessional Collaboration

During his hospitalization, the serial biomarkers showed troponin I decreased below 0.30; so cardiology does not order a cardiac catheterization but will focus on diuretic therapy, hypertension management, and treatment of atrial fibrillation. Due to polypharmacy in the management of heart failure, a clinical pharmacist reviewed his medications to design dosing regimens to achieve goals using evidence-based therapies, especially in light of his decreased renal function and use of nonsteroidal anti-inflammatory drugs (NSAIDs). The pharmacist recommends using acetaminophen instead of ibuprofen for pain due to normal liver function tests.

During the hospital stay, Mr. McNeely was frustrated by his dietary restrictions. During his follow-up visit, he expresses that he does not understand why the nurses did not let him drink tomato juice with his meals. You spend time educating him on foods that contain high sodium, such as deli meats, soups, processed and prepackaged foods, and vegetable juices. Additionally, you refer him to a clinical dietitian and diabetes educator to provide additional education on foods appropriate for his chronic conditions.

Finally, you discuss the progressive and chronic nature of both heart failure and chronic kidney disease with Mr. McNeely. You describe the important goal of well-being, function, and planning care that aligns with his long-term goals. You recommend a referral to cardiac rehab to help him preserve day-to-day functioning. You also begin the discussion of advanced directives and his wishes as his disease progresses. Although he wants to talk with his wife before making any decisions, he agrees to see an outpatient palliative care team to discuss symptom management and to assist with medical decision-making and advance care planning.

You will continue to have regular follow-up with Mr. McNeely to ensure treatment adherence, quality of life, and to prevent hospital readmission. You keep in mind future referrals such as counseling for depression/anxiety, respite for family/caregiver fatigue, clergy for spiritual distress, social worker due to the financial burden of chronic illness, and home health nursing care for symptom and medication management.

Case Study References

Alpert, C. M., Smith, M. A., Hummel, S. L., & Hummel, E. K. (2017). Symptom burden in heart failure: Assessment, impact on outcomes, and management. *Heart Failure Reviews, 22*(1), 25–39. doi:10.1007/s10741-016-9581-4

Bader, F., Atallah, B., Brennan, L. F., Rimawi, R. H., & Khalil, M. E. (2017). Heart failure in the elderly: Ten peculiar management considerations. *Heart Failure Reviews, 22*(2), 219–228. doi:10.1007/s10741-017-9598-3

Boscart, V. M., Heckman, G. A., Huson, K., Brohman, L., Harkness, K. I., Hirdes, J., . . . Stolee, P. (2017). Implementation of an interprofessional communication and collaboration intervention to improve care capacity for heart failure management in long-term care. *Journal of Interprofessional Care, 31*(5), 583–592. doi:10.1080/13561820.2017.1340875

Kavalieratos, D., Gelfman, L. P., Tycon, L. E., Riegel, B., Bekelman, D. B., Ikejiani, D. Z., . . . Arnold, R. M. (2017). Palliative care in heart failure: Rationale, evidence, and future priorities. *Journal of the American College of Cardiology, 70*(15), 1919–1930. doi:10.1016/j.jacc.2017.08.036.

Low Wang, C. C., Hess, C. N., Hiatt, W. R., & Goldfine, A. B. (2016). Clinical update: Cardiovascular disease in diabetes mellitus: Atherosclerotic cardiovascular disease and heart failure in type 2 diabetes mellitus - mechanisms, management, and clinical considerations. *Circulation, 133*(24), 2459–2502. doi:10.1161/circulationaha.116.022194

Ruppar, T. M., Cooper, P. S., Mehr, D. R., Delgado, J. M., Dunbar-Jacob, J. M. (2016). Medication adherence interventions improve heart failure mortality and readmission rates: Systematic review and meta-analysis of controlled trials. *Journal of the American Heart Association, 5*(6), e002606. doi:10.1161/JAHA.115.002606

Stough, W. G., & Patterson, J. H. (2017). Role and value of clinical pharmacy in heart failure management. *Clinical Pharmacology & Therapeutics, 102*(2), 209–212. doi:10.1002/cpt.687

Yancy, C. W., Jessup, M., Bozkurt, B., Butler, J., Casey, D. E., Jr., Colvin, M. M., ... Westlake, C. (2017). 2017 ACC/AHA/HFSA focused update of the 2013 ACCF/AHA guideline for the management of heart failure: A report of the American College of Cardiology/American Heart Association Task Force on Clinical Practice Guidelines and the Heart Failure Society of America. *Journal of Cardiac Failure, 23*(8), 628–651. doi:10.1016/j.cardfail.2017.04.014

REFERENCES

Akhar, S., & Ramani, R. (2015). Geriatric pharmacology. *Anesthesiology Clinics, 33*(2), 457–469. doi:10.1016/j.anclin.2015.05.004

American Heart Association. (2013). Older Americans and cardiovascular disease. Statistical fact sheet: 2013 Update. Retrieved from https://www.heart.org/idc/groups/heart-public/@wcm/@sop/@smd/documents/downloadable/ucm_319574.pdf

Eckel, R. H., Jakicic, J. M., Ard, J. D., de Jesus, J. M., Houston Miller, N., Hubbard, V. S., ... American College of Cardiology/American Heart Association Task Force on Practice Guidelines. (2014). AHA/ACC guideline on lifestyle management to reduce cardiovascular risk: a report of the American College of Cardiology/American Heart Association Task Force on Practice Guidelines. *Circulation, 129*, S76–S99.

Hanlon, J. T., Aspinall, S. L., Semla, T. P., Weisbord, S. D., Fried, L. F., Good, C. B., ... Handler, S. M. (2009). Consensus guidelines for oral dosing of primarily renally cleared medications in older adults. *Journal of American Geriatric Society, 57*(2), 335–340. doi:10.1111/j.1532-5415.2008.02098.x

Harvard C.H. Chan School of Public Health. (2018). *Preventing heart disease*. Nutrition Source. Retrieved from https://www.hsph.harvard.edu/nutritionsource/disease-prevention/cardiovascular-disease/preventing-cvd

Holliman, K. (2018). *Managing the elderly with cardiovascular disease*. ACP Internist. Retrieved from https://acpinternist.org/archives/2011/10/CVD.htm

Jones-Lloyd, D. (2016). Epidemiology of cardiovascular disease. *Goldman-Cecil Medicine, 52*, 257–262.e1

Kannel, W. B., & Levine, B. S. (2003). Coronary heart disease risk in people 65 years of age and older. *Medscape Pharmacist*. Retrieved from https://www.medscape.com/viewarticle/459037

Kleczk, J., & Benjamin, I. (2018). Evaluation of the patient with cardiovascular disease. *Andreoli and Carpenter's Cecil Essentials of Medicine, 3*, 22–36. Retrieved from https://ezproxy.oum.edu.ws:2053/#!/browse/book/3-s2.0-C20100672099

Lewington, S., Whitlock, G., Clarke, R., Sherliker, P., Emberson, J., Halsey, J., ... Collins, R. (2007). Blood cholesterol and vascular mortality by age, sex, and blood pressure: a meta-analysis of individual data from 61 prospective studies with 55,000 vascular deaths. *Lancet, 370*, 1829–1839.

Yazdanyar, A., & Newman, A. (2010). The burden of cardiovascular disease in the elderly: Morbidity, mortality, and costs. *Clinics in Geriatric Medicine, 25*(4), 563–577.

18 Respiratory Disorders

Abimbola Farinde

OBJECTIVES

1. Discuss acute and chronic respiratory conditions that can be identified in older adults
2. Evaluate the preventive and treatment approaches for managing specific respiratory conditions or disorders in older adults
3. Review pharmacological and nonpharmacological interventions that can be used to manage or treat respiratory conditions in older adults

INTRODUCTION

The presence of upper respiratory tract infections (URTIs) in older adults is not considered to be more common when compared to their younger counterparts, but the associated complications are more prevalent in this population (Geffen, 2006). Upper respiratory infections (URIs) can include an aspect of the upper airway and are most commonly attributed to viruses. If an older adult experiences a URTI, this has the potential to significantly impact his or her quality of life and decrease the time to recovery from the presenting illness. Given the dynamic changes that occur with the older population, it is recognized that specific factors can play a major role in the severity of the URI such as decreased immunity and inflammatory issues that can occur in older adults. Older adults may present with atypical symptoms of an infection; so clinicians must be cognizant of this as this is a group that is at high risk for URTIs (Geffen, 2006). The most commonly identified URTIs among the general population and older adults are influenza and respiratory syncytial virus (RSV) (Zachary, 2019). In older adults aged 70 years and above, pneumococcal disease is up to 14 times more common and can be associated with other conditions such as sinusitis and otitis media (Geffen, 2006). These infections have the ability to affect the nose, throat, ears, and sinuses of healthy individuals. The signs and symptom presentation can include chills, fevers, headache, decreased hunger or thirst, and coughing to name a few. Other additional symptoms can include sore throat, clear eye discharge, or general malaise. The clinical symptoms tend to vary without a close link to the specific virus.

TREATMENT

The management of URIs is typically symptomatic in nature. For older adults, nonpharmacological interventions can be the first-line treatment for management such as the use of heated or humidified air. If nonpharmacological interventions fail to produce symptom control, the use of topical nasal decongestants that contain pseudoephedrine or phenylephrine, keeping in mind stable blood pressure, may be helpful with the alleviation of symptoms. Oxymetazoline is a nasal decongestant solution that can be used for short-term symptom control. The use of topical nasal decongestants should be short-term, limiting to 2 to 3 days. Other pharmacological options for symptom management can include intranasal cromolyn or ipratropium bromide. Cromolyn sodium is a mast cell stabilizer that is considered to be less effective than corticosteroids and to be used for only about 1 week in the presence of symptoms to provide relief with minor side effects (Nyenhuis & Mathur, 2013). Cromolyn is considered to be a good option for use in older adults who are not able to tolerate antihistamines or decongestants (Ratner, Ehrlich, Fineman, Meltzer, & Skoner, 2002). Ipratropium bromide is an anticholinergic agent, which can be used to reduce the severity of sneezing, rhinorrhea, and nasal secretions (Meneghetti, 2018). Antihistamines such as diphenhydramine can be used to decrease nasal secretions and improve congestion.

When it comes to pain management, fever, and body aches that can be associated with a URI, the analgesic and antipyretic acetaminophen or nonsteroidal anti-inflammatory agents such as ibuprofen or naproxen can be utilized. The presence of inflammation can also be another aspect of URI, and steroids such as dexamethasone are used to help reduce inflammation within the airway passage and decrease swelling as well as congestion.

In addition to pharmacological treatment, there are nonmedicine interventions that include instructing older adults to rest and to consume liquids, to keep warm and get plenty of sleep, and to wash their hands after blowing their noses. There is also the potential consideration of herbs and supplements to aid with symptom control, but this is only after discussion with the provider. The use of honey has also been proposed to aid with reducing cough.

Either nonpharmacological or pharmacological interventions have been found to be effective in the management of URIs, and they can also be used in combination. Depending on the severity of the infection, a clinician can determine if an older adult may be suited for one or the other or a combination of both options.

ACUTE SINUSITIS

Acute sinusitis or acute rhinosinusitis is known to make the cavities of the nasal passage inflamed and swollen. It is recognized as one of the most common conditions for which older adults may seek medical treatment affecting one in seven adults (Aring & Chan, 2011). Acute sinusitis can be divided into bacterial or viral origin, with most cases being attributed to viral infections, typically from influenza. The management of acute sinusitis can range from the use of analgesics, decongestants, saline irrigation, and antibiotics when deemed appropriate. The natural history of sinusitis is believed to be positive in older adults, and about 85% of individuals can demonstrate a reduction in symptoms with the advent of antibiotics, which are one of the agents that are used for treatment (Rothaus, 2016).

Chronic Sinusitis

Acute sinusitis has the potential to progress to chronic sinusitis in an older adult if symptom relief is not able to be achieved. This form of sinusitis can be divided into two categories, which are chronic rhinosinusitis (CRS) with nasal polyps (CRSwNP) and CRS without nasal polyps (CRSsNP); see Piromchai, Kasemsiri, Laohasiriwong, and Thanaviratananich (2013). CRS with or without nasal polyps is recognized as an inflammation of the nose and the paranasal sinuses. Similar to acute sinusitis, the chronic form is a common health issue that can substantially impact the quality of life. The goal of treatment of chronic sinusitis is to decrease inflammation and remove the associated infection.

Therapeutic Intervention Options
Analgesics
The use of analgesics can be prescribed in conjunction with other treatments to help to alleviate pain, promote much needed rest during recovery, and aid with the resumption of activities of daily living. The choice of an analgesic can be determined by the degree of pain and coexisting conditions that can be identified in an older adult. The use of acetaminophen is well known, or a nonsteroidal anti-inflammatory drug (NSAID) as monotherapy or in conjunction with another agent can be used to manage mild to moderate pain (Aring & Chan, 2011). The decision to initiate an analgesic is to be evaluated on a case-by-case basis in older adults based on symptom presentation, current medication regimen, and the presence of other co-occurring conditions. The decision to initiate an analgesic can be largely dependent on the severity of the pain and the risk versus the benefit of initiation of therapy.

Nasal Decongestants
Another therapeutic option that can be utilized in older adults depending on the status of acute sinusitis is the use of decongestants. The intent of decongestants is to help decrease mucus-associated edema and aid with draining from the sinus. Decongestants have been evaluated by systematic reviews and have been shown to produce only minor short-term beneficial relief of congestion in adults with cold. Along with the use of systemic decongestants that are quick-acting, the use of topical decongestants can also be considered for reducing mucosal edema but for no longer than 3 days due to the potential for rebound nasal congestion (Aring & Chan, 2011; Brook, 2018; Taverner & Latte, 2007).

Antihistamines
The use of antihistamines is another option when treating acute sinusitis due to their ability to produce a drying effect of the sinusitis if it becomes runny. However, to date, antihistamines are not recommended as they have been shown to be not beneficial in aiding with congestion, sneezing, or rhinorrhea (Aring & Chan, 2011; Brooks, 2018).The recommendation is that antihistamines are not to be utilized particularly in patients who have a notable history of allergies.

Saline Nasal Irrigation
The use of nasal irrigation is recommended as adjunctive therapy for acute sinusitis with the goal of improving the movement of mucus. The process of cleansing the nasal cavity with the use of saline nasal irrigation has been shown to be beneficial in relieving the complaints of excessive secretions. Nasal irrigations are considered to be a safe and less costly therapeutic intervention for older adults who seek relief for their symptoms (Aring & Chan, 2011).

Mucolytics
Mucolytics such as guaifenesin and saline lavage can assist with the improvement of nasal drainage as well but they are generally not recommended or used in clinical practice for acute sinusitis, particularly guaifenesin (Aring & Chan, 2011; Brook, 2018).

Corticosteroids
For the management of mild to moderate symptoms, corticosteroids are typically recommended even though the associated benefits are thought to be moderate at best. Systemic, intranasal corticosteroids can be used to decrease inflammation and edema within the nasal mucosa. While there are minimal controlled trials that have definitively supported the use of systemic corticosteroids, they can be utilized in conjunction

with antibiotics to shorten the time to symptom relief (Brook, 2018). In many cases, corticosteroids are used in conjunction for other regimens for management.

Antimicrobial Therapy

Antibiotic therapy is to be utilized in patients who present with signs and symptoms of acute sinusitis if there is no symptom improvement within 7 days or symptoms become increasingly worse with time. The use of antibiotics is noted to help increase the cure date by 15% when compared to placebo at 12 days (Rosenfeld, Singer, & Jones, 2007). At the 14- to 15-day mark, it is established that the use of antibiotics may no longer deliver the same therapeutic benefit to a patient (Aring & Chan, 2011).

When it comes to the selection of an antibiotic for acute sinusitis, most therapeutic guidelines recommend the use of amoxicillin 500 mg by mouth every 8 hours for 10 days or 875 mg every 12 hours for 10 days as first-line. If there is an existing allergy to amoxicillin, the use of a macrolide such as levofloxacin 500 mg by mouth daily for 10 to 14 days or moxifloxacin 400 mg by mouth per day for 10 days can also be prescribed as an alternative. Other options to amoxicillin include trimethoprim/sulfamethoxazole 800 mg/160 mg by mouth twice daily for 10 days or azithromycin 500 mg by mouth daily for 3 days (A. W. Chow et al., 2012). The antibiotic that is prescribed to any older adult should be evaluated on a case-by-case basis taking into consideration safety, tolerability, efficacy, and potential contraindications.

Antibiotic Length of Therapy

For the use of an antibiotic for acute sinusitis, the recommended duration of therapy is typically 10 days based on the results of randomized clinical trials as support (Aring & Chan, 2011; Barclay, 2013). There are cases in which the length of therapy may be lessened if symptom presentation is not severe in a given patient.

Treatment Options for Chronic Sinusitis

The treatment of chronic sinusitis can be similar to that of the acute version, which includes the use of nasal decongestants, steroids, saline irrigations, and antibiotics (Piromchai et al., 2013). However, the treatment approach can diverge when surgical intervention may be selected as an alternative if medical therapy does not produce therapeutic outcomes. An example of such a surgical procedure would be endoscopic sinus surgery (Piromchai et al., 2013).

Summary

Acute sinusitis is recognized as a common condition that can develop in older adults with symptoms ranging from nasal discharge, fever, cough, and facial pain. The immediate identification of symptoms can bring about relief in older adults through proper treatment that can include the use of decongestants, analgesics, corticosteroids, or antibiotics. Based on symptom presentation, treatment can be tailored to each individual patient with ongoing monitoring of therapeutic benefits and effects being performed. There is the potential for acute sinusitis symptoms to reappear; so a clinician who has experience with the identification of signs and symptoms can quickly implement treatment.

ACUTE BRONCHITIS

Acute bronchitis can present in older adults as an inflammatory process in the bronchi that can have a deregulating effect on function and structure. It can be accompanied by a cough that can last up to 3 weeks (Tackett & Atkins, 2012). In an older adult, the condition can present as an inflammatory process of the mucus membrane of the tracheobronchial tree. The manifestation of acute bronchitis in older adults can mimic that of a respiratory infection of the upper respiratory tract, and it can gradually affect the nasopharynx, larynx, and trachea. This infection can also travel to other aspects of the respiratory tract to produce laryngitis, tracheitis, or bronchitis. Within pulmonary tissue, older adults can appear to have sites of atelectasis that can arise from obstruction of the secretions of the lumen of the small bronchi.

Symptom Presentation

Acute bronchitis can present with a cough, which can be an initial symptom. This cough can be dry with mucus production that can range from being clear to cloudy, to yellow or green in color. Other presenting symptoms can include sore throat, wheezing, fatigue, or shortness of breath (Harvard Health Publishing, 2018). The clinical course of acute bronchitis in older adults can be determined by the status of the functionality of respiration and impaired bronchial patency.

Treatment

The treatment of acute bronchitis in older adults can differ depending on the symptom presentation and severity of the course of the disease. In certain cases, the viral infection that serves as the origin of most cases of acute bronchitis can resolve within a few days, but there are cases where symptoms can persist for many more weeks. The symptom presentation of cold and wheezing associated with breathing difficulty can also last for about 2 months even after the infection has disappeared. The treatment of acute bronchitis can include the use of medicine or nonmedicine interventions in combination or as monotherapy.

Nonmedicine Intervention

The combination of bed rest, adequate fluid intake, and breathing in warm air has the ability to provide some relief of symptoms and help to promote quicker recovery. Bed rest can be accompanied by active movement chest massage or raised nose to aid with lung ventilation. In many instances, these therapeutic interventions are strongly recommended as first-line or as adjunctive to other therapies. The use of vaporizers or humidifiers can also assist with loosening of nasal, mucus discharge and relieve the presenting cough. Most of all, there should be an ongoing attempt to avoid irritants; so older adults should be advised to not smoke and to wear a mask if there is air pollution or the avoidance of household irritants that can induce symptoms.

Pharmacological Interventions

Antibiotics

In older adults who are considered to be healthy, antibiotics are rarely utilized in the initial, acute stages of treatment of acute bronchitis that are uncomplicated (Holzinger, Beck, Dini, Stöter, & Heintze, 2014). Clinical trials on the effect of antibiotics in the treatment of acute bronchitis have been mixed. Patients diagnosed with acute bronchitis who have also had symptoms of the cold for less than 1 week did not benefit from antibiotic therapy (Knutson & Braun, 2002).

Bronchodilators

The improvement of airway opening and flow can be achieved with the use of bronchodilators such as albuterol or levalbuterol. When utilizing bronchodilators, clinicians should be aware of the effects of increased heart rate, trouble sleeping, and nervous or shaking feeling and monitor closely. It was identified that patients who used albuterol metered-dose inhalers were less likely to be coughing at week 1 when compared to their placebo counterparts (Hueston, 1994; Knutson & Braun, 2002).

Protussives and Antitussives

Given that acute bronchitis is considered to be caused by a viral infection in many cases, treatment typically also tends to focus on cessation or control of cough (antitussive and protussive) or making the cause more effective in terms of mucus release (protussive therapy). The use of Brethine, amiloride, and hypertonic saline aerosols has been proved to be successful in clearing the airway of mucus buildup. Antitussive therapy may be initiated if an older adult experiences distressful cough, and the type of antitussive that is ultimately utilized can be dependent on the primary cause of the disease. The use of antitussive such as hydrocodone 5 mg by mouth every 4 to 6 hours, dextromethorphan 30 mg by mouth every 12 hours, and codeine 10 to 20 mg by mouth every 4 to 6 hours can assist with suppressing the presenting course.

Summary

Acute bronchitis is an inflammatory process of the mucus membrane that can present with discomforting symptoms of cough, sore throat, low-grade fever, sputum production, or chest discomfort to name a few. The use of bronchodilator, antitussive, and protussive therapies can offer comfort until the viral or bacterial infection disappears.

BACTERIAL PNEUMONIA

The development of bacterial pneumonia is considered to be quite common in older adults, but with its presentation comes the potential for death if not immediately treated. Bacterial pneumonia is described as an inflammation of the lungs as the result of a bacterial infection. The primary causative organism for bacterial pneumonia is *Streptococcus pneumoniae*, with an occurrence rate of about 900,000 individuals per year and 400,000 requiring hospitalization.

Older adults represent a sensitive patient population, and thus they can be susceptible to contracting pneumonia. The signs and symptoms of pneumonia can ultimately present differently in older adults when compared to their younger counterparts. The symptoms that are seen in older adults can be less or not specific in nature but can include confusion, lethargy, or slow deterioration. The symptoms can vary in presentation based on severity and can include fever, chills, shortness of breath or difficulty breathing, headache, confusion or lethargy, and profuse sweating (Chase, Leonard, & Gotter, 2017; Marrie & File, 2016). With bacterial pneumonia, an older adult's temperature rises, and the two hallmark symptom presentations in older adults can be confusion and delirium.

Prevention

In order to prevent the development of bacterial pneumonia, it is best to recommend to an older adult to work to preserve the strength of his or her immune system, and this can entail healthy eating, adequate rest, and good hygiene. Given the fact that bacterial pneumonia can arise as a result of complications of the flu, the administration of a yearly flu shot can help to minimize the development of bacterial pneumonia. For older adults, it is recommended that pneumococcal vaccines PCV13 and PPSV23 can be administered. The status of an older adult can help to determine which vaccination can be administered (S. Chow, 2018).

Treatment

The treatment of bacterial pneumonia can be determined by several factors and can have an impact on the approach that is ultimately taken in older adults. The goal of treatment is to get rid of the infection and to prevent complications. The treatment approach and outcome can be determined by the presenting pneumonia and the severity of the symptoms. The initial antibiotic treatment is based on the type of organism to target the specific type of bacterium that is causing the infection (De Pietro, 2019; Chase, Leonard, & Gotter, 2017). Nonpharmacological interventions can also include drinking plenty of fluids and resting. Additional treatment in the form of over-the-counter (OTC) NSAIDs can also be used to assist with fever or pain reduction in older adults. Older adults who develop more serious complications or severe cases of bacterial pneumonia may require oxygen supplementation or assisted breathing devices.

INFLUENZA

Influenza or the flu is considered to be a viral infection that can be easily contracted with symptoms lasting for at least 7 days. It is known to cause about 200,000 hospitalizations and up to 49,000 deaths each year in the United States (Lindegren et al., 2015). Older adults are viewed to be at higher risk for complications related to flu, given the decline of the functions of the immune system as one advances in age. The development of influenza can increase the risk of heart attack by three to five times and stroke by two to three times during the first 2 weeks of infection (National Foundation for Infectious Diseases, n.d.). When influenza develops, it can be mistaken for the common cold given the similarities in symptom presentation. However, one of the initial signs can be a high fever that can go as high as 102°F to 106°F. The presence of a high fever is a characteristic finding of influenza. The symptoms of the flue in older adults mimic that of other age groups and can also include headache, fatigue, aches and pains, and cough, but older adults can have more extensive problems related to the flu that can include a longer length of stay at the hospital or even the potential for death.

Treatment

The best course of action to prevent influenza according to the Centers for Disease Control and Prevention is to have the annual flu vaccine administered to each older adult who meets the criteria for administration. The administration of the flu vaccine can make the difference between hospitalization and a fatality. There are two types of vaccines for older adults that can aid with boosting the immune system against the flu virus. The high-dose vaccine form has about four times the amount of antigen as the normal flu shot and the adjuvanted vaccine is the typical or normal flu shot with the addition of an adjuvant, which helps to promote a much stronger immune system, particularly in an older adult.

Other methods for preventing the flu in an older adult would be to continuously promote good hygiene, which can help with not getting the virus and also minimizing the spread to others. The ability to practice adequate hygiene can assist with limiting contraction of the flu virus, and this should be communicated to all older adults. The use of zinc is also believed to minimize or prevent the development of viral proteins and can inhibit the replication of rhinoviruses (Arnold, n.d.).

In addition, if it is determined that an older adult is a candidate for antiviral therapy, there is the administration of zanamivir or oseltamivir that can help to reduce the chances of contracting the virus if administered before an outbreak. Oral oseltamivir is generally given as 75 mg twice daily in adults (Arnold, n.d.). Inhaled zanamivir can be given as 10 mg (two 5 mg inhalations twice daily) in an adult (Arnold, 2019). If an older adult does ultimately get the flu virus, he or she can be prescribed antiviral agents (e.g., zanamivir or oseltamivir) that can decrease the length of symptom presentation. The administration of an antiviral drug may help to speed recovery by approximately 1 day. If initiated within 48 hours once symptoms are noticeable, there is the potential for the duration of infection to be reduced but this is not an absolute in every case.

Conclusion

While influenza is a common infection among older adults, it is also a preventable one. Through proper hygiene as well as the administration of the flu vaccination, the threat of the infection can be minimized. In the event that an older adult does contract influenza, there are available therapeutic options, both pharmacological and nonpharmacological, that can help to decrease the duration of symptom presentation.

CHRONIC CONDITIONS
Allergic Rhinitis

Acute rhinitis has the ability to affect any individual regardless of age and has the capacity to affect the quality of life. It is a common allergic disease that can affect about 30% of individuals, but up to 90% of allergic rhinitis may go untreated (Church, Church, & Scadding, 2016).

Rhinitis is defined as an inflammatory reaction or swelling that occurs with the mucus membrane of the nose. Some of its distinct characteristics include a runny and stuffy nose, eye irritation, sore/itchy throat, and sneezing (Spadini, 2016). When it comes to the development of these symptoms, environmental triggers also have the potential to contribute as well; so clinicians should be mindful of their involvement in potentiating rhinitis (Dunlop, Matsui, & Sharma, 2016). Depending on the participating origin of the rhinitis, it can be viewed as a seasonal or perennial presentation (Spadini, 2016).

Treatment

The goal of treating allergic rhinitis is to reduce or eliminate symptoms as a means of improving the quality of life of those who suffer from the condition. The treatment of allergic rhinitis in older adults can include a myriad of agents such as OTC agents (e.g., loratadine, cetirizine, fexofenadine, desloratadine, diphenhydramine, glucocorticoids, oral and nasal antihistamines, leukotriene-receptor antagonists). However, when pharmacological agents are proven to be not effective, immunotherapy may be employed (Wheatley & Togias, 2015). Evidence-based guidelines currently recommend the use of intranasal steroids with intranasal antihistamines and leukotriene-receptor antagonists (Brożek et al., 2017).

OTC Treatment

The use of OTC medications can offer effective treatment with regard to the reduction of nasal itching or sneezing episodes that are observed to be mild in presentation. However, if episodes are viewed to be mild, the use of medications such as triamcinolone or fluticasone that target inflamed tissues or symptoms of nasal congestion is preferred (Spadini, 2016). If these agents prove to be not successful, another suitable alternative that can be utilized is the mast cell stabilizer such as cromolyn sodium or oral decongestants, which should be used only for short-term relief of symptoms.

Legend Medications

If OTC medications do not produce the desired outcome, older adults can be treated with prescription medications in the form of intranasal corticosteroids (mometasone, fluticasone, triamcinolone or budesonide), antihistamines, or decongestants. These medications may be used as monotherapy, combined with existing OTC medications, or used as replacement therapy.

Intranasal corticosteroids can be used longer than antihistamines or decongestants, approximately up to 7 days to achieve full effect. For older adults who are prescribed antihistamines, the use of loratadine or cetirizine may offer less anticholinergic effects

(Spadini, 2016). The use of second- or third-generation antihistamines typically offers less side effects when compared to the first-generation formulations.

The use of decongestants may not be appropriate for all older adults, especially in cases where they present with high blood pressure or cardiovascular conditions. If decongestants are required, they should be used for a short period of time as rebound congestion can develop if used for an extended period of time (Graf, 2005; Spadini, 2016). Older adults should be counseled on the proper use of decongestants and not to exceed the duration of use that has been established for them.

If no therapeutic interventions produce expected outcomes, another line of therapy that may be considered is the use of immunotherapy, which may provide resolution (Cox et al., 2011). Given that not all older adults will achieve success with immunotherapy, they will be administered about 1 to 3 subcutaneous injections per week or sublingual immunotherapy tablets or drops daily for at least 3 to 5 years.

While allergic rhinitis can be viewed as a common ailment that can affect any age group, older adults can be more susceptible to the symptoms and eventual consequences of the condition. There are a variety of OTC and prescription medications that can be used to produce a resolution of the bothersome symptoms that can lead to the restoration of quality of life.

Chronic Obstructive Pulmonary Disease

Chronic Obstructive Pulmonary Disease (COPD) is considered to be a larger term that describes the presence of progressive lung diseases that include emphysema, chronic bronchitis, and refractory asthma. In older adults as well as other members of the population, the condition is incurable but with proper diagnosis, effective management can be achieved. The most commonly identifiable signs and symptoms of COPD can include wheezing, an increase in shortness of breath, or tightness of chest. These specific presentations are typically regarded as cardinal symptoms of COPD. With the presence of co-occurring conditions such as congestive heart failure, the complications of COPD can be worsened (Clini, Beghé, & Fabbri, 2013). In an older adult, it is important for a clinician to be aware of existing conditions and take this into consideration when managing COPD exacerbations.

Emphysema

The damage that is inflicted on the air sacs of the lungs is what causes emphysema. With progressive damage, the walls of the air sacs fade and the numerous small sacs can become larger sacs (Qureshi, Sharafkhaneh, & Hanania, 2014). The development of these larger sacs can make it difficult for oxygen to be absorbed into the bloodstream. The damage to the lungs can cause an expansion and loss of their elasticity. With time, it becomes a challenge to breathe, leading to shortness of breath.

Chronic Bronchitis

The development of chronic bronchitis is the result of damage inflicted to the bronchial tubes, and the tubes can become swollen. The result of this swollenness contributes to shortness of breath as well. If mucus is produced with the cough and the cough can remain for at least 3 months for 2 years in a row, the bronchitis has become chronic bronchitis.

Nonreversible Asthma

In older adults, COPD may also be accompanied by the presence of asthma that does not achieve symptom management with the use of conventional interventions. The pharmacological agents that are designed to provide relief of swelling and tightness that occurs with an asthmatic attack may not work in these cases; so other options must be explored.

Management of COPD

The presentation of COPD in older adults can vary and affect each individual differently, but it is the role of the patient to describe his or her symptoms as specific as possible and the role of the clinician to provide optimal management based on the patient's report. The desired end result of COPD management is to lower the impact of exacerbation while also preventing the development of future exacerbations (Qureshi et al., 2014). The management of COPD can include the use of pharmacological and nonpharmacological interventions, either as monotherapy or in combination. With immediate identification of the signs and symptoms of COPD, there can be an increased likelihood of positive therapeutic outcomes for older adults.

Pharmacological Interventions

There are several pharmacological interventions that exist for the management of COPD exacerbations. One such class that can be used in older adults is the inhaled bronchodilator such as albuterol that works to increase the level of cyclic adenosine monophosphate. The short-acting muscarinic agonists such as ipratropium bromide block the muscarinic receptors of acetylcholine and work to inhibit vagally mediated reflexes that antagonize the action of acetylcholine. Research does not indicate the superior efficacy of one class over another but after 3 hours of use, the therapeutic effects of the bronchodilator can decline (Qureshi et al., 2014).

While the short-acting bronchodilators may decline in effects over time, the long-acting bronchodilators have been reserved for maintenance treatment of COPD. One of the most commonly utilized bronchodilators in this class is formoterol, which has been shown to be well tolerated by users in the event of exacerbation (Qureshi et al., 2014).

Antibiotic Therapies

The development of COPD exacerbations is largely due to bacterial organisms that infect the respiratory tract. Some of the more commonly identified pathogens include *Haemophilus influenzae, Streptococcus pneumoniae,* and *Moraxella catarrhalis.* While antibiotics can be applied, their routine use has not been definitively established. The use of antibiotics has been noted to increase sputum purulence, but the treatment approach is generally empirical in nature and not always based on the results of sputum cultures. The decision to initiate an antibiotic in an older individual can be based on a number of factors that include severity, previous use, use of systemic steroids, and if there is an underlying lung disease (Qureshi et al., 2014).

Corticosteroids

As it currently stands, there is no strong evidence to support appropriate corticosteroid selection in patients and how this is to be administered. The use of systemic corticosteroids offers the benefit of decrease in time to recovery and help to address failures that have been experienced with other treatment options. According to the Global Initiative for Chronic Obstructive Lung Disease (GOLD), a recommended dose of 30 to 400 mg of prednisolone by mouth for 10 to 14 days can be utilized or methylprednisolone 125 mg intravenous four times daily for 3 days followed by 2 or 8 weeks of tapering dose of oral prednisone (60 mg). While it is unclear as to who will respond favorably to corticosteroid therapy, this still continues to be utilized as a means of stabilizing COPD exacerbations (Qureshi et al., 2014).

Mucolytic Agents

The use of mucolytic agents with COPD has generated much debate, but these agents have shown favorable outcomes in some patients, particularly those with significant sputum.

Methylxanthines
Intravenous methylxanthines such as theophylline can also be used in certain cases when therapeutic response has not been achieved by bronchodilators. These classes of agents are recommended for use as second-line therapies and not at the beginning stages of COPD exacerbations.

Adjunctive Therapies
First-line or second-line therapies can be combined with adjunctive treatments depending on an older adult's current clinical status, and these therapies can consist of the use of anticoagulants, diuretics, or treatments specifically aimed at treating other co-occurring conditions with the COPD.

Nonmedicine Interventions
The management of COPD exacerbations can also apply a nonmedicine approach in the form of smoking cessation. The ability to initiate smoking cessation can have a significant impact on COPD exacerbation effect and frequency. Smoking cessation can be promoted by all clinicians who provide care to older adults. The use of influenza and pneumococcal vaccinations is typically recommended for individuals with COPD as this can provide significant benefits that include decreased hospitalization and reduced rate of mortality (Qureshi et al., 2014). Another therapeutic intervention that continues to gain attention in reducing COPD exacerbation frequency is immunostimulatory agents, but additional studies are required to fully understand the mechanism and definitive role that these agents can have on COPD management.

One of the most important nonmedicine interventions is to educate older adults about the importance of disease progression, which can have a significant impact on COPD exacerbation symptoms and reduced frequency of hospitalizations.

Summary
COPD represents a chronic disease that requires continuous management, particularly as it relates to exacerbations. There are a variety of treatment modalities that are available to assist with alleviating the symptom presentation in older adults. The use of pharmacological and nonpharmacological interventions can greatly assist with the management of COPD symptoms.

Asthma
While asthma is commonly considered a disease of childhood, it is also a common condition in individuals who are 65 years of age and older (Rance & O'Laughlen, 2014). The condition is reported to affect about 2 million Americans. The development of asthma in older adults has the potential to contribute to health problems, complications, and a higher rate of morbidity and mortality if not appropriately treated (Dunn & Wechsler, 2017). Asthma is viewed to be a disease of progressively increasing response of the airway due to a variety of stimuli including irritants or allergens that block the airway. The constriction of the muscles that are around the airway as well as inflammation of the lining of the airway can occur, and an individual can have problems with breathing. The classic symptoms of asthma are dyspnea, chest tightness, wheezing, and persistent coughing. In older adults, there are unique features of asthma, and asthma can present with a greater risk for respiratory failure; so close monitoring of symptoms is highly recommended (Mathur & Bernstein, 2018). Unlike their younger counterparts, older adults with asthma can experience periods of remission, but unfortunately it is likely to become an increasing serious condition that can alter the quality of life.

Given that older adults can present with other conditions, it can be difficult to make a diagnosis of asthma and it might go undiagnosed for some time. The symptoms of asthma can present as persistent cough with sputum production, and there can be other illnesses such as a heart disease or emphysema. Effective and efficient diagnosis of the presence of asthma in older adults is through recognition of the symptoms of wheezing and breathing difficulty after exercise. With inactivity in older adults, there is the likelihood that asthma symptoms can surface.

Asthma Treatment

The ability to effectively treat asthma needs to focus on the optimization of respiratory function and control of symptoms (Durham, Fowler, Smith, Whitney, & James, 2017). The treatment of asthma can be addressed in a variety of ways with prescription medications that can provide short-term relief as well as long-term control of the predominant symptoms. The quick relief of asthma symptoms can be managed with the use of either short-acting inhaled beta2-agonists or anticholinergics. Both of these agents work to expand passageways that go into the lungs, which enables more air to come in and out. However, these quick relief agents do not work to control inflammation, which can cause additional symptoms. This is where long-term control medications can come into play, and these are typically taken each day to prevent attacks and symptom presentation. Some examples of long-term control medications include cromolyn sodium, inhaled corticosteroids, leukotrienes or leukotriene modifiers, long-acting inhaled beta2-agonists, methylxanthines, and immunomodulators (American College of Allergy, Asthma, and Immunology, n.d.). All of the agents have been found to be effective in decreasing airway inflammation and improving asthma control. Along with prescription medication, nonpharmacological interventions in the form of lifestyle modifications can assist with management of symptoms. The inclusion of routine vaccinations for pneumonia and influenza is also recommended in older adults with asthma. The combined use of medicine and nonmedicine interventions is considered to be an optimal approach toward the management of the long-term symptoms of asthma and maintaining the quality of life of older adults.

SUMMARY

Although asthma is believed to be a disease of childhood, it has also the potential to develop in older adults. The development of asthma can not only present with specific features in older adults but can also be life-threatening if not properly treated. The use of quick-acting agents, long-term control medications, and nonpharmacological intervention such as lifestyle modification is considered to be the mainstay of asthma management and long-term stability of symptoms.

RESPIRATORY INTERPROFESSIONAL CASE STUDY

Megan Hebdon

Patient Presentation

MT is a 67-year-old woman who presents to your office with a chief complaint of shortness of breath and chest tightness for the past 3 weeks. The symptoms started during a bout of influenza A, from which she is now recovered. In addition to this, she reports night-time coughing episodes that keep her awake. The shortness of breath and chest tightness are pervasive throughout the day, but seem to worsen when she tries to run, go up the stairs, or with other physical activities. She is currently training for a half-marathon, and this has interrupted her training schedule. She reports having frequent URIs over the past year that "go to her chest." She has had issues with asthma on and off throughout her life but has not required medication for the past 20 years. She does not have a rescue inhaler. In addition, she has runny nose and congestion with current spring weather, some dizziness when she becomes really short of breath, and issues with anxiety that she self-treats with exercise and mindfulness.

History

She has a past medical history of asthma as a child, but she "grew out of it." She also had anorexia and bulimia as a young adult. She has had three cesarean sections, but no surgeries otherwise. She is sexually active with one male partner, her spouse, and she has three children. She works as a college professor with no plans to retire in the near future. She has no alcohol, tobacco, or drug use. She drinks 2 to 3 cups of green tea per day, exercises daily, and eats a vegan diet. Her family history is profound for allergic rhinitis, asthma, and mental health issues such as anxiety and depression. Her current medical diagnoses are allergic rhinitis and generalized anxiety disorder.

Medications

Loratadine 10 mg at night and fluticasone nasal spray, 2 sprays in each nostril daily.

She has an allergy to latex.

Physical Exam

Vital signs are: Blood pressure: 110/74 mmHg; Pulse: 74 beats per minute; Respirations: 18 breaths per minute; Temperature: 98.2 degrees F; Oxygen saturation: 96%; Height: 67 inches; Weight: 128 lbs.

Her physical exam is positive for bulging tympanic membranes with no erythema, patent nares with pale mucosa, and a posterior pharynx with mild erythema. Her cardiac exam is within normal limits. She has expiratory wheezes throughout her lung fields with normal respiratory rate and depth and no accessory muscle use.

Diagnostic Testing

Complete blood count (CBC), comprehensive metabolic panel (CMP), chest x-ray, and spirometry.

CBC and CMP were within normal limits. The chest x-ray was clear and spirometry demonstrated evidence of prebronchodilator airway obstruction less than the lower limit of normal. This did improve after administration of a bronchodilator.

Plan of Care

You determine that MT's complaints are related to asthma, of which she has a significant personal and family history. MT states that her goal of care is to be able to continue to run and to have better sleep at night. She reports being inconsistent with taking medication; so she would prefer not to have something she has to remember multiple times per day. Due to this and her relative overall health, it is decided that she will start on montelukast

10 mg at night and she will be prescribed an albuterol HFA inhaler with 1 to 2 puffs every 4 to 6 hours when needed for cough, wheezing, or shortness of breath. She is provided education regarding the potential for headache with montelukast and increased heart rate and feelings of jitteriness with albuterol. You advise her to watch for sustained increased heart rate and to follow up immediately if this occurs. You advise her to try to stop the loratadine and see if her allergy symptoms are managed between the montelukast and fluticasone nasal spray. Together, you develop an asthma action plan for albuterol use and seeking emergency care. You plan a follow-up with her in 1 month to reevaluate her symptoms and then will increase it to every 6 months or as needed for her asthma.

Interprofessional Collaboration

MT has a significant history for anxiety as well as family history for mental health issues. You provide encouragement for her ongoing efforts with exercise and mindfulness and provide her with resources regarding local counseling if the need arises. If her asthma symptoms do not respond to the aforementioned plan, then you may consider adding a steroid inhaler. If her symptoms continue to progress, then a referral to pulmonology may be considered. You review her health maintenance needs including a pelvic exam and pap smear, cardiovascular risk assessment, mammogram, and pneumonia and shingles vaccines. You provide the appropriate orders and referrals and plan follow-up for her annual health exam.

Case Study References

Chhabra, S. K. (2015). Clinical application of spirometry in asthma: Why, when, and how often? *Lung India, 32*(6). 635–637. doi:10.4103/0970-2113.168139

Falk, N. P., Hughes, S. W., & Rodgers, B. C. (2016). Medications for chronic asthma. *American Family Physician, 94*(6), 454–462. Retrieved from https://www.aafp.org/afp/2016/0915/p454.html

Fanta, C. H. (2019). An overview of asthma management. In R. A. Wood, B. S. Bochner, & H. Hollingsworth (Eds.), *UpToDate*. Retrieved from https://www.uptodate.com/contents/an-overview-of-asthma-management

Rance, K., & O'Laughlen, M. (2014). Managing asthma in older adults. *The Journal for Nurse Practitioners, 10*(1), 1–9. doi:10.1016/j.nurpra.2013.11.009

Schichilone, N., Battaglia, S., Benfante, A., & Bellia, V. (2013). Safety and efficacy of montelukast as adjunctive therapy for treatment of asthma in elderly patients. *Clinical Interventions in Aging, 8*, 1329–1337. doi:10.2147/cia.s35977

REFERENCES

American College of Allergy, Asthma, and Immunology. (n.d.). Asthma treatment. Retrieved from https://acaai.org/asthma/asthma-treatment

Aring, A., & Chan, M. (2011). Acute rhinosinusitis in adults. *American Family Physician, 83*(9), 1057–1063. Retrieved from https://www.aafp.org/afp/2011/0501/p1057.html

Arnold, S. (n.d.). Treating patients infected with influenza virus in the urgent care setting. *The Journal of Urgent Care Medicine*. Retrieved from https://www.jucm.com/treating-patients-infected-with-influenza-virus-in-the-urgent-care-setting

Barclay, L. (2013). Acute bacterial sinusitis addressed in new AAP guidelines. *Medscape Medical News*. Retrieved from http://www.medscape.com/viewarticle/806791

Brook, I. (2018). Acute sinusitis treatment and management. In M. S. Bronze (Ed.), *Medscape*. Retrieved from https://emedicine.medscape.com/article/232670-treatment

Brożek, J. L., Bousquet, J., Agache, I., Agarwal, A., Bachert, C., Bosnic-Anticevich, S., . . . Schünemann, H. (2017). New guidelines in allergic rhinitis and impact on asthma. *Journal of Allergy and Clinical Immunology, 140*(4), 950–958. doi:10.1016/j.jaci.2017.03.050

Chase, C., Leonard, M., & Gotter, A. (2017). Bacterial pneumonia: Symptoms, treatment, and prevention. *Healthline*. Retrieved from https://www.healthline.com/health/bacterial-pneumonia

Chow, A. W., Benninger, M. S., Brook, I., Brozek, J. L., Goldstein, E. J., Hicks, L. A., . . . Wald, E. R. (2012). IDSA clinical practice guideline for acute bacterial rhinosinusitis in children and adults. *Clinical Infectious Disease, 54*(8), e72–e112. doi:10.1093/cid/cir1043

Chow, S. (2018). Pneumonia epidemiology. *News Medical Life Sciences*. Retrieved from https://www.news-medical.net/health/Pneumonia-Epidemiology.aspx

Church, D., Church, M., & Scadding, G. (2016). Allergic rhinitis: Impact, diagnosis, treatment and management. *The Pharmaceutical Journal*. Retrieved from https://www.pharmaceutical-journal.com/research/review-article/allergic-rhinitis-impact-diagnosis-treatment-and-management/20201509.fullarticle?firstPass=false

Clini, E., Beghé, B., & Fabbri, L. (2013). Chronic obstructive pulmonary disease is just one component of the complex multimorbidities in patients with COPD. *American Journal of Respiratory Critical Care Medicine, 187*, 668–671. doi:10.1164/rccm.201302-0230ed

Cox, L., Nelson, H., Lockey, R, Calabria, C., Chacko, T., Finegold, I., . . . Blessing-Moore, J. (2011). Allergen immunotherapy: A practice parameter third update. *Journal of Allergy and Clinical Immunology, 127*(Suppl 1), S1–S55. doi:10.1016/j.jaci.2010.09.034

De Pietro, M. (2019). What to know about bacterial pneumonia. *Medical News Today*. Retrieved from https://www.medicalnewstoday.com/articles/312565.php

Dunlop, J., Matsui, E., & Sharma. H. P. (2016). Allergic rhinitis: Environmental determinants. *Immunology and Allergy Clinics of North America, 36*, 367–377. doi:10.1016/j.iac.2015.12.012

Dunn, R., & Wechsler, B. (2017). Asthma in the elderly and late-onset asthma. *European Journal of Allergy and Clinical Immunology, 73*(2), 284–294. doi:10.1111/all.13258

Durham, C., Fowler, T., Smith, T., Whitney, S., & James, S. (2017). Adult asthma: Diagnosis and treatment. *Nurse Practitioner, 42*(111), 16–24. doi:10.1097/01.npr.0000525716.32405.eb

Geffen, L. (2006). Common upper respiratory tract problems in the elderly: A guide to clinical diagnosis and prudent prescription. *South African Family Practice, 48*(5), 20–23. doi:10.1080/20786204.2006.10873390

Graf, P. (2005). Rhinitis medicamentosa: A review of causes and treatment. *Treatments in Respiratory Medicine, 4*(1), 21–29. doi:10.2165/00151829-200504010-00003

Harvard Health Publishing. (2018). Acute bronchitis. Retrieved from https://www.health.harvard.edu/lung-health-and-disease/acute-bronchitis

Holzinger, F., Beck, S., Dini, L., Stöter, C., & Heintze, C. (2014). The diagnosis and treatment of acute cough in adults. *Deutsches Ärzteblatt Online, 111*(20), 356–363. doi:10.3238/arztebl.2014.0356

Hueston, W. J. (1994). Albuterol delivered by metered-dose inhaler to treat acute bronchitis. *Journal of Family Practice, 39*, 437–440. Retrieved from https://mdedge-files-live.s3.us-east-2.amazonaws.com/files/s3fs-public/jfp-archived-issues/1994-volume_38-39/JFP_1994-11_v39_i5_albuterol-delivered-by-metered-dose-inha.pdf

Knutson, D., & Braun, C. (2002). Diagnosis and management of acute bronchitis. *American Family Physician, 65*, 2039–2044. Retrieved from https://www.aafp.org/afp/2002/0515/p2039.html

Lindegren, M. L., Griffin, M. R., Williams, J. V., Edwards, K. M., Zhu, Y., Mitchel, E., . . . Talbot, H. P. (2015). Antiviral treatment among older adults hospitalized with influenza 2006–2013. *PLOS One, 10*(3), e0121952. doi:10.1371/journal.pone.0121952

Marrie, T. J., & File, T. M. (2016). Bacterial pneumonia in older adults. *Clinics in Geriatric Medicine, 32*(3), 459–477. doi:10.1016/j.cger.2016.02.012

Mathur, S., & Bernstein, D. (2018). On the road to improving asthma outcomes in older adults: The phenotypes of asthma in older adults. *The Journal of Allergy and Clinical Immunology: In practice, 6*(1), 250–251. doi:10.1016/j.jaip.2017.08.038

Meneghetti, A. (2018). Is ipratropium bromide effective in treating upper respiratory tract infections (URI)? In Z. Mosenifar (Ed.), *Medscape*. Retrieved from https://www.medscape.com/answers/302460-86994/is-ipratropium-bromide-effective-in-treating-upper-respiratory-tract-infections-uri

National Foundation for Infectious Diseases. (n.d.). Flu in adults age 65 years and older: What are the risks? Adult vaccination. Retrieved from http://www.adultvaccination.org/vpd/influenza/influenza-65-infographic

Nyenhuis, S., & Mathur, S. (2013). Rhinitis in older adults. *Current Allergy and Asthma Reports, 13*(2), 171–177. doi:10.1007/s11882-013-0342-3

Piromchai, P., Kasemsiri, P., Laohasiriwong, S., & Thanaviratananich, S. (2013). Chronic rhinosinusitis and emerging treatment options. *International Journal of General Medicine, 6*, 453–464. doi:10.2147/ijgm.s29947

Qureshi, H., Sharafkhaneh, A., & Hanania, N. (2014). Chronic obstructive pulmonary disease exacerbations: Latest evidence and clinical implications. *Therapeutic Advances in Chronic Disease, 5*(5), 212–227. doi:10.1177/2040622314532862

Rance, K., & O'Laughlen, M. (2014). Managing asthma in older adults. *The Journal for Nurse Practitioners, 10*(1), 1–9. doi:10.1016/j.nurpra.2013.11.009

Ratner, P. H., Ehrlich, P. M., Fineman, S. M., Meltzer, E. O., & Skoner, D. P. (2002). Use of intranasal cromolyn sodium for allergic rhinitis. *Mayo Clinic Proceedings, 77*(4), 350–354. doi:10.4065/77.4.350

Rosenfeld, R. M., Singer, M., & Jones, S. (2007). Systematic review of antimicrobial therapy in patients with acute rhinosinusitis. *Otolaryngology Head Neck Surgery, 137*(Suppl. 3), S32–S45. doi:10.1016/j.otohns.2007.06.724

Rothaus, C. (2016). Acute sinusitis in adults. *NEJMResident 360*. Retrieved from https://resident360.nejm.org/clinical-pearls/acute-sinusitis-in-adults

Spadini, F. (2016). Allergic rhinitis: Counseling points for better patient outcomes. *Contemporary Clinic*. Retrieved from https://contemporaryclinic.pharmacytimes.com/journals/issue/2016/april2016/allergic-rhinitis-counseling-points-for-better-patient-outcomes

Tackett, K., & Atkins, A. (2012). Evidence-based acute bronchitis therapy. *Journal of Pharmacy Practice, 25*(6), 586–590. doi:10.1177/0897190012460826

Taverner, D., & Latte, G. J. (2007). Nasal decongestants for the common cold. *Cochrane Database Systematic Review*, (1), CD001953. doi:10.1002/14651858.cd001953.pub3

Wheatley, L., & Togias, A. (2015). Allergic rhinitis. *The New England Journal of Medicine, 372*, 456–463. doi:10.1056/nejmcp1412282

Zachary, K. (2019). Treatment of seasonal influenza in adults. In M. S. Hirsch (Ed.), *UptoDate*. Retrieved from https://www.uptodate.com/contents/treatment-of-seasonal-influenza-in-adults

19 Gastrointestinal Disorders

Megan Hebdon

OBJECTIVES
1. Describe the major gastrointestinal complaints in the geriatric population that may be encountered in primary care
2. Identify pharmacologic considerations for gastrointestinal disease that are unique to the geriatric population
3. Outline pharmacologic and nonpharmacologic treatments for gastrointestinal complaints in older adults

INTRODUCTION
Gastrointestinal complaints, especially constipation, are frequent issues in the elderly population. Nurse practitioners working in primary care need to be aware of how to evaluate and diagnose these conditions, and they need to understand the unique issues that may affect pharmacologic management of gastrointestinal complaints in older adults. This chapter provides an overview regarding management of constipation, diarrhea, diverticulosis/diverticulitis, and irritable bowel syndrome (IBS). Inflammatory bowel conditions, chronic pancreatitis, and gallbladder issues are also important for nurse practitioners to identify, but management generally occurs in specialty care settings. Therefore, only a brief overview is provided.

CONSTIPATION
Constipation is a frequent complaint in older adults, and it is more commonly encountered in women (De Giorgio et al., 2015; Schuster, Kosar, & Kamrul, 2015). It may be intermittent or chronic and can affect the quality of life. It may be associated with other conditions such as urinary tract infections and may be worsened by illnesses such as neurodegenerative disorders (De Giorgio et al., 2015). There are Rome criteria that help support the diagnosis of constipation, but for many patients, decreased stool frequency in addition to the character of the stool is important to consider (De Giorgio et al., 2015; Rao, 2019). The subtypes of constipation include the following:

- Slow transit constipation
- Outlet obstruction
- Constipation in IBS (this is addressed later in this chapter; De Giorgio et al., 2015)

In older adults, there are many complicating factors contributing to constipation including comorbid conditions, medication use, limited mobility, nutritional deficits, and decreased fluid intake. Although constipation is common, it is important for nurse practitioners to complete a full history and physical exam to ensure secondary causes are identified. Secondary causes include the following:

- Neuropathic and myopathic disorders
- Cancer
- Electrolyte imbalances
- Organic intestinal diseases
- Endocrine causes
- Psychological causes
- Other: age, kidney disease, lack of privacy/time (De Giorgio et al., 2015; Schuster et al., 2015)

Diagnosis of constipation is made based on history, physical exam, and exclusion of alarm features (rapid weight loss, blood in stool, family history of colorectal cancer or inflammatory bowel disease [IBD], positive fecal occult blood test, anemia, and new-onset symptoms); see De Giorgio et al. (2015) and Schuster et al. (2015). The Rome III criteria include:

- Two or more of the following:
  - Straining during 25% or more of defecations
  - Lumpy or hard stools in 25% or more of defecations
  - Sensation of incomplete evacuation in 25% or more defecations
  - Sensation of anorectal obstruction or blockage in 25% or more defecations
  - Manual maneuvers to facilitate 25% or more defecations (digital evacuation, support of the pelvic floor, etc.)
  - Fewer than three defecations per week
- Loose stools are rarely present without laxative use
- Do not meet criteria for IBS (De Giorgio et al., 2015; Schuster et al., 2015)

Management of constipation in older adults is key due to the quality-of-life issues and risk of bowel obstruction. Lifestyle changes may help improve constipation, including increased water intake (if possible), increased fiber, increased physical activity, and removing functional barriers. In older adults, research does not necessarily support a dramatic change in bowel frequency with the addition of physical activity, but it will help with the patient's health overall (Mounsey, Raleigh, & Wilson, 2015). Having a toileting schedule may help, and patients are most successful when attempting defecation in the morning and after meals (De Giorgio et al., 2015; Schuster et al., 2015). Probiotics have also been used to promote regular bowel movements, but the research is insufficient at this time (De Giorgio et al., 2015; Rao, 2019). Biofeedback is another useful tool for patients who struggle with defecation effort (De Giorgio et al., 2015).

If there are medications that may be contributing to constipation, the nurse practitioner should address this with the patient and family with some suggested alternative treatments, either pharmacologic or lifestyle. Examples of these medications include nonsteroidal anti-inflammatory drugs (NSAIDs) and opioids, anticholinergic agents, anti-Parkinson agents, anticonvulsants, antidepressants, antidiarrheals, antiemetics, antihistamines, antihypertensives, antispasmodics, chemotherapy (vincristine, cyclophosphamide), and cholestyramine (Schuster et al., 2015). Opioids are one of the most common agents that contribute to constipation, and their use is already fraught with side effects in older adults. The lowest effective dose should be targeted, and a bowel regimen should be initiated at the same time as opioid initiation in older adults (Schofield, 2016).

Medications that may be used to treat constipation are outlined in Table 19.1. As a general rule, stimulant laxatives and enemas should be avoided as first-line agents for maintenance therapy due to potential side effects. Fecal impaction may be treated with a mineral oil and warm water enema (Mounsey et al., 2015; Rao, 2019). Stepwise treatment includes starting with a bulk-forming agent (psyllium), followed by an osmotic agent (polyethylene glycol), and then a stimulant laxative up to three times a week if there is no response to other treatments (Schuster et al., 2015).

TABLE 19.1 Pharmacotherapy for Constipation in Older Adults

Agent	Mechanism of Action	Side Effects/Considerations
Natural or semisynthetic fibers (psyllium, methylcellulose)	Bulk-forming, binding with intraluminal water	Bloating, flatulence Patients need adequate fluid intake for these to be effective
Polyethylene glycol		Bloating, flatulence Avoid in patients prone to aspiration, risk of electrolyte imbalances. Avoid in creatinine clearance <30 mL/min or congestive heart failure
Disaccharides and alditols (lactulose, sorbitol)	Interstitial H_2O binding	Bacterial fermentation (bloating, flatulence) Not as effective in slow transit constipation
Osmotic laxatives (magnesium hydroxide, magnesium citrate, magnesium sulfate, sodium phosphate)	Interstitial H_2O binding	Electrolyte abnormalities, avoid in cardiac or renal disease
Docusate sodium	Intraluminal H_2O binding, bulk-forming	Cramping, abdominal pain Lacks evidence for use
Bisacodyl	Stimulating action on intestinal mucosa and increasing peristalsis	Abdominal pain, cramping
Senna	Decreases colonic absorption of water and electrolytes	Abdominal pain, cramping
Linaclotide	Increases water in the intestine and intestinal motility	Resistant constipation, cost-prohibitive, diarrhea, abdominal pain, and nausea Long-term risks in older adults are unknown

(continued)

TABLE 19.1 Pharmacotherapy for Constipation in Older Adults (*continued*)

Agent	Mechanism of Action	Side Effects/Considerations
Lubiprostone	Moves water into the intestinal lumen	Severe constipation Nausea, may be cost-prohibitive
Methylnaltrexone, alvimopan, and naloxegol	Decrease the gastrointestinal effects of opioids	Diarrhea and abdominal pain, used in opioid-induced constipation

Sources: Data from De Giorgio, R., Ruggeri, E., Stanghellini, V., Eusebi, L. H., Bazzoli, F., & Chiaroni, G. (2015). Chronic constipation in the elderly: A primer for the gastroenterologist. *BMC Gastroenterology, 15*(13). doi:10.1186/s12876-015-0366-3; Mounsey, A., Raleigh, M., & Wilson, A. (2015). Management of constipation in older adults. *American Family Physician, 92*(6), 500–504. Retrieved from https://www.aafp.org/afp/2015/0915/p500.html; Rao, S. S. C. (2019). Constipation in the older adult. In N. J. Talley, K. E. Schmader, & S. Grover (Eds.), *UpToDate*. Retrieved from https://www.uptodate.com/contents/constipation-in-the-older-adult; Schuster, B. G., Kosar, L., & Kamrul, R. (2015). Constipation in older adults: Stepwise approach to keep things moving. *Canadian Family Physician, 61*(2), 152–158. Retrieved from https://www.cfp.ca/content/61/2/152

DIARRHEA

Acute or chronic diarrhea in older adults is of concern due to the risk of dehydration and nutritional deficiencies that may coincide with the conditions. Acute diarrhea in first-world countries is most often attributable to infectious causes (LaRocque & Harris, 2019). Generally, acute diarrhea is self-limiting and will resolve with non-pharmacologic management. Nurse practitioners need to determine when to do stool testing and initiate empiric antimicrobial therapy (LaRocque & Harris, 2019). Acute diarrhea is considered when a patient presents with three or more loose stools in 24 hours, and remains acute for up to 14 days.

The most common causes of acute diarrhea include norovirus, rotavirus, adenovirus, *Escherichia coli*, *Clostridioides difficile* (*C. difficile*), *Campylobacter*, *Salmonella*, and protozoa like *Giardia* and *Cyclospora*. Most cases of acute diarrhea are of viral origin, and most stool cultures are negative. History and physical exam will help providers determine mild versus more serious cases of diarrhea. Reasons for greater concern include persistent fever, bloody diarrhea, severe abdominal pain, and evidence of volume depletion. Patients may need to be hospitalized in these cases. Providers should determine stool frequency, quality, food history, and exposures. Laboratory tests are not needed in mild cases, but stool cultures should be considered in patients with severe illness, symptoms of inflammatory diarrhea, high-risk host features (older age and comorbidities), persistent symptoms (over 1 week), and public health concerns (institutionalized patients); see LaRocque and Harris (2019).

Management of acute diarrhea includes maintaining fluid balance, advancing diet as tolerated, and empiric antibiotic therapy for severe disease, symptoms suggestive of bacterial infection, or high risk for complications such as older age, comorbid conditions, or immunocompromised state. Box 19.1 provides an overview of antibiotics and medications used for symptomatic treatment of acute diarrhea (LaRocque & Harris, 2019).

Chronic diarrhea may be related to malabsorption syndromes (celiac disease or lactose intolerance), chronic conditions (IBD or hyperthyroidism), IBS, chronic infections, or medication side effects (metformin); see Asaradnam et al. (2018) and Bonis and Lamont (2019). An effective history and physical exam will help delineate the cause and guide treatment decision-making. Examples include mucosal inflammation (IBD), abdominal

BOX 19.1 Medications With Indications for Management of Acute Diarrhea in Older Adults

Medications for Empiric Antibiotic Therapy and Indication
Azithromycin—fever or bloody diarrhea, patients at risk for fluoroquinolone resistance
Fluoroquinolones—ciprofloxacin or levofloxacin (consider dose adjustments and risks in older adults)
Treatment of *Clostridioides difficile* (*C. difficile*): oral vancomycin (risk of nephrotoxicity) or metronidazole (disulfiram-like effect with alcohol)

Symptomatic Treatment
Loperamide: in afebrile patients without bloody stool, not for use in *C. difficile*
Lomotil: not optimal in older adults due to central opiate effects, controlled substance
Bismuth salicylate: watch dose for salicylate toxicity
Probiotics: effectiveness with Lactobacillus and Saccharomyces boulardii has been established

Source: Data from LaRocque, R., & Harris, J. B. (2019). Approach to the adult with acute diarrhea in resource-rich settings. In S. B. Calderwood & A. Bloom (Eds.), *UpToDate*. Retrieved from https://www.uptodate.com/contents/approach-to-the-adult-with-acute-diarrhea-in-resource-rich-settings

masses (cancer), wasting (malabsorption), lymphadenopathy (HIV infection), and anal sphincter function (fecal incontinence); see Bonis and Lamont (2019). Nurse practitioners must be careful not to attribute patient-reported symptoms of watery stool to diarrhea if there is a bowel obstruction. Treating patients with an antimotility agent in the presence of a bowel obstruction increases complications and the risk of mortality.

The workup of chronic diarrhea is based on the history and physical exam. If diarrhea is intermittent and seems food related, patients may need to keep a food diary to see if there is an offending agent. Most cases of chronic diarrhea require further testing, and a good baseline approach is a complete blood count (CBC), metabolic panel, C-reactive protein and sedimentation rate, thyroid testing, total protein and albumin, and fecal occult blood (Asaradnam et al., 2018; Bonis & Lamont, 2019). Examples include the following:

- Serologic testing for celiac disease or hydrogen breath testing for lactose intolerance
- Stool tests for inflammation
- Colonoscopy for symptoms of IBD or colorectal cancer
- Imaging of the pancreas and small bowel for inflammation or pancreatic insufficiency (Asaradnam et al., 2018; Bonis & Lamont, 2019)

Many cases of chronic diarrhea are self-limiting and idiopathic. In a case with an identified cause, the management of chronic diarrhea may involve a multifaceted approach including removal of offending agents (foods/medications), treating organic cause (hyperthyroidism), and management of symptoms (Asaradnam et al., 2018; Bonis & Lamont, 2019). Antimotility agents (loperamide) may be used in some patients, but this should be weighed with the risks of inducing constipation in elderly patients (Bonis & Lamont, 2019). Frequent reassessment and good patient education can help with this issue. Nurse practitioners should also be aware of the potential for nutritional deficiencies (calcium, potassium, magnesium, and zinc); see Ochoa and Surawicz (2012).

DIVERTICULOSIS AND DIVERTICULITIS

Diverticulosis is a structural change in the bowel that occurs most often after the age of 40 (American Society for Gastrointestinal Endoscopy [ASGE], n.d.). Pockets or pouches form in the wall or lining of the digestive tract when the inner layer pushes through weak spots in the outer layer of the intestinal wall (Pemberton, 2019b). These are generally found in the large intestine and may be caused by a low-fiber diet (ASGE, n.d.). Patients are generally asymptomatic with diverticulosis, but the pouches or pockets are found on colonoscopy (ASGE, n.d.). Diverticulosis can place patients at greater risk for intestinal blockages or diverticulitis, which is an infection of the diverticulum.

Diverticulitis is the main complication that arises from diverticulosis. When the pouches become infected or inflamed, patients develop diverticulitis. Patients may present to the clinic with localized pain (often left lower quadrant), chills or fever, nausea and vomiting, and constipation or diarrhea (ASGE, n.d.; Pemberton, 2019b). Blood work may show elevated white blood cells (WBCs), and a diagnostic confirmation comes from an abdominal CT scan with contrast (Pemberton, 2019b). Other labs to consider include a metabolic panel, urinalysis, amylase, lipase, and alkaline phosphatase to rule out other causes of abdominal pain. Stool studies can help rule out infectious agents such as *C. difficile*.

Complications of diverticulitis include abscess formation, bowel obstruction, fistula formation, and bowel perforation. Uncomplicated diverticulitis can be treated noninvasively in most cases (Pemberton, 2019a). Patients should be treated in the inpatient setting if they have the following characteristics:

- Complicated disease (signs of perforation, abscess, etc.)
- Signs of sepsis
- Immunosuppression (diabetes)
- High fever and significant leukocytosis
- Older age
- Severe abdominal pain
- Multiple or significant comorbid conditions
- Poor adherence (Pemberton, 2019a)

Outpatient treatment includes rest, following a clear liquid or BRAT (bananas, rice, applesauce, toast) diet depending on the patient's symptoms, and medication management (Pemberton, 2019a). Medication management is focused on infection control with the use of antibiotic combinations listed in Box 19.2. Pain control should start out conservatively and progress as needed.

Patient follow-up should occur after 2 to 3 days to assess treatment response with outpatient treatment. Weekly follow-up after the initial follow-up appointment will provide ongoing support until symptoms resolve (Pemberton, 2019a).

IRRITABLE BOWEL SYNDROME

IBS is becoming more common with the increasing aging population. Symptoms most often start before 45 years of age, and IBS is more common in women (Cedars-Sinai, n.d.; Wald, 2019a). IBS is classified as a functional bowel disease because there is no presence of inflammation with diagnostic testing. The pathophysiology for this diagnosis is poorly understood but has been linked to diet, mental health, and gut flora. The symptoms of IBS such as diarrhea, constipation, both diarrhea and constipation, urgency, and incomplete emptying (tenesmus) may overlap with other diagnoses

BOX 19.2 Medication Regimens for Outpatient Treatment of Acute Diverticulitis

Ciprofloxacin (500 mg every 12 hours) plus metronidazole (500 mg every 8 hours)
Levofloxacin (750 mg daily) plus metronidazole (500 mg every 8 hours)
Trimethoprim–sulfamethoxazole DS (1 twice daily) plus metronidazole (500 mg every 8 hours)
Augmentin 875/125 (every 8 hours) or XR (2 tablets every 12 hours)
Moxifloxacin (400 mg daily); in patients intolerant of metronidazole and beta-lactam agents

Source: Adapted from Pemberton, J. H. (2019). Acute colonic diverticulitis: Medical management. In M. Weiser, & W. Chen (Eds.), *UpToDate.* Retrieved from https://www.uptodate.com/contents/acute-colonic-diverticulitis-medical-management

(Wald, 2019a). Other symptoms include bloating, gassiness, and cramping (Harvard Health Publishing, 2018).

Usually, the diagnosis is made after a careful history, physical exam, and symptom-directed workup. Patients do not need blood work or diagnostic testing to receive the diagnosis of IBS, although the blood work and diagnostic testing may rule out other conditions, such as celiac disease or IBD (Wald, 2019a). The Rome IV criteria include recurrent abdominal pain related to two or more of the following: defecation, associated with a change in stool frequency and stool form. Subtypes of IBS can be classified according to predominant bowel habits and stool consistency with the Bristol stool form scale. The Manning scale includes relief of pain with bowel movements, looser and more frequent stools with the onset of pain, passage of mucus, and a sense of incomplete emptying (Wald, 2019a). When completing the workup for IBS, nurse practitioners should be aware of alarm features that require either referral or further workup including: age of onset after 50 years (concern for cancer), rectal bleeding or melena, nocturnal diarrhea, progressive abdominal pain, unexplained weight loss, laboratory abnormalities, and patients with a family history of IBD or colorectal cancer (Wald, 2019a).

Once the diagnosis of IBS has been established, management of the condition consists of both behavioral change and medications if needed. Dietary changes and physical activity are the primary behavioral approaches. Some patients respond well to the low FODMAP diet; so this can be trialed. For some patients, an elimination diet based on a food diary may also be used (patients may be sensitive to wheat, dairy, and gas-producing foods); see Wald (2019b). Medications for IBS are focused on symptom control. Table 19.2 provides an overview of medications, the symptom target, and side effects of the medications. Patients with IBS may experience high levels of distress related to their condition, and coinciding mental health issues may be present. Nurse practitioners must be supportive with education and time in addition to providing a treatment plan for these patients (Wald, 2019b).

INFLAMMATORY BOWEL CONDITIONS, CHRONIC PANCREATITIS, AND GALLBLADDER COMPLAINTS

Inflammatory Bowel Conditions

The incidence of inflammatory bowel conditions is increasing in older adults due to the growing aging population. IBD generally occurs between the ages 20 and 39, but a second peak occurs between ages 50 and 70 (Nimmons & Limdi, 2016). Ulcerative colitis (UC) and Crohn's disease (CD) are the most common IBDs in older adults

TABLE 19.2 Medications Used to Treat IBS

Medication	Symptom Type	Considerations
Soluble fiber	Constipation	Adequate fluid intake
PEG	Constipation	Bloating, abdominal pain
Lubiprostone	Constipation after treatment with PEG	Nausea, limited data in older adults
Guanylate cyclase agonists (linaclotide and plecanatide)	Constipation despite treatment with PEG	Long-term risks unknown
Loperamide	Diarrhea	Limited doses, as needed basis, risk for constipation, does not improve global IBS symptoms
Eluxadoline	Diarrhea	Limited data, avoid use in patients with biliary disease, no gallbladder, pancreatitis, liver impairment, or heavy alcohol use
Bile acid sequestrants	Diarrhea	Use limited by bloating, flatulence, abdominal pain, and constipation
Alosetron (5-HT3 antagonist)	Severe diarrhea	Prescribed under restricted conditions due to risk of ischemic colitis and severe constipation
Antispasmodics (dicyclomine and hyoscyamine)	Abdominal bloating and pain	Anticholinergic activity may limit use in older adults
Antidepressants (TCAs, SSRIs, and SNRIs)	Abdominal pain	Anticholinergic activity of TCAs
Rifaximin	Moderate to severe IBS without constipation (bloating)	Modest improvement in randomized trials
Probiotics	Global IBS symptoms	Limited research to support use

IBS, irritable bowel syndrome; PEG, polyethylene glycol; SNRI, serotonin and norepinephrine reuptake inhibitor; SSRI, selective serotonin reuptake inhibitor; TCA, tricyclic antidepressant.

Source: Adapted from Wald, A. (2019). Treatment of irritable bowel syndrome in adults. In N. J. Talley, & S. Grover (Eds.), *UpToDate*. Retrieved from https://www.uptodate.com/contents/treatment-of-irritable-bowel-syndrome-in-adults

(Rawla, Sunkara, & Raj, 2018). Older onset UC is more common in older adults, and rates are higher in older men (Taleban, Columbel, Mohler, & Fain, 2015). UC affects only the colon, but CD is characterized by skip lesions from the mouth to the anus (Peppercorn & Cheifetz, 2019).

Patients may present with symptoms such as weight loss, diarrhea, abdominal pain, and anemia. Other symptoms may include poor bowel control, blood in the stool, nausea, and constitutional symptoms if acutely ill. For UC, the symptoms (bleeding, diarrhea, and abdominal pain) may be subtle in older patients, and distal disease is more common (Nimmons & Limdi, 2016). In CD, the mean time to diagnosis may be longer in older patients, and they experience more colonic involvement with greater inflammatory disease (Nimmons & Limdi, 2016). History and physical exam help determine the frequency of symptoms, triggers, and location of pain. Colonoscopy with biopsy is the definitive test for diagnosing IBD, although diagnosis may be supported with labs (CBC, inflammatory markers, biomarkers), x-ray, barium enema, and CT scan (Cleveland Clinic, 2019; Crohn's & Colitis Foundation, 2010).

Treatment of both conditions in older patients requires some important considerations such as decreased immune function and polypharmacy. In addition, older patients with new-onset disease generally have less progression (Nimmons & Limdi, 2016; Taleban et al., 2015). The drug-efficacy trials are limited in older adults, especially with immunosuppressive agents (Taleban et al., 2015). Treatment decisions should balance these issues with the goals of clinical and endoscopic remission, prevention of disease complications, and better quality of life (Arnott, Rogler, & Halfvarson, 2017; Nimmons & Limdi, 2016; Taleban et al., 2015). Treatment includes stress management, smoking cessation, limiting dietary triggers, use of anti-inflammatory agents listed in Table 19.3, and surgery for serious disease or complications.

TABLE 19.3 Medications Used for IBD

Medication	Considerations in Older Adults
5-Aminosalicylates	Combination (oral and topical) therapy in UC is more effective, although complex dosing regimens are of concern; physical limitations may affect topical use in older adults; interacts with warfarin
Antibiotics (ciprofloxacin and metronidazole)	Mild–moderate CD restricted to the colon; fluoroquinolones increase risk of *Clostridioides difficile* infection; CNS abnormalities, QT prolongation, and tendon rupture with ciprofloxacin; both interact with warfarin; metronidazole associated with neuropathy; nausea, anorexia, and metallic taste with metronidazole may affect nutrition status in frail adults
Corticosteroids	Used to induce remission in UC and CD; risks of long-term use: elevated glucose, osteoporotic fractures, fluid retention, and mental health; may interact with anticoagulants, phenytoin, phenobarbital, and rifampin

(*continued*)

TABLE 19.3 Medications Used for IBD (*continued*)

Medication	Considerations in Older Adults
Thiopurines (azathioprine and 6-mercaptopurine)	Preserve remission of CD and UC; idiosyncratic reactions: fever, pancreatitis, hepatitis; myelosuppression (test thiopurine methyltransferase, CBC, and metabolic panel); risk of nonmelanoma skin cancer and non-Hodgkin's lymphoma; bone marrow toxicity in combination with allopurinol
Methotrexate	Treatment in CD; increased renal toxicity with concomitant NSAID use; side effects: nausea, fatigue, rash, and stomatitis (folic acid supplements may help); interacts with tetracycline, penicillin, theophylline, and loop diuretics
Cyclosporine	Limited use in IBD currently, may be used as rescue treatment in fulminant colitis; older adults experience significant side effects; interacts with gentamicin, vancomycin, NSAIDs, H2-receptor antagonists, verapamil, allopurinol, phenytoin, carbamazepine, and phenobarbital
Biologic therapies TNF-alpha (infliximab, adalimumab, certolizumab, and golimumab) Integrins (vedolizumab and natalizumab) IL-12 and IL-23 antagonists (ustekinumab)	TNF-alpha: serious infections (pneumonia, septic arthritis, cellulitis, pyelonephritis, and diverticulitis) due to immunosuppression, risk of malignancies (nonmelanoma skin cancer, lymphoma, breast, colon, lung, melanoma, and prostate cancers), and demyelinating neurological disease Integrins: infusion reactions, infections (including herpes), fatigue, progressive multifocal leukoencephalopathy (natalizumab) IL-12 and IL-23 antagonists: nasopharyngitis, injection site redness, vulvovaginal candidiasis, serious infections (abscess, gastroenteritis, and pneumonia), hypersensitivity reactions

CBC, complete blood count; CD, Crohn's disease; CNS, central nervous system; IBD, inflammatory bowel disease; NSAID, nonsteroidal anti-inflammatory drug; UC, ulcerative colitis.

Source: Data from Nimmons, D., & Limdi, J. K. (2016). Elderly patients & inflammatory bowel disease. *World Journal of Gastrointestinal Pharmacology & Therapeutics, 7*(1), 51–65. doi:10.4292/wjgpt.v7.i1.51; Rawla, P., Sunkara, T., & Raj, J. P. (2018). Role of biologics and biosimilars in inflammatory bowel disease: Current trends & future perspectives. *Journal of Inflammation Research, 11*, 215–226. doi:10.2147/jir.s165330; Taleban, S., Columbel, J. F., Mohler, M. J., & Fain, M. J. (2015). Inflammatory bowel disease and the elderly: A review. *Journal of Crohn's & Colitis, 9*(6), 507–515. doi:10.1093/ecco-jcc/jjv059

Pancreatitis

Primary care nurse practitioners may see older patients with acute or chronic pancreatitis. Chronic pancreatitis generally occurs between the ages of 30 and 40 and is more common in men (The National Pancreas Foundation [NPF], n.d.). Excessive alcohol use is a risk factor along with smoking, cystic fibrosis, autoimmune conditions, family history, and conditions that cause a blocked pancreatic duct (Forsmark,

2013; Forsmark, Freedman, & Lewis, 2019; NPF, 2019). Symptoms may include nausea, vomiting, weight loss, diarrhea, and oily, fatty, or clay-colored stools. Diagnosis may be made based on history, physical exam, imaging (MRI, magnetic resonance cholangiopancreatography [MRCP], endoscopic ultrasound [EUS], CT), and pancreatic enzyme levels (Forsmark, 2013; NPF, n.d.).

While the onset of chronic pancreatitis is less common in older patients, the aging nature of the population means that nurse practitioners will see more older adults with chronic pancreatitis. It is characterized by fibroinflammatory changes over time, which results in permanent damage to the pancreas (Forsmark et al., 2019). Over time patients experience pancreatic failure, and they may require medication to help with exocrine and endocrine pancreatic function (Forsmark, 2013; Forsmark et al., 2019; NPF, n.d.). Additionally, patients with chronic pancreatitis may experience a great deal of pain. Pain management may be where primary care nurse practitioners will interface the most with older patients diagnosed with chronic pancreatitis (Forsmark, 2013; NPF, n.d.). Like any pain management regimen, it is best to start with nonopioids such as acetaminophen (no more than 2,000 mg/day), followed by mild opioids (tramadol or hydrocodone), and then strong opioids (morphine); see NPF (n.d.) and Schofield (2016). Nurse practitioners must balance pain and symptom management in geriatric patients with the risks related to opioid therapy such as constipation and central nervous system depression that complicates respiratory illness and contributes to falls (Schofield, 2016).

Acute pancreatitis occurs when there is an acute inflammatory process involving the pancreas and possibly surrounding tissues, and it is generally self-limiting (Forsmark et al., 2019; Zagaria, 2011). The most common cause of acute pancreatitis in older adults is gallstones (Zagaria, 2011). Issues that increase the risk of mortality in these patients include older age, alcohol use, and diabetes. Being female is associated with better survival rates. Patients may present to primary care with severe upper abdominal pain that radiates to the back and may be associated with a recent alcohol binge or fatty meal (Zagaria, 2011). Medication such as estrogens, infectious disease such as cytomegalovirus, trauma, hypertriglyceridemia, and hypotensive ischemia can all be precursors to acute pancreatitis (Zagaria, 2011). Along with pain, patients experience nausea, vomiting, abdominal tenderness, elevated temperature, elevated WBCs, and toxic appearance.

Nurse practitioners in primary care may suspect a diagnosis based on history and physical exam alone. Serum pancreatic enzyme levels, CBC, inflammatory markers, and a metabolic panel may also contribute to the clinical picture. If acute pancreatitis is suspected, patients should be rapidly transferred to the ED for further evaluation and disposition. Depending on severity, patients may be managed on the medical floor or the ICU. Fasting, fluid resuscitation, management of nausea and vomiting, and pain management until pancreatic inflammation subsides are the primary goals of care (Zagaria, 2011).

Gallbladder Disease

Gallbladder disease in older adults includes stones and gallbladder dysfunction. Gallstones are common in adults, and patients are often asymptomatic. They may be found incidentally with abdominal imaging (Zakko, 2018). Complicated gallstone disease occurs when patients experience acute cholecystitis, gallstone pancreatitis, or gallstone ileus. Acute cholecystitis is the most common complication of gallstones, and patients present with classic symptoms such as nausea, right upper quadrant pain that radiates to the back, sweating, fever, elevated WBCs, and possibly diarrhea and clay-colored stools. These may be less distinct in older patients. Symptom onset may follow a fatty meal but is not always associated with meals (Zakko, 2018). Risk factors for gallstone disease in older adults include older age, female gender, White/

Mexican American/Native American ethnicity, female hormones for contraception or replacement, or treatment of prostate cancer, rapid weight loss, obesity, and dyslipidemia (Zagaria, 2010).

Diagnosis can be made based on history and physical exam for uncomplicated cholelithiasis, but if there are leukocytosis and elevated liver or pancreatic enzymes, complications should be considered (Zakko, 2018). Diagnostic testing includes ultrasound initially although a CT scan may demonstrate evidence of stones, sludge, or gallbladder inflammation (Zagaria, 2010).

If a patient does not present with gallstone complications, such as cholecystitis, then no intervention is needed. Most patients presenting with complicated disease should proceed with laparoscopic cholecystectomy (Zagaria, 2010; Zakko, 2018). There are risks in older adults, such as higher mortality, although rates remain low overall. Another risk of cholecystectomy in geriatric patients is common bile duct injury (Nassar & Richter, 2019). Another treatment strategy is endoscopic cholangiopancreatography (ECRP), although this is less effective when compared to surgery. Studies have demonstrated some benefit with cholecystectomy with ECRP although the risk of proceeding to an open versus endoscopic procedure is higher (Nassar & Richter, 2019). Some patients may be considered for stone dissolution with ursodiol if gallstones are composed of cholesterol. There have been no studies addressing ursodiol use in older patients; so the lowest dose should be initiated. Monitoring includes liver enzymes and alkaline phosphatase at the start of therapy and 1, 3, and 6 months thereafter. Individuals should avoid aluminum-based antacids while on ursodiol (Zagaria, 2010). Finally, pain management is a primary concern in all patients with complicated cholelithiasis, and this should be addressed similarly to pain management with pancreatitis.

Functional gallbladder disease is relatively rare and is generally a diagnosis of exclusion in patients with biliary colic in the absence of gallstones, sludge, or microcrystals. Patients may present with constant right upper quadrant pain, sweating, nausea, and vomiting (Zakko & Zakko, 2018). Attacks generally last about 6 hours. Pain may be associated with a fatty meal but not always. History and physical exam can help establish the diagnosis of gallbladder dysfunction. Laboratory tests and abdominal imaging are normal. In selected patients, cholecystokinin-stimulated cholescintigraphy will be considered to evaluate gallbladder ejection fraction. If it is below 35% to 40%, it is considered low. False-positive results may occur due to conditions such as diabetes, celiac disease, obesity, cirrhosis, and medications listed in Box 19.3 (Zakko & Zakko, 2018).

Symptoms of functional gallbladder disease may resolve spontaneously; so using behavioral management is generally the best initial approach with a low-fat diet. If individuals have low gallbladder ejection fraction and over 3 months of persistent biliary pain, they may be considered for surgery (Zakko & Zakko, 2018). Again, symptomatic patients may have significant pain; so they should be treated starting with nonopioid pain medications and then stepped up to mild and then strong opioids. These decisions should be made in consideration of comorbid conditions and the potential for medication interactions (Schofield, 2016).

SUMMARY

Bowel conditions are common and result in pain and functional limitations in older adults. Primary care nurse practitioners must be aware of the presenting symptoms, diagnostic workup, and pharmacologic treatment of these conditions. Of particular note in older adults is the management of chronic constipation, which can improve quality of life.

BOX 19.3 Medications Implicated in False-Positive Cholescintigraphy

Calcium channel blockers
Oral contraceptives
Progesterone
H2-receptor antagonists
Opioids
Benzodiazepines
Atropine
Octreotide
Theophylline

Source: Data from Zakko, S. F., & Zakko, W. F. (2018). Functional gallbladder disorder in adults. In S. Chopra & S. Grover (Eds.), *UpToDate*. Retrieved from https://www.uptodate.com/contents/functional-gallbladder-disorder-in-adults

GASTROINTESTINAL INTERPROFESSIONAL CASE STUDY

Megan Hebdon

Patient Presentation

Mrs. L, an 80-year-old female, presents to the clinic reporting acute abdominal tenderness to her left lower abdomen that is radiating to her back. She states the pain started yesterday and she has been feeling hot and cold in waves starting this morning. She has had diarrhea all morning, although there is some form to the stool. She has not eaten more than a few crackers and had a small amount of water due to nausea. She denies vomiting. She denies body aches, headache, or other associated symptoms. She has a past medical history of diverticulosis but has never had diverticulitis or IBD. She has no gallbladder or appendix.

History

She has a past history of alcoholism, and she has been sober for 15 years. She has no history of tobacco or illicit drug use. She is married to her second husband, and she has no children. She has no siblings, and her parents passed away over 20 years ago—she believes of "old age." She has high cholesterol, blood pressure, atrial fibrillation, chronic back and knee pain, depression, insomnia, type 2 diabetes, and peripheral neuropathy. She has what she suspected to be a ministroke last year. She has had both knees replaced, an appendectomy, a cholecystectomy, and a breast reduction. She does not exercise due to her chronic arthritis pain. She eats whatever she wants. She does not drive; her husband brought her to the appointment. She has a do-not-resuscitate (DNR) order.

Medications

Metoprolol 50 mg daily, simvastatin 40 mg at night, aspirin (ASA) 81 mg daily, oxycodone–acetaminophen (APAP) 5/325 one every 6 hours for arthritis pain, acetaminophen 325 mg every 6 hours for arthritis pain, ibuprofen 400 mg every 8 hours for pain, gabapentin 600 mg three times a day, zolpidem 10 mg at night, paroxetine 20 mg daily, Lantus 40 units at night, and metformin 500 mg twice a day.

No medication allergies.

Physical Exam

Vital signs are Blood pressure: 108/60 mmHg; Pulse: 108 beats per minute; Respirations: 22 breaths per minute; Temperature: 99.2 degrees F; Oxygen saturation: 98%.

She is ill-appearing, and her skin is sweaty. She has tachycardia with irregular rhythm. Her lungs are clear in all fields. On abdominal exam, she has hyperactive bowel sounds and point tenderness to the left lower quadrant.

Diagnostic Testing

Complete blood count (CBC), comprehensive metabolic panel (CMP), urinalysis, and abdominal ultrasound. CT scanning is not available at the clinic site.

CBC shows mild leukocytosis, CMP with calculated creatinine clearance of 32 mL/min, the urinalysis has high specific gravity and presence of WBC with no blood or leukocyte esterase, and the abdominal ultrasound shows bowel wall thickening over the area of tenderness and surrounding diverticula.

Plan of Care

Based on history, physical examination, and diagnostic testing results, you determine that the patient has acute diverticulitis. There is no current evidence of complications such as a perforation or abscess. She is also dehydrated, and you are concerned about her ability to restore fluid balance without intravenous (IV) fluids. She is hemodynamically stable right now, but she may not remain that way with ongoing nausea and diarrhea. Due to her other chronic conditions and age, you are inclined to admit her to the hospital. When you discuss this with the patient, she refuses. With the patient and her spouse, you review the risks of outpatient therapy and you develop a plan to ensure adequate hydration, antibiotic therapy, and watching for worsening signs or symptoms that would prompt evaluation in the ED. The patient is started on Bactrim DS every 12 hours and metronidazole 500 mg every 8 hours for 10 days. The patient is on abundant pain medication; so pain management will focus on behavioral strategies such as rest, a liquid to advance to the BRAT diet when symptoms improve, use of heat/ice, and mindfulness. A short-term follow-up is planned in 2 days to reevaluate her diverticulitis. You also plan to call her tomorrow to check in.

Interprofessional Collaboration

The patient's medication list is concerning for multiple pain medication, high doses of Ambien, ASA for her age, simvastatin for her age, use of paroxetine, which has more anticholinergic side effects, and her desires for DNR. You plan to consult a pharmacist regarding medication optimization and harm reduction. A 4-week follow-up is planned to start optimizing and reducing the number of medications she is taking. If needed, she will be referred to pain management, an acupuncture provider, and/or physical therapy for evaluation based on mutually agreed upon goals at her next visit. A follow-up with her gastroenterologist will be planned if she has persistent gastrointestinal symptoms.

Case Study References

American Geriatric Society Beers Criteria Update Expert Panel. (2019). American Geriatrics Society 2019 updated AGS Beers Criteria for potentially inappropriate medication use in older adults. *Journal of the American Geriatrics Society, 67*(4), 674–694. doi:10.1111/jgs.15767

Baum, J. A., & Companioni, R. A. C. (2018). Colonic diverticulitis. *Merck manual: Professional version*. Kenilworth, NJ: Merck & Co. Retrieved from https://www.merckmanuals.com/professional/gastrointestinal-disorders/diverticular-disease/colonic-diverticulitis

Epocrates. (April 2, 2019). Bactrim DS. [Electronic App].

Pemberton, J. H. (2019a). Acute colonic diverticulitis: Medical management. In M. Weiser & W. Chen (Eds.), *UpToDate*. Waltham, MA.

Pemberton, J. H. (2019b). Clinical manifestations and diagnosis of acute diverticulitis in adults. In J. T. Lamont & S. Grover (Eds.), *UpToDate*. Retrieved from Waltham, MA.

REFERENCES

American Society for Gastrointestinal Endoscopy. (n.d.). Understanding diverticulosis Retrieved from https://www.asge.org/home/for-patients/patient-information/understanding-diverticulosis

Arnott, I., Rogler, G., & Halfvarson, J. (2017). The management of inflammatory bowel disease in elderly: Current evidence & future perspectives. *Inflammatory Intestinal Disease, 2*, 189–199. doi:10.1159/000490053

Asaradnam, R. P., Brown, S., Forbes, A., Fox, M. R., Hungin, P., Kelman, L., . . . Walters, J. R. F. (2018). Guidelines for the investigation of chronic diarrhea in adults: British Society of Gastroenterology, 3rd edition. *Gut, 67*(8), 1380–1399. doi: 10.1136/gutjnl-2017-315909

Bonis, P. A. L., & Lamont, J. T. (2019). Approach to the adult with chronic diarrhea. In P. Rutgeerts & S. Grover (Eds.), *UpToDate*. Retrieved from https://www.uptodate.com/contents/approach-to-the-adult-with-chronic-diarrhea-in-resource-rich-settings

Cedars-Sinai. (n.d.). Irritable bowel syndrome (IBS). Retrieved from https://www.cedars-sinai.org/health-library/diseases-and-conditions/i/irritable-bowel-syndrome-ibs.html

Cleveland Clinic. (2019). Inflammatory bowel disease (IBD). Retrieved from https://my.clevelandclinic.org/health/diseases/17126-inflammatory-bowel-disease-ibd

Crohn's & Colitis Foundation. (2010). Diagnosing Crohn's disease and ulcerative colitis. Retrieved from https://www.crohnscolitisfoundation.org/sites/default/files/legacy/assets/pdfs/diagnosingibd.pdf

De Giorgio, R., Ruggeri, E., Stanghellini, V., Eusebi, L. H., Bazzoli, F., & Chiarioni, G. (2015). Chronic constipation in the elderly: A primer for the gastroenterologist. *BMC Gastroenterology, 15*(13). doi:10.1186/s12876-015-0366-3

Forsmark, C. E. (2013). Management of chronic pancreatitis. *Gastroenterology, 144*, 1282–1291. doi:10.1053/j.gastro.2013.02.008

Forsmark, C. E., Freedman, S. D., & Lewis, M. D. (2019). Etiology and pathogenesis of chronic pancreatitis in adults. In D. C. Whitcomb & S. Grover (Eds.), *UpToDate*. Retrieved from https://www.uptodate.com/contents/etiology-and-pathogenesis-of-chronic-pancreatitis-in-adults/print

Harvard Health Publishing. (2018). Irritable bowel syndrome (IBS). Retrieved from https://www.health.harvard.edu/a_to_z/irritable-bowel-syndrome-ibs-a-to-z

LaRocque, R., & Harris, J. B. (2019). Approach to the adult with acute diarrhea. In S. B. Calderwood & A. Bloom (Eds.), *UpToDate*. Retrieved from https://www.uptodate.com/contents/approach-to-the-adult-with-acute-diarrhea-in-resource-rich-settings

Mounsey, A., Raleigh, M., & Wilson, A. (2015). Management of constipation in older adults. *American Family Physician, 92*(6), 500–504. Retrieved from https://www.aafp.org/afp/2015/0915/p500.html

Nassar, Y., & Richter, S. (2019). Management of complicated gallstones in the elderly: Comparing surgical and non-surgical treatment options. *Gastroenterology Report, 7*, 205–211. doi:10.1093/gastro/goy046

The National Pancreas Foundation. (n.d.). About chronic pancreatitis. Retrieved from https://pancreasfoundation.org/patient-information/chronic-pancreatitis

Nimmons, D., & Limdi, J. K. (2016). Elderly patients & inflammatory bowel disease. *World Journal of Gastrointestinal Pharmacology & Therapeutics, 7*(1), 51–65. doi:10.4292/wjgpt.v7.i1.51

Ochoa, B., & Surawicz, C. M. (2012). Diarrheal diseases—Acute and chronic. *American College of Gastroenterology*. Retrieved from https://gi.org/topics/diarrhea-acute-and-chronic

Pemberton, J. H. (2019a). Acute colonic diverticulitis: Medical management. In M. Weiser & W. Chen (Eds.), *UpToDate*. Retrieved from https://www.uptodate.com/contents/acute-colonic-diverticulitis-medical-management

Pemberton, J. H. (2019b). Clinical manifestations and diagnosis of acute diverticulitis in adults. In J. T. Lamont & S. Grover (Eds.), *UpToDate*. Retrieved from https://www.uptodate.com/contents/clinical-manifestations-and-diagnosis-of-acute-diverticulitis-in-adults

Peppercorn, M. A., & Cheifetz, A. S. (2019). Definitions, epidemiology, and risk factors for inflammatory bowel disease in older adults. In P. Rutgeerts & K. M. Robson (Eds.), *UpToDate*. Retrieved from https://www.uptodate.com/contents/definitions-epidemiology-and-risk-factors-for-inflammatory-bowel-disease-in-adults/print

Rao, S. S. C. (2019). Constipation in the older adult. In N. J. Talley, K. E. Schmader, & S. Grover (Eds.), *UpToDate*. Retrieved from https://www.uptodate.com/contents/constipation-in-the-older-adult

Rawla, P., Sunkara, T., & Raj, J. P. (2018). Role of biologics and biosimilars in inflammatory bowel disease: Current trends & future perspectives. *Journal of Inflammation Research, 11*, 215–226. doi:10.2147/jir.s165330

Schofield, P. (2016). Pain management in older adults. *Medicine in Older Adults, 45*(1), 42–45. doi:10.1016/j.mpmed.2016.10.005

Schuster, B. G., Kosar, L., & Kamrul, R. (2015). Constipation in older adults: Stepwise approach to keep things moving. *Canadian Family Physician, 61*(2), 152–158. Retrieved from https://www.cfp.ca/content/61/2/152

Taleban, S., Columbel, J. F., Mohler, M. J., & Fain, M. J. (2015). Inflammatory bowel disease and the elderly: A review. *Journal of Crohn's & Colitis, 9*(6), 507–515. doi:10.1093/ecco-jcc/jjv059

Wald, A. (2019a). Clinical manifestations and diagnosis of irritable bowel syndrome in adults. In N. J. Talley & S. Grover (Eds.), *UpToDate*. Retrieved from https://www.uptodate.com/contents/clinical-manifestations-and-diagnosis-of-irritable-bowel-syndrome-in-adults

Wald, A. (2019b). Treatment of irritable bowel syndrome in adults. In N. J. Talley & S. Grover (Eds.), *UpToDate*. Retrieved from https://www.uptodate.com/contents/treatment-of-irritable-bowel-syndrome-in-adults

Zagaria, M. A. E. (2010). Gallstones: Aging and medications increase risk. *US Pharmacist, 35*(12), 21–24. Retrieved from https://www.uspharmacist.com/article/gallstones-aging-and-medications-increase-risk

Zagaria, M. A. E. (2011). Acute pancreatitis: Risks, causes, and mortality in older adults. *US Pharmacist, 36*(1), 20–24. Retrieved from https://www.uspharmacist.com/article/acute-pancreatitis-risks-causes-and-mortality-in-older-adults

Zakko, S. F. (2018). Overview of gallstone disease in adults. In S. Chopra & S. Grover (Eds.), *UpToDate*. Retrieved from https://www.uptodate.com/contents/overview-of-gallstone-disease-in-adults

Zakko, S. F., & Zakko, W. F. (2018). Functional gallbladder disorder in adults. In S. Chopra & S. Grover (Eds.), *UpToDate*. Retrieved from https://www.uptodate.com/contents/functional-gallbladder-disorder-in-adults

20 Central Nervous System Impairments

Lisa C. Hutchison

OBJECTIVES
1. Describe the changes commonly seen as the brain ages
2. Design a plan to prevent, identify, and treat delirium in an older adult
3. Contrast etiology, symptoms, and therapies for mild cognitive impairment (MCI), Alzheimer's disease (AD), and Parkinson's disease
4. Design a treatment plan for cognitive and noncognitive symptoms associated with dementia
5. Identify treatments for motor symptoms, wearing off, dyskinesias, and nonmotor symptoms of Parkinson's disease

INTRODUCTION
The specter of cognitive impairment leads many people to fear and dread growing old, given the prospect of losing independence and functionality. While cognitive change is a normal component of aging, cognitive impairment is not. Clinicians must be aware of the expected changes seen with normal aging and differentiate those signs and symptoms seen with neurocognitive impairment diseases such as delirium or dementia. This helps us to provide the best care for patients and guide them to strive for successful aging.

THE AGING BRAIN
Structure
The structural changes typically found in the aging brain begin with a reduction in size and weight. On average, the brain is 11% smaller in older adults over the age of 60 as compared to the young adult although this varies with head size and body weight. Gray matter is where neurons are located and white matter is where the nerve fibers are located. Gray matter loss tends to be less than white matter; so normal older adults maintain the majority of their neurons. So, the losses are not from neuron death as much as they are from decreased neuron size and connectivity. Volume losses are more apparent in the cerebral cortex, hippocampus, and cerebral white matter. The ventricles start to enlarge as the brain shrinks, as do the sulci (grooves between the gyri). Cerebral blood flow diminishes in relation to the size alterations (Harada, Love, & Triebel, 2013).

Neurons and Neurotransmitters

As a corollary of the diminished size and weight, the number of neurons has been reported to decline by as much as 10% over the life span. However, some studies refute this finding when improved techniques and better control of subject variables were applied.

Chemical messengers that are released by the neuron to elicit a response in the postsynaptic neuron are called "neurotransmitters." Common neurotransmitters are acetylcholine, dopamine, serotonin, norepinephrine, glutamate, and gamma-aminobutyric acid (GABA). Some example changes in neurotransmitters are seen with acetylcholine and dopamine. Acetylcholine is important in learning and memory, and a decline in the cholinergic neurons that produce acetylcholine is often seen with aging. Pharmacologic inhibition of the acetylcholine receptors has been shown to contribute to delirium, and medications that reduce the degradation of acetylcholine are shown to improve cognition in patients with dementia. Dopamine receptors are associated with motor control, and excess stimulation of dopamine receptors causes hallucinations. Dopamine levels, transporters, and receptors are reduced with aging; so it takes a smaller dose of dopamine antagonists (e.g., antipsychotic medications) to cause motor dysfunction like extrapyramidal symptoms (Puglielli & Mattson, n.d.).

Function

Because of these changes, in many adults the reserve capacity of the brain is reduced with aging, and a reduction in function may occur with fewer neurologic or physiologic insults than would be needed in a younger patient. Typical age-related changes for cognition are evident primarily with fluid memory, which includes sometimes forgetting names but remembering them later, trouble finding the right word, misplacing things from time to time, and needing extra help to use new equipment (Alzheimer's Association, 2018). While the fluid memory is less effective in aging, crystallized memory such as vocabulary, accumulated knowledge, and the ability to see patterns remains intact and continues to expand (Harada et al., 2013).

DISORDERS OF COGNITION
Delirium
Definitions

Delirium is defined as an acute state of confusion that tends to fluctuate and requires a disturbance in attention. Other terms have been used including "altered mental status," "metabolic encephalopathy," and "acute brain failure" (Marcantonio, 2017). A key difference is that the change in cognition and other symptoms occur acutely, fluctuate, and, if the underlying condition resolves, are expected to abate, although growing evidence reveals some cases persist for months. Currently, the pathophysiology underlying delirium is not understood.

Prevalence

Delirium is commonly seen in hospitalized older adults, especially after surgery where it has been reported in as high as 50% of high-risk patients undergoing high-risk procedures (Marcantonio, 2017). One-third of older adults hospitalized for medical problems have delirium. Half of these are admitted with delirium and the other half develop it during admission. At the end of life, delirium occurs in over 80% of individuals. Nonetheless, delirium is underrecognized and undertreated in older adults (Inouye, Westendorp, & Saczynski, 2014).

Risk Factors

Risk factors for delirium are categorized as predisposing factors and precipitating factors. For predisposing factors, older age, dementia, reduced functional status, and multiple comorbidities are most commonly identified. Often the dementia was not diagnosed prior to the onset of delirium, but is identified as the clinician interviews family or friends regarding the patient's premorbid state. Other data also identify male sex, poor vision, reduced hearing, depression, MCI, alcohol abuse, and electrolyte abnormalities (sodium, calcium) as possible predisposing factors. The predisposing factors are characteristics that the patient has amassed during his or her life before he or she arrives at the hospital or clinic. The more predisposing factors being present reduces the number of precipitating factors needed for the patient to develop delirium (Marcantonio, 2017).

Precipitating factors are numerous. Drugs are especially common causes of delirium. The 2015 American Geriatrics Society (AGS) Beers Criteria lists include anticholinergics, antipsychotics, benzodiazepines, corticosteroids, histamine-2 blocking agents, meperidine, and sedative hypnotics as drugs to avoid in delirium (AGS, 2015a). Other opioid analgesics and anesthesia are also implicated as precipitating agents. Surgery, infections, anemia, and high pain levels are examples of nonpharmacologic precipitating actors (Marcantonio, 2017; Oh, Fong, Hshieh, & Inouye, 2017).

It is helpful to identify the predisposing factors that a patient has so that diligent efforts may be implemented to prevent delirium.

Screening Tools and Diagnosis

The criteria published in the *Diagnostic and Statistical Manual of Mental Disorders* (5th ed.; [DSM-5] American Psychiatric Association, 2013) are considered the gold standard for delirium screening. These criteria are the following:

- There is a disturbance in attention and awareness.
- Disturbance develops acutely and fluctuates in severity.
- Disturbances are not explained by a preexisting dementia, nor do they occur in the context of arousal or coma.
- There is evidence of an underlying organic cause.

The Confusion Assessment Method (CAM) is a commonly used screening tool, which is based on the *DSM-5*. It has been used for over 20 years and has adaptations for critical care and other settings (Inouye et al., 1990; Oh et al., 2017). It is composed of four elements as shown in Table 20.1 along with its adaptation for intensive care settings (Ely & Vanderbilt University, 2016). Many other screening tools exist, including the Nursing Delirium Symptom Checklist (NuDESC); see De and Wand (2015). The NuDESC is arranged as a continuous monitor so that trained nurses from each shift can document patient symptoms of disorientation, inappropriate behavior, inappropriate communication, illusions/hallucinations, and psychomotor retardation, thus providing a way to follow trends and fluctuation in symptoms (Gaudreau, Gagnon, Harel, Tremblay, & Roy, 2005). It is compared to the CAM and CAM-Intensive Care Unit (CAM-ICU) in Table 20.1.

While larger concern and attention is placed on patients with hyperactive delirium because of risk of self-harm or harm, only 25% of patients experience this form while the remaining 75% have hypoactive symptomatology (Inouye et al., 2014). Because patients with hypoactive symptoms are less commonly a concern, overall probably only 12% to 35% of delirium cases are recognized. Over 20 different screening tools have been published in the literature (Oh et al., 2017). The CAM-ICU modifies the method for assessing attention, given that patients who are intubated are not able to

TABLE 20.1 Delirium Assessment Tools

Feature	CAM	CAM-ICU	NuDESC
Acute-onset and fluctuating course	Is there evidence of an acute change in mental status from patient baseline? Did the abnormal behavior fluctuate during the day?	Is the patient's mental status different than at baseline? Has there been any fluctuation in mental status seen on a consciousness scale (e.g., RASS), GCS or previous assessment in the past 24 hours?	Not a specific item on the list; checklist is performed every shift, which would document changes
Inattention	Did patient have: Difficulty focusing attention? Easily distractible? Difficulty keeping track of what was being said?	Use Letters Attention Test—patient to squeeze hand of tester when he or she hears letter "A." Tester reads a series of 10 letters (SAVEAHAART, CASABLANCA, or ABADBADAAY)	Assesses inappropriate behavior, pulling at tubes, getting out of bed when contraindicated, hallucinations present, delayed responses
Altered level of consciousness	Rated as alert, vigilant/hyperalert, lethargic, stuporous or in a coma	Uses RASS score to assess	Assesses psychomotor retardation, patient unarousable
Disorganized thinking	Was patient's thinking rambling, incoherent, unclear, or illogical?	Asks yes/no questions for thinking (e.g., Will a stone float on water?) and gives a command to hold up two fingers with each hand consecutively	Assess patient orientation to time, place, and persons in the room

CAM, Confusion Assessment Method; CAM-ICU, Confusion Assessment Method-Intensive Care Unit; GCS, Glasgow Coma Score; NuDESC, Nursing Delirium Symptom Checklist; RASS, Richmond Agitation–Sedation Scale.

Source: Data from De, J., & Wand, P. F. (2015). Delirium screening: A systematic review of delirium screening tools in hospitalized patients. *Gerontologist, 55,* 1079–1099. doi:10.1093/geront/gnv100; Ely, E. W., & Vanderbilt University. (2016). *Confusion Assessment Method for the ICU (CAM-ICU): The complete training manual.* Retrieved from https://uploads-ssl.webflow.com/5b0849daec50243a0a1e5e0c/5bacedc24b30f7738581bd39_RASS.pdf; Gaudreau, J. D., Gagnon, P., Harel, F., Tremblay, A., & Roy, M. A. (2005). Fast, systematic, and continuous delirium assessment in hospitalized patients: The nursing delirium screening scale. *Journal of Pain and Symptom Management, 29,* 368–375. doi:10.1016/j.jpainsymman.2004.07.009; Inouye, S. K., van Dyck, C. H., Alessi, C. A., Balkin, S., Siegal, A. P., & Howitz, R. I. (1990). Clarifying confusion: The confusion assessment method. A new method for detection of delirium. *Annals of Internal Medicine, 113,* 941–948. doi:10.7326/0003-4819-113-12-941

respond verbally to the interviewer. The use of the CAM or the CAM-ICU by clinicians is encouraged in order to increase the recognition and diagnosis of delirium; so appropriate measures can be adopted in the effort to improve outcomes (Ely & Vanderbilt University 2016; Oh et al., 2017).

Guidelines for Prevention and Treatment

Guidelines for prevention and treatment of postoperative delirium have been promulgated by the AGS (AGS Expert Panel on Postoperative Delirium in Older Adults, 2015b; Inouye et al., 2015). These guidelines may also be applied to medical and surgical patients. First and foremost is the recommendation to educate healthcare professionals about delirium. Education has been shown to reduce the prevalence of delirium and reduce length of stay in hospitalized patients. Nonpharmacologic interventions are recommended for both prevention and management. Pain management is essential but preferably achieved without the use of opioid analgesics. As long as it is not contraindicated, scheduled acetaminophen should be initiated for patients with pain. Other nonopioid agents can be considered such as gabapentin, nonsteroidal anti-inflammatory drugs, and topical lidocaine. However, control of severe pain is warranted even if opioid analgesics are required. Caution should be exercised in the older adult if nonsteroidal anti-inflammatory drugs are used, given the risk for gastric bleeding and renal insufficiency. In some cases, topical diclofenac may be an option that reduces the risk for these complications. As noted earlier, medications highly associated with the incidence of delirium should be avoided unless drug withdrawal concerns are present (AGS, 2015a).

When delirium has been diagnosed, efforts to identify and manage the cause (precipitating factors) are imperative. A medical/laboratory evaluation and assessment of medications and environmental contributors should be performed with the initiation of appropriate treatment. A physical examination may identify causes. Laboratory tests should include electrolytes, complete blood count (CBC), urinalysis, and possibly blood and urine cultures (Oh et al., 2017).

Nonpharmacologic Measures

Nonpharmacologic measures are indicated for prevention and treatment of delirium. Ensuring the patient has adequate sleep is a key precipitating factor that is difficult to accomplish in the hospital setting. Reducing medical or nursing procedures performed during nighttime hours, reducing noise and light levels at night, and scheduling medication administration during waking hours are simple measures that can aid sleep hygiene. In addition, the use of massage and warm drinks (noncaffeinated) has been employed as a nonpharmacologic means to aid with inducing sleep (AGS Expert Panel on Postoperative Delirium in Older Adults, 2015b, Inouye et al., 2015, Oh et al., 2017).

It is important to provide orientation to time, place, and person to the patient. Family members are frequently called upon to keep the patient oriented. Hearing aids and glasses should be provided so that patients can participate in normal conversations. Early mobilization after surgery, removing catheters and other lines as quickly as possible, and having patients sit up for meals help convey a normal routine for the patient (Inouye et al., 2015).

Medications

For the prevention of delirium, psychoactive medications such as anticholinergics, opioids, benzodiazepines, and sedative/hypnotics should be avoided unless the patient is at risk for withdrawal. If a patient has developed delirium, both nonpharmacologic and pharmacologic methods for prevention should be implemented. There is no medication with an indication for the treatment of delirium. If a patient is in a hyperactive delirium, the preferred treatment is nonpharmacologic reassurance and reorientation. In the event that the patient begins pulling out lines or striking at caregivers, small doses of second-generation antipsychotics such as risperidone, olanzapine, and quetiapine may be used to help sedate and calm the patient (Oh et al., 2017). Intramuscular haloperidol has also been used if a patient cannot take oral medications. It is recommended to avoid lorazepam or other benzodiazepines for sedation if alcohol or benzodiazepine withdrawal is suspected as a precipitating factor as these agents may cause further disorientation and confusion (AGS Expert Panel on Postoperative Delirium in Older Adults, 2015b).

MCI and Dementia

Definitions

MCI is defined as a modest decline in one or more cognitive domains, but the decline is not to the level of interfering with a patient's independence in everyday activities. In contrast, dementia is a more significant decline of one or more cognitive domains, which does interfere with independence when performing everyday activities. A diagnosis of either MCI or dementia requires that delirium is not a cause of the decline and no other mental disorder would explain the symptoms. MCI often precedes the development of dementia although not in all patients (Alzheimer's Association, 2018, Hugo & Ganguli, 2014).

Dementia can be further designated according to type. AD is the most common type of dementia occurring both as early-onset (age 50–65) and late-onset (>65). Dementia with Lewy bodies has motor features of parkinsonism identified concurrently with the change in mental status. This is in contrast to dementia of advanced Parkinson's disease, which occurs years after the diagnosis of Parkinson's disease. Vascular dementia occurs within 6 months of a stroke and is closely associated with cerebrovascular risk. There are other causes of dementia, including frontotemporal dementia, Creutzfeldt–Jakob disease, and normal pressure hydrocephalus, but these account for less than 10% of cases (Hugo & Ganguli, 2014).

Prevalence and Risk Factors

MCI has recently been studied to identify its prevalence, which is estimated at 15.8% of adults in the United States over age 60. Not everyone with MCI will progress to AD, but approximately 12% will progress each year to AD. Some have proposed MCI as a preclinical stage of AD, but this has yet to be proven, and patients with MCI may have other causes (Alzheimer's Association, 2018).

It is estimated that 14% of adults over the age of 70 have some type of dementia (Alzheimer's Association, 2018). AD is the most common type at 60% to 80% of cases, as compared to dementia with Lewy bodies (4%–22%) and vascular dementia (10%); see Alzheimer's Association (2018) and Vann Jones and O'Brien (2014).

Of utmost concern is the increase in absolute numbers of patients with dementia and associated financial burden expected over the next decades. Currently, an annual cost of $277 billion is estimated for the United States. This is expected to grow exponentially as the prediction is that every 65 seconds a new individual develops AD, leading to an estimated 88 million sufferers by 2050 (Alzheimer's Association, 2018). No cure or prevention has been discovered to curb this growth although researchers are working diligently.

Risk factors identified for dementias are specific to the type of dementia. For MCI, usually increasing age and low educational attainment are identified as increasing risk. Some believe that MCI is a precursor to AD, but this has been shown only in a subset of patients.

For AD, the most important risk factor is also increasing age. It is the only risk factor that continues to be identified for individuals after the eighth decade. Prevalence at ages 65 to 74 runs about 3%, rising to 32% in those over age 85 (Hugo & Ganguli, 2014).

If an individual has a parent, brother, or sister with AD, the risk increases. Genetics may play a role. The presence of the Apolipoprotein E4 allele as a component of Chromosome 19 increases the risk, and an individual with two copies (homozygous) for the allele has an even greater risk. Only 2% of the population is homozygous for Apolipoprotein E4; these individuals have an 8- to 12-fold increased risk of developing AD. Having one copy (heterozygous) only increases risk by threefold. However, neither of these is a guarantee for developing AD (Alzheimer's Association, 2018). It is interesting that the presence of Apolipoprotein E4 is also a risk factor for the other major dementias, including vascular dementia and dementia with Lewy bodies. As this protein is responsible for the transport of cholesterol in the bloodstream, this process may provide a common trigger for different types of dementia.

Another genetic association is seen with individuals born with Down syndrome. These patients are born with an additional copy of Chromosome 21, which increases the risk of AD. Approximately 50% of individuals with Down syndrome will develop AD in their lifetimes (Alzheimer's Association, 2018).

Other risk factors for AD identified are modifiable. These include chronic cardiovascular diseases, low educational level, low social/cognitive engagement, midlife obesity, tobacco abuse, and traumatic brain injury. Given the paucity of treatment choices, clinicians may help patients address and control these risk factors in order to avoid the development of AD and other dementias.

The risk for dementia with Lewy bodies is also associated with advanced age, but family history is limited to Parkinson's disease. Vascular dementia is associated with the same risk factors as cerebrovascular disease (Hugo & Ganguli, 2014).

Screening Tools and Diagnosis

There are multiple tools used for dementia screening. The Mini-Cog is one of the quickest and easiest to administer. It includes a three-item recall and a clock-drawing test and takes approximately 3 minutes to administer for a maximum score of 5. Scores below 3 have been validated for dementia screening, but greater sensitivity can be achieved with a cut point of 4. It has a sensitivity of 76% to 99% and a specificity of 89% to 93%. It is available in several languages (Borson, Scanlan, Chen, & Ganguli, 2003; Borson, Scanlan, Watanabe, Tu, & Lessiq, 2005).

Further evaluation can be performed with the Mini-Mental State Exam (MMSE), the Saint Louis University Mental Status (SLUMS) Examination, or the Montreal Cognitive Assessment (MoCA). These three screening tools offer the advantage of assessing more domains of cognition and helping to stage dementia. In addition, the SLUMS and the MOCA have adjustments for individuals with low educational levels. The SLUMS is used often by institutions because it does not have copyright issues (Tariq, Tumosa, Chibnall, Perry, & Morley, 2006). The MOCA is available in 13 languages, is available for electronic administration, and has a method for testing individuals who are blind (www.mocatest.org).

More extensive neuropsychological testing conducted by a trained neuropsychologist may be indicated and can be used to help differentiate between neurocognitive disorders and depression, anxiety, or other disorders. A battery of tests are conducted to evaluate intelligence, language, memory, visuospatial function, and executive function. However, this testing is not required for diagnosis (Galvin & Sadowsky, 2012).

Diagnosis of dementia is usually based on the criteria published in the *DSM-5* for major neurocognitive disorders (e.g., AD, Lewy body disease, vascular dementia, or other causes of dementia). These criteria include identification of cognitive decline that interferes with daily activities and cannot be explained by delirium or other causes.

The diagnosis can further be specified as to behavioral disturbance (present or not) and current severity (mild, moderate, or severe); see American Psychiatric Association (2013).

AD is the most common cause of dementia, and diagnosis is often based on the National Institute on Aging-Alzheimer's Association guidelines (McKhann et al., 2011). These guidelines first stipulate that the patient must meet the criteria for dementia. Then the signs and symptoms exhibited by the patient must have an insidious onset, showing a clear-cut history of worsening cognition. In addition, there must be initial deficits of either amnestic presentation with impairment in learning and recall plus one other cognitive dysfunction or nonamnestic presentation with deficits in word-finding, spatial cognition, or executive dysfunction. Last, there should be no evidence of other substantial active neurological or non-neurological diseases with effect on cognition (Galvin & Sadowsky, 2012; McKhann et al., 2011). These guidelines include whether the diagnosis of AD is probable or possible based on the clinical criteria. Additional evidence from biomarkers, imaging, or nuclear scans, if available, can also support the level of certainty.

Biomarkers, imaging, and nuclear scans have been developed with the principal purpose of helping to diagnose AD in the preclinical state so as to facilitate research into ways to prevent or slow progression of the disease. Beta-amyloid proteins and tau proteins are hallmarks of AD found at autopsy, and the cerebrospinal fluid (CSF) can be tested to determine the presence of these proteins. Low levels of beta-amyloid protein in CSF and high levels of tau protein are consistent with AD pathology in the brain. Brain imaging with magnetic resonance showing the presence of medial temporal lobe atrophy and reduced glucose metabolism on PET are other methods to diagnose AD. At present, third-party payers do not pay for these tests except in special circumstances; so they are seldom performed for the clinical diagnosis of AD, but this may change in the future (Alzheimer's Association, 2018; Hugo & Ganguli, 2014).

Other types of dementia have different features. Dementia with Lewy bodies seems to have symptoms of sleep disturbance, well-formed visual hallucinations, and movement features similar to Parkinson's disease like slowness, gait imbalance, and tremor. Vascular dementia features include impaired judgment, inability to plan, and slow gait and poor balance. Evidence of cerebrovascular disease on imaging studies (e.g., stroke) is frequently used to support the diagnosis of vascular dementia. Some patients may have signs and symptoms that point to more than one type of dementia. This is especially common in people aged 85 and older (Alzheimer's Association, 2018).

No matter what type of dementia a patient has, he or she can be staged with the Functional Assessment Staging tool (FAST) . It has seven stages with five subsets to further describe stages 6 and 7. Staging a patient is helpful to understand life expectancy and to aid in understanding the progression of the disease. Individuals in the FAST 7 stage are eligible for hospice (Sclan & Reisberg, 1992).

Guidelines for Prevention and Treatment

Older adults should be evaluated for complaints of memory impairment. If MCI or dementia is suspected, reversible causes should be investigated. Other diseases can present with symptoms consistent with dementia and should be ruled out. Hypothyroidism, anemia, depression, hyponatremia, hypercalcemia, and hepatic encephalopathy could be underlying causes of cognitive impairment. In addition, vitamin B12 deficiency without significant anemia may be present. The current level of folic acid supplementation in breads and cereals in the United States can mask the anemia if vitamin B12 levels in tissue are depleted. Higher ranges for serum concentrations of vitamin B12 are recommended for older adults (300–500 pg/mL); see Blaszczyk and Hutchison (2015). Also, the potential effect of medications that can cause delirium must be considered. The 2015 AGS Beers Criteria lists common agents that should be avoided in patients because they contribute to delirium and dementia, but other medications have case reports in the literature (AGS, 2015a).

In addition, a healthy lifestyle is recommended as a way to prevent AD. Regular physical exercise increases blood and oxygen flow to the brain. Social engagement and intellectual activity help keep individuals mentally active as they age. Prevention of head trauma and traumatic brain injury through home assessment for risk of falls, use of seat belts while traveling, and wearing helmets during sports activity is also suggested as a way to prevent insults to the brain (Alzheimer's Association, n.d.).

Vitamin E, gingko, huperzine A, and turmeric have been proposed as possible natural remedies to prevent neurocognitive decline. Despite multiple studies, no clear evidence in support of their benefit has been published.

Nonpharmacologic Measures

If a patient is diagnosed with AD, the healthy lifestyle measures that we hope will prevent dementia can be implemented so as to help prevent progression of the disease. Avoidance of alcohol should be recommended. In addition, modifiable risk factors for dementia like cardiovascular disease can be addressed. Correcting any visual or hearing deficits may help optimize sensory input for the patient, allowing optimal communication between the patient, family, friends, and caregivers. Advance directives and durable power of attorney documents can be prepared, easing family and caregiver concerns as the disease progresses. As the disease progresses and the patient requires more aid for activities of daily living, it is useful to know his or her wishes for feeding tube placement and long-term care.

Caregivers of patients with AD have been shown to have increased stress, healthcare costs, and mortality. It is important to provide assistance to caregivers in order to provide optimal care for patients with AD. Support groups, respite, counseling, training in effective/efficient caregiving, case management, and psychotherapy have been shown independently and as components of intensive support strategies to provide benefit (Alzheimer's Association, 2018).

Medications

Acetylcholinesterase Inhibitors (ACIs)

The first line of treatment for AD is the ACIs donepezil, rivastigmine, and galantamine. These agents work by inhibiting the enzyme acetylcholinesterase so that the acetylcholine released by the neuron is not inactivated. Table 20.2 shows the different agents and their dosing information. Not all patients will respond to ACIs, and for those who do respond, the results are modest with an improvement on the MMSE of about two points on average. The drugs are not shown to stop progression of the disease although they may delay changes in functional status. Donepezil has been on the market for the longest time period and is dosed once a day. It comes in both oral tablets and an orally disintegrating tablet, which may aid in administration. Rivastigmine comes in capsules, solution, and a transdermal patch. Dosing is twice a day except for the transdermal patch. Galantamine is available in tablets and solution and is given twice a day or for extended release tablets, once a day. A 23 mg dose of donepezil and a 13.3 mg patch of rivastigmine are also available and may be indicated for individuals who seem to have quit responding to the lower doses. However, a high dropout rate is seen with these doses due to adverse effects; so many

TABLE 20.2 Pharmacology and Dosing of Medications for Alzheimer's Disease

Generic Drug (Trade Name)	Serum Half-Life	Protein Binding	Metabolism; Renal Excretion	Initial Dose	Recommended Maintenance Dose	Renal Dosing Adjustment
Acetylcholinesterase Inhibitors						
Donepezil (Aricept)	70–80 hours	96%	CYP 2D6, 3A4; 17% excreted as unchanged drug	5 mg/day	10 mg/day	No
Galantamine (Razadyne)	5–7 hours	10%–20%	CYP 2D6, 3A4; 20%–32% excreted as unchanged drug	IR: 4 mg BID ER: 8 mg/day	24 mg/day	Yes
Rivastigmine (Exelon)	2–3 hours	40%	Hydrolysis, D-methylation, or sulfation; insignificant excretion	Oral: 1.5 mg BID Patch: 4.6 mg/day	Oral: 12 mg/day Patch: 9.5–13.3 mg/day	No
N-Methyl-D-Aspartate Receptor Antagonist						
Memantine (Namenda)	60–80 hours	45%	Glucuronidation, reduction, hydrolysis; 52%–80% excreted as unchanged drug	IR: 5 mg/day XR: 7 mg/day	IR: 20 mg/day XR: 28 mg/day	Yes
Combination Product						
Donepezil/Memantine (Namzaric)	See donepezil and memantine	See donepezil and memantine	See the donepezil and memantine	10/7* mg/day	10/28 mg/day	Yes

*Patient should be titrated on donepezil to 10 mg daily before switching to combination product.

BID, two times per day; CYP, cytochrome P450.

Source: Data from Wolters Kluwer Clinical Drug Information, Inc. (2019, October 23). Lexicomp. Retrieved from https://www.wolterskluwercdi.com/lexicomp-online/

patients are unable to utilize them (Blaszczyk & Hutchison, 2015; Hugo & Ganguli, 2014; Wolters Kluwer Clinical Drug Information, 2018).

Adverse effects of the ACIs are generally a class effect. Nausea, vomiting, diarrhea, and anorexia are seen in 5% to 20% of patients due to actions on peripheral cholinergic receptors in the gut. For this reason, doses are started at the lowest level and then increased as tolerated, usually at 2- to 4-week intervals. Insomnia is reported in 1% to 14%; so it is best to dose early in the day. Other systems with parasympathetic innervation may be affected including the bladder and the heart. Incontinence is often seen. Clinicians should avoid treating this symptom with anticholinergic drugs like oxybutynin or tolterodine since they may reduce the effectiveness of the ACIs. Bradycardia may occur with stimulation of the parasympathetic system in the heart; so the agents are listed as potentially inappropriate medications in patients with syncope on the AGS 2015 Beers Criteria (AGS, 2015a).

Memantine

Memantine is an N-methyl-D-aspartate receptor antagonist that is indicated for moderate–severe AD. It is thought to work by modulating the influx of calcium over the neuron membrane. Memantine comes in regular release tablets, solution, and extended release capsules. These are dosed twice a day for the tablets and solution, and once a day for the capsules. Improvement documented in clinical trials was only a mean of 3 points out of a 100-point scale of the Severe Impairment Battery. Because of this, many clinicians do not believe a clinically significant improvement will occur. The most recent evidence does not support adding it to an ACI, but it may be used in place of these agents if they are not tolerated. Adverse effects include dizziness, headache, constipation, and somnolence (Blaszczyk & Hutchison, 2015; Wolters Kluwer Clinical Drug Information, 2018).

While the ACIs and memantine have been studied primarily in AD, they are sometimes used in other types of dementia. Donepezil is prescribed for dementia with Lewy bodies and dementia associated with advanced Parkinson's disease although these are off-label uses. Rivastigmine is indicated for AD and dementia in advanced Parkinson's disease and used for dementia with Lewy bodies as well. Memantine is sometimes used in vascular dementia (Hugo & Ganguli, 2014).

Behavioral and Psychological Symptoms of Dementia (BPSD)

BPSD include depression, anxiety, insomnia, apathy, paranoia, wandering, delusions, hallucinations, disinhibition, and aggression. Estimates indicate that 80% to 97% of patients with dementia will have one or more BPSD symptoms (Galvin & Sadowsky, 2012; Kales, Gitlin, & Lyketsos, 2015). These symptoms, if not managed effectively, will frequently lead to nursing home placement. If a behavior is new, undiagnosed medical conditions should be explored as a contributing factor. Untreated pain, infection, or other undiagnosed problems may be underlying the patient's behavior. A change in caregiver or environmental factors has also been identified as causative (Alzheimer's Association, 2018). If a patient has an unrecognized and unmet need that cannot be communicated in typical fashion, behavioral symptoms may be the best he or she can do to communicate this need. Overstimulation can be addressed with calming music and elimination of noise and activity.

Understimulation may be addressed by regular exercise or interesting (to the patient) things to look at or talk about. Generally, an established routine is preferred and shows positive effects (Kales et al., 2015).

Nonpharmacologic Measures

Nonpharmacologic strategies are preferred for BPSD. Methods run the gamut and include reminiscence therapy, music therapy, validation therapy, aromatherapy, light therapy, and others. The choice may be directed by what is known about the patient before dementia was diagnosed (Kales et al., 2015). If insomnia or nighttime behaviors are present, implementation of good sleep hygiene, providing exercise and lights during the day, using a routine for meals and activities, and providing warm milk or decaffeinated tea at bedtime may prevent the need for pharmacologic interventions, which can sometimes be hazardous. A medication regimen review to identify agents that may cause agitation or medications that may be contributing to the problem is useful. For example, levetiracetam and memantine have agitation listed as common side effects. Administering a diuretic in the evening for a patient who is awakening at night to wander could be contributing to the behavior.

Medications

No medications are approved specifically for BPSD. If a patient is not on an ACI, it may be appropriate to try one of these agents, particularly for patients with agitation. Depression and anxiety in patients without dementia are treated with selective serotonin reuptake inhibitors or serotonin–norepinephrine reuptake inhibitors. Therefore, clinicians attempt to provide relief with these agents for patients with dementia and similar symptoms. Most commonly selected because of their safety profiles are sertraline, citalopram, escitalopram, and duloxetine. Evidence is sparse that they provide similar relief as in younger adults. Benzodiazepines and tricyclic antidepressants should be avoided as they may cause additional problems such as disinhibition, delirium, and constipation.

For insomnia, the safest sedative–hypnotic agents are melatonin and ramelteon. Trazodone, an antidepressant, has been used at low doses (doses inadequate for effect as an antidepressant) as one of its major side effects is sedation. For patients with both depression and insomnia, mirtazapine may be preferred.

Attempts to treat apathy should focus on nonpharmacological options, but investigators are evaluating methylphenidate with some results. However, many patients cannot tolerate the cardiovascular toxicity of this agent.

For most of the other symptoms, clinicians have tried different antipsychotic agents although they are not indicated and, in fact, bear a box warning that use has been shown to increase mortality in patients with dementia. Therefore, the risk and benefit must be carefully considered with the caregiver(s) in order to respect the patient's autonomy. If the behaviors create a harm to the patient and/or caregiver, such as injury from physical altercations or nursing home placement, then the benefit to the patient may make the risk acceptable. If decision to treat with an antipsychotic is made, the atypical antipsychotics are preferred and one may be selected based on its known side-effect profile. Table 20.3 provides a comparison for some agents used in treatment of BPSD. Of note, wandering is not shown to respond to any pharmacologic agent unless the patient is sedated to the point that he or she cannot get up. Providing a safe place (e.g., a courtyard or fenced area) for him or her to wander is the best remedy.

SUMMARY

Cognitive and central nervous system disorders seen in older adults tend to be progressive, chronic illnesses with unknown etiology and no preventive treatments. Some medications are available for the treatment of symptoms, which help maintain a patient's function and quality of life such as cholinesterase inhibitors for AD and levodopa/carbidopa for Parkinson's disease.

TABLE 20.3 Medications Used Off-Label in BPSD

Symptom	Medication Used After Nonpharmacological Treatment Fails	Comments
Anxiety	SSRI/SNRI Gabapentin Buspirone	Avoid benzodiazepines
Apathy	Acetylcholinesterase inhibitors	Investigational agent: methylphenidate
Depression	SSRI or mirtazapine	Tend to have lower response rate than in patients without dementia
Insomnia	Melatonin, ramelteon trazodone Gabapentin if patient has anxiety Mirtazapine if patient has depression	Avoid medications that cause insomnia, diuretics or alcohol near bedtime Avoid benzodiazepines and nonbenzodiazepine receptor agonists
Paranoia, hallucinations	Risperidone, olanzapine, quetiapine	May need informed consent for use because of box warning of increased risk of mortality in adults with dementia Avoid antipsychotics in patients with Lewy body dementia
Agitation, aggression	Risperidone, olanzapine, quetiapine	May need informed consent for use because of box warning of increased risk of mortality in adults with dementia Investigational agents: citalopram, prazosin, dextromethorphan/quinidine

BPSD, behavioral and psychological symptoms of dementia; SNRI, serotonin and norepinephrine reuptake inhibitor; SSRI, selective serotonin reuptake inhibitor.

CENTRAL NERVOUS SYSTEM DISORDERS AND COGNITION INTERPROFESSIONAL CASE STUDY

Megan Hebdon

Patient Presentation

Ms. Rice, an African American woman, presents to the clinic with her daughter to be evaluated for "my memory." She is 72 years old, and she has been in relatively good health up to this point. She notes difficulty remembering upcoming events, where she puts her keys, and most concerning, she is having more challenges paying her bills. Her daughter reports that when she does not remember something, she becomes very frustrated. That is not her baseline behavior. She has had issues in the past with word-finding or remembering people's names, but she feels like this is different. Her mother had "dementia of some sort" when she died. Her father had no memory issues when he passed away. She currently lives near her daughter. She denies feeling unsafe or being disoriented to her setting. She reports increased stress due to an upcoming event she is planning at her church.

History

Ms. Rice is single, not currently sexually active, but has had both male and female partners in the past. She has no other children, besides her daughter. She lives near her daughter and helps with her three grandchildren. She states, "they keep me busy!" She is not currently being treated for any chronic conditions. She does not like coming to the doctor and has not been seen for the past 2 years. She had a broken arm when she was 12; otherwise she had no major injuries or surgery. She "likes a drink," and drinks 1 to 2 alcoholic beverages per week. She has a history of tobacco use, but she stopped smoking when she became pregnant with her daughter 40 years ago. She denies illicit drug use. She is a retired education professor. She stays active by taking care of her grandchildren and volunteering with her church. She "could eat better."

Medications

She takes a daily multivitamin, acetaminophen 500 mg as needed for pain, diphenhydramine 50 mg as needed for allergies or sleep, and she started ginkgo biloba for her memory about 6 months ago.

Physical Exam

Vital signs are Blood pressure: 140/82 mmHg left arm; Pulse: 88 beats per minute; Respirations: 20 per minute; Oxygen saturation: 96%; Height: 68 inches; Weight: 180 pounds; Body mass index (BMI): 27.4.

Patient is cooperative and pleasant, her clothing is clean and appropriate, and her shoes are tied; patient is wearing makeup applied well. Fundoscopic exam, cranial nerves, cardiac, and pulmonary assessment are within normal limits. You administer the MMSE and the MoCA. Her scores are 22 and 23, respectively. Her Geriatric Depression Scale and Generalized Anxiety Disorder 7-item scale are both within normal limits. You screen for sleep apnea using the STOP-BANG questionnaire. She is positive for snoring, tiredness, high blood pressure, and age over 50.

Repeat blood pressure: 142/78 right arm.

Diagnostic Testing

No current labs, positive screening for hypertension, and has never been tested for HIV or hepatitis C; so you order a CBC, comprehensive metabolic panel (CMP), lipid panel, Hgb A1C, vitamin D, thyroid-stimulating hormone (TSH) and T4, B12, HIV, hepatitis C virus (HCV) antibody, urinalysis, and an EKG.

Plan of Care

On exam, Ms. Rice had a positive screening for MCI with both the MMSE and MoCA. In addition to these findings, there were other significant clinical findings including elevated blood pressure and a positive sleep apnea screen. When you evaluate her medications, diphenhydramine is a culprit for cognitive impairment. You discuss these concerns with Ms. Rice and her daughter. Together, you develop a treatment plan including home blood pressure monitoring for 1 week. If elevated blood pressure is sustained and there is evidence of either diabetes and/or kidney disease with laboratory testing, then you will start Ms. Rice on lisinopril 10 mg daily. If there is no diabetes or kidney disease, then amlodipine 5 mg daily will be initiated.

You recommend that Ms. Rice be evaluated for sleep apnea with a sleep study. You also recommend stopping Benadryl for allergy symptoms and sleep issues. You offer a prescription for Astelin nasal spray for the allergy symptoms and discuss sleep hygiene techniques, such as having a bedtime routine, avoiding naps, avoiding caffeine after 3 p.m., and using the bed only for sleep and sex. If needed, you discuss using melatonin at 1 to 2 mg for intermittent sleep issues.

Finally, you recommend dietary changes including decreased sodium, 6 to 7 fruits and vegetables per day, whole grains, lean meats, and limited added sugars or animal fats. You also discuss a walking program that is available at the church community center. Stress management is emphasized with deep breathing and mindfulness handouts.

Due to the multiple changes discussed, you and Ms. Rice establish two goals for the next 2 weeks: not watching TV in her bed and walking for 20 minutes three times per week. You plan a follow-up appointment in 2 weeks to discuss labs, reevaluate Ms. Rice's symptoms, and address established goals. You provide Ms. Rice with a discharge summary that outlines the treatment plan and identifies the two goals.

Interprofessional Collaboration

Ms. Rice will be referred for a sleep study to determine if that is a contributing factor to her elevated blood pressure and cognitive issues. There are multiple factors that could contribute to her current cognitive impairment including stress, poor sleep, poorly managed health, and possible sleep apnea. Once these issues are fully addressed, then ongoing cognitive symptoms will need to be evaluated with a neuropsychological exam. You plan to refer Ms. Rice for this with her next appointment because there is a 6-month waiting period for these evaluations. Ms. Rice has identified her daughter as her power of attorney; so you also plan to have ongoing conversations with Ms. Rice and her daughter about goals of care if her cognitive symptoms progress to dementia.

Case Study References

American Geriatric Society Beers Criteria Update Expert Panel. (2019). American Geriatrics Society 2019 updated AGS Beers Criteria for potentially inappropriate medication use in older adults. *Journal of the American Geriatrics Society, 67*(4), 674–694. doi:10.1111/jgs.15767

Centers for Disease Control & Prevention. (n.d.). *HIV testing in clinical settings*. Retrieved from https://www.cdc.gov/hiv/testing/clinical/index.html

McDade, E. M. (2019). Mild cognitive impairment: Epidemiology, pathology, and clinical assessment. In. S. T. DeKosky & J. L. Wilterdink (Eds.), *UpToDate*. Retrieved from https://www.uptodate.com/contents/mild-cognitive-impairment-epidemiology-pathology-and-clinical-assessment

National Heart, Lung, and Blood Institute. (n.d.). Calculate your body mass index. Retrieved from https://www.nhlbi.nih.gov/health/educational/lose_wt/BMI/bmicalc.htm

Popa, A. (2002). Ginkgo biloba & memory. *Pharmacotherapy Update Newsletter*, V(V). Retrieved from https://www.clevelandclinicmeded.com/medical pubs/pharmacy/sepoct02/ginkgo.htm

Sheehan, B. (2012). Assessment scales in dementia. *Therapeutic Advances in Neurological Disorders*, 5(6), 349–358. doi:10.1177/1756285612455733

Singh, J., & Mims, N. (2015). Screening tools for the obstructive sleep apnea for the cardiovascular clinician. Retrieved from https://www.acc.org/latest-in-cardiology/articles/2015/07/14/11/04/screeing-tools-for-the-obstructive-sleep-apnea-for-the-cardiovascular-clinician

Spach, D. H. (2018). Hepatitis C diagnostic testing. Retrieved from https://www.hepatitisc.uw.edu/go/screening-diagnosis/diagnostic-testing/core-concept/all

Whelton, P. K., Carey, R. M., Aronow, W. S., Casey, D. E., Collins, K. J., Himmelfarb, C. D., . . . Wright, J. T. (2017). 2017 guideline for the prevention, detection, evaluation, and management of high blood pressure in adults. *Journal of the American College of Cardiology*, 70(4), 1785–1822. doi:10.1016/j.jacc.2017.07.745

REFERENCES

Alzheimer's Association. (n.d.). Prevention. Retrieved from https://alz.org/alzheimers-dementia/research_progress/prevention

Alzheimer's Association. (2018). 2018 Alzheimer's disease facts and figures. *Alzheimer's & Dementia*, 14, 367–429. doi:10.1016/j.jalz.2018.02.001

American Geriatrics Society Expert Panel on Postoperative Delirium in Older Adults. (2015a). American Geriatrics Society 2015 updated Beers Criteria for potentially inappropriate medication use in older adults. *Journal of the American Geriatrics Society*, 63, 2227–2246. doi:10.1111/jgs.13702

American Geriatrics Society Expert Panel on Postoperative Delirium in Older Adults. (2015b). American Geriatrics Society abstracted clinical practice guideline for postoperative delirium in older persons. *Journal of the American Geriatrics Society*, 63, 142–150. doi:10.1111/jgs.13281

American Psychiatric Association. (2013). *Diagnostic and statistical manual of mental disorders* (5th ed.). Arlington, VA: American Psychiatric Publishing. doi:10.1176/appi.books.9780890425596

Blaszczyk, A. T., & Hutchison, L. C. (2015). Central nervous system disorders. In L. C. Hutchison & R. B. Sleeper (Eds.), *Fundamentals of geriatric pharmacotherapy* (2nd ed., pp. 333–375). Bethesda, MD: American Society of Health-System Pharmacists.

Borson, S., Scanlan, J. M., Chen, P., & Ganguli, M. (2003). The Mini-cog as a screen for dementia: Validation in a population-based sample. *Journal of the American Geriatrics Society*, 51, 1451–1454. doi:10.1046/j.1532-5415.2003.51465.x

Borson, S., Scanlan, J. M., Watanabe, J., Tu, S. P., & Lessiq, M. (2005) Simplifying detection of cognitive impairment comparison of the Mini-cog and Mini-Mental State Examination in a multiethnic sample. *Journal of the American Geriatrics Society, 53*, 871–874. doi:10.1111/j.1532-5415.2005.53269.x

De, J., & Wand, P. F. (2015). Delirium screening: A systematic review of delirium screening tools in hospitalized patients. *Gerontologist, 55*, 1079–1099. doi:10.1093/geront/gnv100

Ely, E. W., & Vanderbilt University. (2016). *Confusion Assessment Method for the ICU (CAM-ICU): The complete training manual.* Retrieved from https://uploadsssl.webflow.com/5b0849daec50243a0a1e5e0c/5bacedc24b30f7738581bd39_RASS.pdf

Erickson, C. A., & Barnes, C. A. (2003). The neurobiology of memory changes in normal aging. *Experimental Gerontology, 38*, 61–69. doi:10.1016/s0531-5565(02)00160-2

Galvin, J. E., & Sadowsky, C. H. (2012). Practical guidelines for the recognition and diagnosis of dementia. *Journal of the American Board of Family Medicine, 25*, 367–382. doi:10.3122/jabfm.2012.03.100181

Gaudreau, J. D., Gagnon, P., Harel, F., Tremblay, A., & Roy, M. A. (2005). Fast, systematic, and continuous delirium assessment in hospitalized patients: The nursing delirium screening scale. *Journal of Pain and Symptom Management, 29*, 368–375. doi:10.1016/j.jpainsymman.2004.07.009

Harada, C. N., Love, M. C., & Triebel, K. (2013). Normal cognitive aging. *Clinics in Geriatric Medicine, 29*, 737–752. doi:10.1016/j.cger.2013.07.002

Hugo, J., & Ganguli, M. (2014) Dementia and cognitive impairment: Epidemiology, diagnosis, and treatment. *Clinics in Geriatric Medicine, 30*, 421–442. doi:10.1016/j.cger.2014.04.001

Inouye, S. K., Robinson, T., Blaum, C., Busby-Whitehead, J., Boustani, M., Chalian, A., . . . Richter, H. (2015). Postoperative delirium in older adults: Best practice statement from the American Geriatrics Society. *Journal of the American College of Surgeons, 220*, 136–148.e1. doi:10.1016/j.jamcollsurg.2014.10.019

Inouye, S. K., van Dyck, C. H., Alessi, C. A., Balkin, S., Siegal, A. P., & Howitz, R. I. (1990). Clarifying confusion: The confusion assessment method. A new method for detection of delirium. *Annals of Internal Medicine, 113*, 941–948. doi:10.7326/0003-4819-113-12-941

Inouye, S. K., Westendorp, R. G. J., & Saczynski, J. S. (2014). Delirium in elderly people. *Lancet, 383*, 2045. doi:10.1016/S0140-6736(14)60994-6

Kales, H. C., Gitlin, L. N., & Lyketsos, C. G. (2015). Assessment and management of behavioral and psychological symptoms of dementia. *British Medical Journal, 350*, h369. doi:10.1136/bmj.h369

Marcantonio, E. R. (2017). Delirium in hospitalized older adults. *The New England Journal of Medicine, 377*(15), 1456–1466. doi:10.1056/NEJMcp1605501

McKhann, G. M., Knopman, D. S., Chertkow, H., Hyman, B. T., Jack Jr., C. R., Kawas, C. H . . . Phelps, C. H. (2011). The diagnosis of dementia due to Alzheimer's disease: Recommendations from the National Institute on Aging-Alzheimer's Association workgroups on diagnostic guidelines for Alzheimer's disease. *Alzheimers Dementia, 7*, 263–269. doi:10.1016/j.jalz.2011.03.005

Oh, E. S., Fong, T. G., Hshieh, T. T., & Inouye, S. K. (2017). Delirium in older persons: Advances in diagnosis and treatment. *Journal of the American Medical Association, 318*, 1161–1174. doi:10.1001/jama.2017.12067

Puglielli, L., & Mattson, M. P. (n.d.). Cellular and neurochemical aspects of the aging brain. In J. B. Halter, J. G. Ouslander, S. Studenski, K. P. High, S. Asthana, M. A. Supiano, & Ritchie, C. (Eds.), *Hazzard's geriatric medicine and gerontology* (7th ed.) New York, NY: McGraw-Hill. Retrieved from http://accessmedicine.mhmedical.com/content.aspx?bookid=1923&sectionid=144523231

Sclan, S. G., & Reisberg, B. (1992). Functional assessment staging (FAST) in Alzheimer's disease: Reliability, validity, and ordinality. *International Psychogeriatrics, 4*(3), 55–69. doi:10.1017/s1041610292001157

Tariq, S. H., Tumosa, N., Chibnall, J. T., Perry, M. H., & Morley, J. E. (2006). Comparison of the Saint Louis University mental status examination and the mini-mental state examination for detecting dementia and mild neurocognitive disorder: A pilot study. *The American Journal of Geriatric Psychiatry, 14*(11), 900–910. doi:10.1097/01.jgp.0000221510.33817.86

Vann Jones, S. A., & O'Brien, J. T. (2014). The prevalence and incidence of dementia with Lewy bodies: A systematic review of population and clinical studies. *Psychological Medicine, 44*(4), 673–683. doi:10.1017/S0033291713000494

Wolters Kluwer Clinical Drug Information, Inc. (2019, October 23). Lexicomp. Retrieved from https://www.wolterskluwercdi.com/lexicomp-online

21

Mental Disorders

Megan Hebdon

OBJECTIVES

1. Identify common mental health concerns in geriatric patients
2. Describe identification procedures and treatment implications for depression, anxiety, sleep disorders, and substance use disorders
3. Outline risks and benefits of psychoactive medications in older adults

INTRODUCTION

Mental health in the aging population is as much of a priority as in other age groups (World Health Organization, 2017). Approximately 20% of individuals aged 55 and older experience some mental health issue such as anxiety or mood disorders. Mental health issues are risk factors for suicide, and suicide rates are highest in older men (Centers for Disease Control and Prevention [CDC] and National Association of Chronic Disease Directors [NACDD], 2008, 2009). Mental health conditions such as depression can complicate other chronic diseases due to self-care activities such as sleep, stress management, medication adherence, diet, and physical activity that might be affected by depression (National Institute of Mental Health [NIMH], 2018). Mental health issues may be mistaken for frailty; so they should be adequately evaluated and treated (NIMH, 2018). This chapter focuses on major depressive disorder, generalized anxiety disorder (GAD), screening for substance use disorders, screening and referral for psychosis, and sleep disorders. The primary care nurse practitioner will most often be treating depression, anxiety, and sleep disorders, but must be able to identify and refer patients for substance use disorders and psychosis.

DEPRESSIVE DISORDERS

Mood disorders are prevalent in older age and include both unipolar depression and bipolar disorder (Valiengo, Stella, & Forlenza, 2016). Bipolar disorder is characterized by both episodes of depression and mania, and it may require more complex evaluation and treatment by psychiatric professionals (Valiengo et al., 2016). In primary care, older individuals may be screened, evaluated, and even treated for bipolar depression, but this is best done in consultation and collaboration with mental health professionals. Unipolar depression may often be successfully managed in outpatient primary care, but nurse practitioners should consider consultation with mental health professionals if patients are at high risk or their symptoms have been resistant to traditional treatment (Valiengo et al., 2016). For the purposes of this discussion, the diagnosis and treatment of unipolar depression, depressive disorder, or as it is generally known, "depression," are emphasized.

Background

Unipolar depression or depressive disorder is one of the most common mental health issues in aging individuals (CDC & NACDD, 2008, 2009). Depressive disorder adversely affects daily functioning, and it can have deleterious effects on chronic disease outcomes. Late-life depression can connote either onset of symptoms in later life or long-standing depression in aging adults (Espinoza & Unützer, 2017). Like so many mental health conditions, depression is often underdiagnosed and undertreated in older adults. Some may attribute depressive symptoms to normal aging due to loss, grief, and multiple life transitions, but depression is a significant health issue requiring appropriate diagnosis and treatment. It is a complex disorder with both genetic and social risk factors. Some predisposing issues to consider are as follows:

- Female sex
- Social isolation
- Being widowed, divorced, or separated
- Poverty
- Comorbid chronic disease
- Pain
- Sleep disturbances
- Functional and cognitive impairment (Espinoza & Unützer, 2017)

Of great concern when considering depression in older adults is the risk of suicide. Elderly patients attempt suicide less frequently than younger counterparts, but they have greater success with suicide attempts. Certain factors may place them at higher risk, including hopelessness, active psychosis, alcohol use, insomnia, untreated and severe pain, physical illness, terminal or worsening physical illness, social isolation, personality disorders, personal history of suicide attempts, and family history of suicide (Espinoza & Unützer, 2017).

Diagnosis

Diagnostic criteria for major depressive disorder include five or more of the following symptoms during the same 2-week period. These must represent a change from prior functioning. At least one of the symptoms must include depressed mood or anhedonia, and symptoms cannot be attributable to a medical condition.

- Depressed for most of the day every day by observation or self-report
- Diminished pleasure or interest in almost all activities
- Weight loss or weight gain
- Insomnia or hypersomnia
- Psychomotor agitation or retardation
- Fatigue or loss of energy
- Feelings of worthlessness or excessive guilt
- Diminished ability to think or concentrate
- Recurrent thoughts of death or recurrent suicidal ideation, plan, or attempt (Espinoza & Unützer, 2017)

These symptoms must cause significant distress and impair daily functioning. Symptoms cannot be attributable to a drug, medical condition, or another mental health disorder. It is important for nurse practitioners to rule out treatable medical conditions such as hypothyroidism, which may have coinciding symptoms.

Individual response to loss may include the aforementioned symptoms, and it is up to the nurse practitioner to determine whether major depression is coinciding with bereavement. The decision to treat is based on clinical judgment and shared decision-making with the patient and family members (Espinoza & Unützer, 2017). In frail older adults, the diagnosis of depression should emphasize mood change, interest change, social regression, and incapacity for at least 2 weeks. If the patient is responding to family and caregivers, continues to find humor, and enjoys social visits, then the diagnosis of depression is less likely (Espinoza & Unützer, 2017). There are many instruments available for depression screening, but these should always be followed by a clinical interview to determine whether criteria have been met and if treatment is needed.

- Two-question screener: During the past month, have you been bothered by feeling down, depressed, or hopeless; have you been bothered by little interest or pleasure in doing things?
- Geriatric Depression Scale: This addresses life satisfaction, boredom, helplessness, desire to stay at home, and worthlessness. Two out of five responses suggest a diagnosis of depression.
- *Patient Health Questionnaire-9* (PHQ-9): This covers all *Diagnostic and Statistical Manual of Mental Disorders* (5th ed.; *DSM-5*; American Psychiatric Association, 2013) criteria and can be used to establish a diagnosis of depression. It is also useful for the assessment of treatment response. The *Patient Health Questionnaire-2* (PHQ-2) version is also effective at identifying individuals with depressive symptoms.
- Cornell Scale for Depression in Dementia: This incorporates observer- and informant-based information for patients who have cognitive impairment.
- The Center for Epidemiologic Studies Depression Scale: This is commonly used in primary care and community settings (Blackburn, Wilkins-Ho, & Wiese, 2017; Espinoza & Unützer, 2017).

Treatment

The first-line treatment for depression includes psychotherapy and/or pharmacotherapy (Blackburn et al., 2017). Researchers have noted particular patient benefit with programs that offer medication and psychotherapy alone or in combination with community outreach by a care manager (Espinoza & Ulützer, 2017). Psychotherapy may involve a range of individual or family engagements adopted in the community or with home-based programs and may be cognitive behavioral, interpersonal, problem-solving, psychodynamic, or life review (Blackburn et al., 2017; Espinoza & Unützer, 2017). All have demonstrated benefit in aging patients. Lifestyle changes such as sleep, exercise, nutrition, and stress management can also contribute to improved mood (Espinoza & Unützer, 2017).

When addressing pharmacologic therapy in older adults, nurse practitioners should keep a few key considerations in mind. First, it may take 8 to 12 weeks for patients to fully respond to antidepressant therapy. Second, side-effect profiles of tricyclic antidepressants (TCAs) and some selective serotonin reuptake inhibitor (SSRI) and serotonin and norepinephrine reuptake inhibitor (SNRI) medications may limit patient treatment. Third, monotherapy is preferred to reduce side effects and drug interactions (Espinoza & Unützer, 2017). Starting low and going slow is important when initiating antidepressant therapy. Initial dosing for older adults should be half of the starting dose that would be used in younger counterparts to minimize side effects and promote adherence (Blackburn et al., 2017; Espinoza & Unützer, 2017). The same therapeutic dosage range should be targeted to ensure adequate treatment.

Short-term follow-up should occur by phone or office visit to address depressive symptoms, suicidal ideation, medication side effects, and other ongoing concerns. The duration of therapy should be based on patient response and goals of care, but 6 to 12 months for the first depressive episode promotes remission. The following agents may be used:

- SSRIs: first-line treatment
  - Escitalopram starting at 5 mg, generally well tolerated, good initial choice in older adults
  - Citalopram starting at 10 mg, also well tolerated, but risk of QT prolongation
  - Sertraline starting at 10 mg, more frequent gastrointestinal (GI) symptoms
  - Fluoxetine starting at 5 to 10 mg, activating for low-energy patients, but has significant drug interactions
  - Paroxetine starting at 10 mg, weakly anticholinergic, useful for patients with insomnia
  - Fluvoxamine starting at 25 mg in the evening, significant drug interactions and discontinuation symptoms
- SNRIs: first-line therapy
  - Venlafaxine extended release starting at 37.5 mg once daily, may cause dose-dependent increase in pulse and blood pressure, prominent GI side effects, activating for low-energy patients and useful for comorbid pain
  - Desvenlafaxine starting at 50 mg in the morning, may cause dose-dependent increase in pulse and blood pressure, prominent GI side effects, activating for low-energy patients and useful for comorbid pain
  - Duloxetine starting at 10 to 20 mg daily, significant drug interactions, useful for comorbid pain
- Atypical antidepressants: second-line treatment
  - Mirtazapine starting at 7.5 mg every evening, long half-life and risk of accumulation in renal and hepatic disorders, weight gain, risk of agranulocytosis, appetite stimulant, and helpful in patients with insomnia
  - Bupropion starting at 75 mg in the morning, avoid in patients with seizure disorders, may increase diastolic blood pressure and worsen insomnia, low risk of cognitive issues
  - Trazodone starting at 12.5 to 25 mg 30 to 60 minutes before bedtime, orthostatic hypotension, nausea, daytime sedation, risk of hyponatremia and cognitive impairment, may be useful for patients with insomnia
- TCAs: second-line treatment, higher risk in older patients due to anticholinergic effects
- Atypical antipsychotics: aripiprazole starting at 2 mg per day as adjunctive therapy may be useful in treatment-resistant depression although the risks of weight gain and parkinsonism inherent to this drug class may limit its use (Blackburn et al., 2017; Espinoza & Unützer, 2017)

Neurostimulation through electroconvulsive therapy, transcranial magnetic stimulation, deep brain stimulation, and vagus nerve stimulation may be considered if patients fail to respond to psychotherapy or pharmacotherapy for depressive symptoms. Electroconvulsive therapy is well studied and should be considered in patients with life-threatening depression that significantly impairs daily functioning. Patients at this point should have been referred to psychiatry for evaluation or collaboration with psychiatry should occur to proceed down this treatment path. The other modalities have less current evidence to support their use (Espinoza & Unützer, 2017).

Depression is a significant health concern for elderly patients, and nurse practitioners can partner with patients to determine an optimal treatment plan with medications and/or psychotherapy, lifestyle changes, and other modalities as needed.

ANXIETY DISORDERS

GAD is common in ambulatory care, and it is the most common anxiety disorder in the elderly population (Baldwin, 2018). The rates of GAD are higher in women than in men (Baldwin, 2018). Other anxiety disorders include:

- Panic disorder: sudden periods of intense fear with abrupt onset. Often triggered by objects or situations. Symptoms include heart palpitations, sweating, trembling, shortness of breath, sense of impending doom, and feeling out of control. Individuals may avoid certain situations to prevent an attack (NIMH, 2018).
- Phobia-related disorder: an intense fear or aversion to objects or situations. The feared object or situation may be reasonable, but the fear is disproportionate to the danger caused by them. Individuals may have excessive worry about encountering the feared object or situation, will actively avoid encounters, experience immediate and intense anxiety if encounters occur, and endure unavoidable objects or situations with high anxiety levels (NIMH, 2018).

Background

The identification and treatment of GAD are emphasized here. GAD is often comorbid with depressive disorders, substance use disorders, posttraumatic stress disorder, and obsessive-compulsive disorder. GAD is a multifactorial disorder with genetic patterns, neuropsychological features, and developmental risk factors (Baldwin, 2018). Clinical manifestations of GAD include the following:

- Excessive or persistent worry
- Hyperarousal
- Autonomic hyperactivity
- Muscle tension, neck pain, and headaches
- Poor sleep
- Fatigue
- High levels of worry over small matters (Baldwin, 2018; NIMH, 2018)

Nurse practitioners may be treating elderly patients with existing GAD or late-onset GAD. Risk factors to consider include the following:

- Female sex
- Low socioeconomic status
- Recent adverse life experiences
- Chronic illness
- Other mental disorders
- Parental loss
- Low emotional support in childhood
- Family history of mental health (Baldwin, 2018; Mental Health America, n.d.)

GAD may result in greater physical health risks including cardiovascular disease and mortality. Individuals suffering from GAD may have functional impairment, and this should be a point of consideration if an elderly patient is showing physical or functional decline (Baldwin, 2018).

Diagnosis

When working up a patient for GAD, validated scales such as the Generalized Anxiety Disorder 7-item (GAD-7), the Hospital Anxiety and Depression Scale (HADS), and the Penn State Worry Questionnaire can be used as part of the history and physical exam. Family history, social history, medical history, and substance abuse history may reveal predisposing factors. Additionally, physical causes of anxiety symptoms should be evaluated such as weight loss, late-onset anxiety, or cognitive impairment. Tests to evaluate anemia, electrolyte imbalances, thyroid disease, drug use, or cardiovascular disease should be considered. These may include a complete blood count (CBC), comprehensive metabolic panel (CMP), thyroid-stimulating hormone (TSH), urinalysis (UA), and EKG (Baldwin, 2018).

Diagnosis is made based on alignment of symptoms with *DSM-5* diagnostic criteria and ruling out physical causes of symptoms (American Psychiatric Association, 2013). The *DSM-5* criteria include:

- A. Excessive anxiety or worry is present most days of the week for at least 6 months.
- B. Individual has trouble not worrying.
- C. Anxiety and worry coincide with three or more of the following symptoms:
  - Restlessness
  - Fatiguing easily
  - Difficulty concentrating
  - Irritability
  - Muscle tension
  - Sleep disturbances
- D. Anxiety and worry cause distress for the individual and result in significant functional impairment.
- E. Anxiety and worry are not due to a medical diagnosis or prescribed or unprescribed substance.
- F. Anxiety and worry are not better explained by another mental health diagnosis. (Baldwin, 2018)

Additional questions to consider when diagnosing an elderly patient include:

- How do you feel during stressful times?
- How well do you control your worries? (Baldwin, 2018)

Treatment

Treatment of anxiety disorders is most successful with the combination of behavioral and pharmacologic therapies. Cognitive behavioral therapy has been shown to be an effective treatment approach alone or in combination with medication. Response to this therapy may be complicated by co-occurring cognitive issues or GAD symptoms so severe that patients cannot engage in therapy. In those cases, initial treatment with medication may be optimal (Craske & Bystritsky, 2019).

Table 21.1 has an overview of medications used to treat GAD. SSRIs and SNRIs are first-line therapy for GAD. Buspirone and pregabalin may be used adjunctively or as

TABLE 21.1 Pharmacologic Treatment for Generalized Anxiety Disorder

Medication	Starting Dose/ Dosage Range	Side Effects	Special Considerations	Other
Citalopram	10 mg 10–40 mg	Nausea, diarrhea, insomnia, somnolence, hyponatremia, and sexual function impairment	QT prolongation, CYP3A4, 2C19 metabolism	SSRI first-line
Escitalopram	5–10 mg 10–20 mg	Nausea, diarrhea, insomnia, somnolence, hyponatremia, and sexual function impairment	CYP3A4, 2C19 metabolism	
Sertraline	25–50 mg 50–200 mg	Nausea, diarrhea, insomnia, somnolence, hyponatremia, and sexual function impairment	Inhibits CYP2B6, 2C19, 2D6 Higher risk of insomnia, agitation, and GI complaints	
Paroxetine	10–20 mg 20–50 mg	Nausea, diarrhea, insomnia, somnolence, hyponatremia, and sexual function impairment	CYP2D6 metabolism, inhibits CYP2D6 and 2C19, weakly anticholinergic, sedating, withdrawal symptoms if not tapered	
Fluoxetine	10–20 mg 20–60 mg	Nausea, diarrhea, insomnia, somnolence, hyponatremia, and sexual function impairment	CYP2D6 and 2C9 metabolism, inhibits CYP2D6 and 2C19, long half-life, no withdrawal symptoms, risk of insomnia/agitation	
Fluvoxamine	50 mg 100–300 mg	Nausea, diarrhea, insomnia, somnolence, hyponatremia, and sexual function impairment	CYP1A2 and 2D6 metabolism, inhibits CYP1A2 and 2C19, significant drug interactions and withdrawal symptoms if not tapered	

(continued)

TABLE 21.1 Pharmacologic Treatment for Generalized Anxiety Disorder (continued)

Medication	Starting Dose/ Dosage Range	Side Effects	Special Considerations	Other
Duloxetine	30 mg 60–120 mg	Nausea, diarrhea, insomnia, somnolence, hyponatremia, and sexual function impairment	CYP1A2 and 2D6 metabolism, inhibits CYP2D6, higher risk of insomnia/ agitation, useful for comorbid pain, withdrawal if not tapered	SNRI first-line
Venlafaxine extended release	75 mg 75–225 mg	Nausea, diarrhea, insomnia, somnolence, hyponatremia, and sexual function impairment	CYP2D6 and CYP3A4 metabolism, risk of insomnia, agitation, increased blood pressure and heart rate with higher doses, useful for comorbid pain, withdrawal symptoms without tapering	
Buspirone	10 mg divided 10–60 mg divided	Dizziness, drowsiness, nausea, headache, fatigue, insomnia, dry mouth, diarrhea	CYP3A4 metabolism, slow onset and modest efficacy, ineffective for comorbid depression	Nonbenzodiazepine anxiolytic
Pregabalin	50 mg divided 50–300 mg divided	Sedation, dizziness, dry mouth, edema and weight gain, abnormal thinking, constipation, tolerance, dependence and withdrawal	Dependent on renal function for metabolism, schedule V controlled substance in the United States, useful for comorbid pain	GABA analog calcium channel modulator anticonvulsant
Mirtazapine	15 mg 15–60 mg	Sedation and increased appetite (may be good for weight loss and sleep disturbances)	CYP1A2, 2D6, and 3A4 metabolism	Atypical antidepressant

Hydroxyzine	50 mg at bedtime 25–50 mg 3–4 times daily as needed	Sedating, anticholinergic side effects with higher doses	Anticholinergic effects may limit safety in elderly patients, augmentation for co-occurring sleep issues	Antihistamine
Quetiapine	25–50 mg 50–300 mg	Sedation, EPS, weight gain, metabolic side effects, rare TD	CYP3A4 metabolism, EPS and sedating effects may limit use in older adults	Second-generation antipsychotic

EPS, extrapyramidal symptoms; GABA, gamma-aminobutyric acid; GI, gastrointestinal; SNRI, serotonin and norepinephrine reuptake inhibitor; SSRI, selective serotonin reuptake inhibitor.

Source: Data from Craske, M., & Bystritsky, A. (2019). Approach to treating generalized anxiety disorder in adults. In M. B. Stein & R. Hermann (Eds.), *UpToDate*. Retrieved from http://www.epocrates.ccm/mobile; Epocrates. (2019a). Buspirone. Epocrates Essentials [Mobile application software]. Retrieved from http://www.epocrates.com/mobile; Epocrates. (2019b). Pregabalin. Epocrates Essentials [Mobile application software]. Retrieved from http://www.epocrates.com/mobile)

monotherapy if there is partial response to SSRIs or SNRIs. Other medications such as mirtazapine, benzodiazepines, and hydroxyzine may be considered. Benzodiazepines and hydroxyzine should be prescribed with caution in older adults due to sedating and dependence effects and anticholinergic effects, respectively (Craske & Bystritsky, 2019).

Patients with GAD may also respond well to alternative approaches such as mindfulness, yoga, deep breathing techniques, and acupuncture. Understanding patient and family preferences and expectations of care will guide the nurse practitioner in these decisions.

SUBSTANCE USE DISORDERS

Older adults are just as vulnerable to substance use disorders as other age groups although there may be aging and chronic disease–related issues that increase risk such as mental health disorders, loneliness, pain, and poor sleep (Kuerbis, Sacco, Blazer, & Moore, 2014). Alcohol is the most commonly used substance in older adults, and illicit substance use is more common in older adults in the United States than in other countries. Opioid and other prescription drug use disorders are relatively common as well (Kuerbis et al., 2014). With the changes in regulations and availability for cannabis and cannabis-related products throughout the United States, increased uptake has occurred (Lloyd & Striley, 2018). Risk factors for substance use include male gender for alcohol, female gender for prescription drugs, race (Caucasian), pain, physical disability, transitions, poor health status and chronic illness, polypharmacy, psychiatric illness, history of alcohol issues, affluence, grief, unexpected retirement, and social isolation (Kuerbis et al., 2014). Nurse practitioners should be aware of these risk factors as well as signs of substance use disorders such as poor hygiene, change in cognition, nutritional issues, idiopathic seizures, dizziness or falls, mood swings, and running out of medication or borrowing medication (Kuerbis et al., 2014).

Older adults can be screened for substance use issues using multiple screening tools: CAGE-AID, the Michigan Alcohol Screening Test-Geriatric version (MAST-G), the Alcohol Use Disorders Identification Test (AUDIT), the Alcohol, Smoking, and Substance Involvement Screening Test (ASSIST), and the Comorbidity-Alcohol Risk Evaluation Tool (CARET); see Kuerbis et al. (2014). In addition, the Screening, Brief Intervention, and Referral to Treatment (SBIRT) approach provides a simple way to incorporate substance use screening and referrals into routine practice (Substance Abuse and Mental Health Services Administration-Health Resources and Services Administration Center for Integrated Health Solutions, n.d.). Prompt referrals for further evaluation at inpatient or outpatient treatment programs should be made once a substance use disorder is identified. A warm hand-off generally results in reassurance for the patient and greater continuity of care.

PSYCHOSIS IN OLDER ADULTS

New-onset hallucinations and delusions in elderly patients can be distressing for patients, challenging for family caregivers, and difficult for providers to assess. Nurse practitioners should keep in mind that new-onset psychosis in late life is most often related to dementia, stroke, or other neurologic diseases, rather than schizophrenia (American Geriatrics Society [AGS], 2011). New-onset schizophrenia and bipolar disorder are uncommon in older adults although a missed diagnosis may be a possibility. In the presence of new-onset psychosis, a delirium assessment should always be conducted to identify a modifiable root cause (AGS, 2011).

Risk factors for developing psychosis in older adults include bed rest, cognitive impairment, female gender, sensory disorders, and social isolation. Physical health factors such as thyroid disease, glucose or electrolyte imbalances, sleep deprivation, or B12 deficiency should be ruled out through history, physical exam, and diagnostic testing (AGS, 2011). In mood disorders, psychotic symptoms are generally congruent with the patient's mood such as delusions of death in depression or grandiose delusions in mania. Late-onset schizophrenia is characterized by paranoid delusions and hallucinations framed in complaints. Delirium, cognitive disorders, mood disorders, and physical health issues must be ruled out before schizophrenia should be considered. However, nurse practitioners should keep in mind that suicidal thoughts and behavior are more common in older adults with schizophrenia (AGS, 2011).

If patient safety is a concern, antipsychotics may be initiated. During the workup, referrals to neurology and psychiatry can be made (AGS, 2011). Antipsychotics should be used judiciously in older adults because any use corresponds to increased mortality risk. First choice medications due to lower risk of adverse events include aripiprazole, olanzapine, quetiapine, and risperidone (AGS, 2011; Hauk, 2018). Lower doses should be initiated, and dose titrations should occur judiciously with awareness of drug-induced parkinsonism, akathisia, hypotension, sedation, tardive dyskinesias, weight gain, and QT prolongation (AGS, 2011).

SLEEP DISORDERS

Sleep disorders are a major issue in older adults with over 50% of elderly individuals experiencing insomnia (Xiong, 2019). Sleep issues are more common in women, and often go under- or unrecognized in older adults (Xiong, 2019). Changes in sleep patterns may be attributable to normal aging, with older adults needing 7 to 8 hours of sleep, but disease processes should be evaluated and treated (Albert et al., 2017; Xiong, 2019). Older individuals tend to spend more time in bed without attempting to sleep or being unable to sleep at night (Xiong, 2019). Additionally, older individuals experience more periods of arousal during sleep, possibly related to nocturia, pain, restless legs, or difficulty breathing (Xiong, 2019). Sleep disorders decreases quality of life and increases mortality risk (Xiong, 2019).

Background

Normal sleep occurs in different stages that cycle throughout the night starting with four stages of non-rapid eye movement (non-REM) followed by REM sleep (American Sleep Association, n.d.; Xiong, 2019). Stages 3 and 4 of non-REM sleep are considered deep sleep or slow wave sleep, where delta waves are prominent on EEG. Individuals spend less time in slow wave sleep as they age and more time in stage 2 (ASA, 2019). REM sleep or stage 5 of the sleep cycle has brain activity that resembles wake time although the body is atonic. Each step of the sleep cycle is essential for restoration of the brain and body; so deprivation in any of these stages may result in adverse health effects (ASA, 2019).

Common Sleep Disorders in Older Adults

Sleep Apnea

Sleep apnea is characterized by periods of apnea during sleep. This can be central, obstructive, or of mixed origin. Individuals may wake up gasping, thrash during sleep, or snore. Sleep apnea may result in daytime sleepiness, hypertension, cardiac arrhythmias, cor pulmonale, or abrupt death (Xiong, 2019). Risk factors for sleep apnea include older age, obesity, structural deformities that may cause airway obstruction, alcohol or substance use, and neurological disorders (ASA, 2019). This can be screened for using tools such as the Epworth Sleepiness Scale (Singh & Mims, 2015). Diagnosis occurs following a physical exam to identify structural issues and with a sleep study—either a traditional polysomnography or home sleep study (ASA, 2019). A primary approach to treatment is lifestyle change through diet and physical activity, followed by continuous positive airway pressure (CPAP) as first-line treatment. Additionally, bilevel positive airway pressure (BiPAP), dental appliances, surgery, or neurostimulation may be used (ASA, 2019). Pharmacologic measures are rarely used for sleep apnea.

Periodic Limb Movements in Sleep (PLMS)

PLMS is characterized by repetitive leg jerks that may cause patient arousal during sleep. It may cause no disturbance to patients, but it can coincide with restless legs syndrome (RLS), which can cause the urge to move legs or cramping, shooting pains in the legs (Comella, 2014; National Sleep Foundation, n.d.). Walking or moving legs may periodically improve symptoms (Comella, 2014). The risk for PLMS increases with age, and both PLMS and RLS are associated with poor sleep outcomes (Comella, 2014; Xiong, 2019). RLS may be associated with iron-deficiency anemia; so patients should be screened for this prior to other interventions, and other causes of symptoms should be ruled out (Comella, 2014). Diagnosis of either disorder generally occurs through a careful health history and physical exam. PLMS may not require any treatment if patients are not symptomatic although if it coincides with RLS, pharmacologic therapy along with nonpharmacologic options should be considered. Nonpharmacologic options may include focused leg exercises, yoga, acupuncture, leg compressions, and cognitive behavioral therapy (Comella, 2014). Two medication options that can be considered for elderly patients are ropinirole and pramipexole although providers should be aware of the risk of falls related to possible hypotension and fatigue (Comella, 2014). Augmentation of symptoms should also be considered with these medications.

Insomnia Related to Cognitive or Psychiatric Illnesses

Sleep impairment may be associated with dementia, depression, anxiety, bipolar disorders, and schizophrenia. It is important for providers to identify and treat cognitive and psychiatric disorders because these may result in improved sleep patterns for elderly patients (Xiong, 2019). Additionally, sleep hygiene (which is discussed in the following) should be emphasized.

Other Causes of Impaired Sleep

Medications

Certain medications can affect sleep and wake cycles including sedating antidepressants and neuroleptics and sedative–hypnotics (Xiong, 2019). Nurse practitioners should note the presence of these medications, the pattern and reasons for use, and work with patients and families to determine long-term need and behavioral or pharmacologic alternatives.

Substance Use

The use of caffeine, alcohol, nicotine, and controlled substances may affect sleep–wake cycles and sleep quality in older adults. Caffeine intake with diet or medications may have a more pronounced effect on wakefulness in elderly patients due to liver clearance. Nicotine also has a stimulating effect that increases wakefulness. Alcohol use may initially cause sleepiness, but patients may have more nighttime wakening once the alcohol has metabolized. Other substances may induce more daytime sleepiness affecting sleep quality at night or increase wakefulness at night, depending on their mechanisms of action. Individuals should be screened for patterns of substance use and be counseled or referred depending on the type of substance and patterns of use.

Chronic Pain

Chronic pain related to arthritis or cancer may escalate with movement at night, increase wakefulness, and reduce overall sleep quality (Xiong, 2019). A behavioral and pharmacologic plan for pain should account for pain symptoms at night.

Chronic Disease

Multiple chronic diseases can affect sleep quality due to difficulty breathing at night with heart failure or chronic obstructive pulmonary disease (COPD), nocturia and urinary frequency due to lower urinary tract symptoms (LUTS) or Parkinson's disease, and discomfort due to reflux, constipation, or pruritic skin disorders (Xiong, 2019). Providers should account for the effect of these conditions on sleep and develop a treatment plan that includes sleep hygiene measures, deprescribing or prescribing pharmacologic support, and acknowledgment of patient distress with these conditions and sleep.

Sleep Hygiene

Education can be provided to patients regarding expected age-related changes with sleep and sleep hygiene practices that can improve sleep quality. Sleep hygiene should always be the first-line treatment, once serious medical conditions have been excluded.

Sleep hygiene practices include the following:

- Maintain a regular nighttime sleep schedule and have a standard bedtime routine.
- Reduce or eliminate naps during the day.
- Exercise daily, but not right before bedtime.
- Use the bed only for the two Ss (sleep and sex).
- Avoid screens or reading in bed.
- Avoid heavy foods before bedtime.
- Limit or eliminate alcohol, caffeine, and nicotine before sleep.
- Ensure an environment that is optimal for sleep (temperature, quiet, and darkness).
- Get adequate daytime exposure to bright light.
- Avoid worry right before bed and if sleep does not come within 30 minutes, perform a soothing activity.
- Use mindfulness, progressive relaxation, deep breathing, or other meditative practices to promote sleep. (Xiong, 2019)

Sometimes patients require other measures such as cognitive behavioral therapy, acupuncture, and yoga to help with sleep. Nurse practitioners should offer the full range of treatment options to patients to support positive sleep practices and improve sleep quality.

Pharmacologic Therapies

The use of pharmacologic therapies to treat insomnia can be difficult because options such as first-generation antihistamines, some TCAs, benzodiazepines, and z-drugs place older adults at greater risk for adverse health outcomes (Matheson & Hainer, 2017). In older adults, first-line therapy includes controlled-release melatonin and doxepin. Rozerem is a melatonin agonist that is mildly effective, but it has a good safety profile. Controlled-release melatonin is lower in cost and may produce the same benefits (Matheson & Hainer, 2017). Doses of 0.1 to 5 mg may be used, but the adage of starting low and going slow should always be used in elderly patients. Providers must keep in mind that melatonin is not regulated by the Food and Drug Administration (FDA); so purity and consistency may be a concern in over-the-counter products (Matheson & Hainer, 2017). Doxepin at low doses (3 mg) may be used in older adults, but nurse practitioners should remember the class-related side effects with TCAs in older adults (Matheson & Hainer, 2017).

SUMMARY

Mental health disorders, substance use, psychotic symptoms, and sleep are significant issues in the aging population. Identification may be difficult due to comorbid conditions, and treatment options may be affected by age-related metabolic changes and co-occurring health disorders. Approaching these issues with respect and a holistic treatment approach will help patients, families, and providers navigate these challenging health concerns.

MENTAL HEALTH INTERPROFESSIONAL CASE STUDY
Jerusalem Walker

Patient Presentation

Arlene is a 72-year-old female patient who is new to your primary care practice. She is accompanied to the clinic by her daughter, after her last provider retired. She is being seen for multiple chronic diseases. Review of systems is positive for fatigue/low energy, insomnia (early morning awakening), unintentional weight loss of 6 pounds over the past 2 months, and balance problems leading to two falls in the past 5 weeks. She has also not been driving much since she had a "fender bender" 3 weeks ago. She has some concerns about her memory though she is independent with activities of daily living (ADLs)/instrumental activities of daily living (IADLs). Review of systems is negative for headache/tinnitus, blurred vision/vision change, chest pain/palpitations, shortness of breath, diarrhea/constipation, urinary incontinence, and numbness/tingling in extremities. The patient states, "I just don't feel right. I just can't put my finger on it."

History

Arlene has a past medical history of hypertension, hypercholesterolemia, gastroesophageal reflux disease (GERD), hypothyroidism, vitamin B12 deficiency, osteopenia, and insomnia. Two years ago, she lost her husband of 48 years. She is a breast cancer survivor, and underwent lumpectomy followed by chemotherapy 8 years ago. In addition, she had a cholecystectomy 15 years ago and a tonsillectomy as a child. She has a pension as a retired schoolteacher as well as Social Security benefits and describes her finances as adequate. She does not drink alcohol and has never smoked. She used to volunteer at the local elementary school as a reading tutor, but she stopped when her husband fell ill. The patient describes mostly sedentary activities. Her daughter and her family live 20 minutes away and visit about once a month.

Medications

She is allergic to sulfa drugs and penicillin (PCN). Her current medications include: lisinopril 10 mg once daily, propranolol 40 mg twice daily, atorvastatin 20 mg daily at bedtime, levothyroxine 50 mcg daily, ranitidine 75 mg twice daily as needed, vitamin B12 injection monthly, calcium/vitamin D supplement, and diazepam 5 mg every night at bedtime.

Physical Exam and Mental State Exam

PHQ-9 triggered on intake yields a score of 10 (moderate depression). Vitals for today's visit: Blood pressure: 102/65 mmHg; Heart rate: 64 beats per minute; Respirations: 16 breaths per minute; temperature: 98 degrees F; body mass index (BMI): 20.9; Oxygen saturation: 96%. Patient denies pain. Montreal Cognitive Assessment (MoCA) score today is 27/30 (negative for mild cognitive impairment).

Physical exam is unremarkable, including focused neuro exam for evaluation of falls. Mental state exam is as follows:

Appearance: alert, neatly dressed, well-groomed, thin female, appears stated age

Speech: clear, fluent

Behavior: cooperative, conversant

Orientation: to person, place, time, and situation

Mood: depressed

Affect: briefly tearful during interview

Thought process: logical, clear

Thought content: no thoughts of harm to self/others; no paranoia, delusions, or hallucinations

Memory: intact (see MoCA score)

Judgment: good

Insight: good

Diagnostic Testing

Recent labs available: CMP, CBC, TSH, and vitamin D, B12 are unremarkable. Urine dipstick done today is negative, with normal specific gravity. You decide to do a point of care A1c, which is 5.5.

Plan of Care

You determine that this patient should be followed closely over the next several months to monitor medications and response to therapy. Medication review shows a number of contributing factors for the recent falls and depressive symptoms (and possibly the car accident). First, the patient's hypertension is overcorrected. Since beta-blockers can contribute to feelings of fatigue, depression, and precipitate falls, you discuss tapering the propranolol 40 mg to 1 tablet daily for 1 week, then once every other day for 1 week to avoid rebound hypertension, and then discontinuing. The patient is encouraged to monitor her blood pressures at home and report to the clinic regarding trends of high or low blood pressures. You also discuss that diazepam can contribute to falls and depressed mood. With the patient, you identify sleep hygiene measures such as a bedtime routine, avoiding screens in bed, and limiting naps during the day as well as a meditation app to help her with sleep. In addition, you discuss the benefits of switching to a shorter-acting benzodiazepine, such as lorazepam, and plan to taper her over the next 3 months. For depressive symptoms, you offer psychotherapy and information about a support group, but the patient declines. However, she is open to receiving physical therapy for an evaluation for the falls and to initiate an exercise program for her mood and sleep. She is also willing to be referred for occupational therapy for an evaluation of driving, following medication adjustments. You identify social isolation as contributing to her depressive symptoms and work with the patient to identify social activities. These include volunteering at the school again and possibly taking a pottery class with a couple of her friends who have also lost spouses as ways to socialize and "get outside herself."

The patient is amenable to a trial of mirtazapine 15 mg to address the mood symptoms, sleep difficulties, and appetite problems. You recommend a follow-up in 1 month for medication review, or sooner as needed.

Interprofessional Collaboration

A team-based approach would be most helpful for Arlene, as it is for many community-dwelling elders with chronic health conditions complicated by mood disorders. While Arlene is not amenable to psychotherapy, physical therapy consultation may be helpful to establish an exercise regimen that may enhance her mood and alleviate the sleep disturbances, in addition to reducing the risks associated with low bone density. Because the patient has identified multiple plans for health behavior changes, it will be important to support her through this process. In addition, having someone she can "check in" with may be a motivating factor. You discuss a social work consult to help the patient stay on track with her plans to improve her health. The patient agrees, and you provide a "warm hand-off" to a licensed clinical social worker integrated within your clinic.

A consult with a registered dietitian is also indicated for the patient's unintentional weight loss and osteopenia. While the mirtazapine should stimulate her appetite, the patient may need higher calorie finger foods and a meal plan to help her regain the weight she has lost.

Because the patient's medication regimen and sleep disturbance may have contributed to the auto accident, timing the occupational therapy consult for her driving evaluation is important. If the evaluation is within normal limits, it may help the patient gain lost confidence in her driving abilities. If not, this patient will likely need social work support to identify resources for transportation so that she can maintain her level of independence.

Because of the risks associated with mental health problems in older adults, it is important that Arlene understands and agrees to communicate with her healthcare team if any changes are noted, including adverse effects of medications, worsening of mood, or thoughts of harm to self or others. As always, if a patient experiences worsening of mood, an urgent consultation with a psychiatric mental health professional is warranted. Arlene verbalizes understanding of the plan of care and agrees to contact the clinic with any changes.

Case Study References

Blackburn, P., Wilkins-Ho, M., & Wiese, B. S. (2017). Depression in older adults: Diagnosis and management. *British Columbia Medical Journal*, 59(3), 171–177. Retrieved from https://www.bcmj.org/articles/depression-older-adults-diagnosis-and-management

Coventry, P., Lovell, K., Dickens, C., Bower, P., Chew-Graham, C., McElvenny, D., . . . Gask, L. (2015). Integrated primary care for patients with mental and physical multimorbidity: Cluster randomised controlled trial of collaborative care for patients with depression comorbid with diabetes or cardiovascular disease. *British Medical Journal*, 350, h638. doi:10.1136/bmj.h638

Flett, J. A., Hayne, H., Riordan, B. C., Thompson, L. M., & Conner, T. S. (2018). Mobile mindfulness meditation: A randomised controlled trial of the effect of two popular apps on mental health. *Mindfulness, 10,* 1–14. doi:10.1007/s12671-018-1050-9

Hashimoto, T., Shiina, A., Hasegawa, T., Kimura, H., Oda, Y., Niitsu, T., . . . Iyo, M. (2016). Effect of mirtazapine versus selective serotonin reuptake inhibitors on benzodiazepine use in patients with major depressive disorder: A pragmatic, multicenter, open-label, randomized, active-controlled, 24-week trial. *Annals of General Psychiatry, 15*(1), 27. doi:10.1186/s12991-016-0115-1

Hikichi, H., Kondo, N., Kondo, K., Aida, J., Takeda, T., & Kawachi, I. (2015). Effect of a community intervention programme promoting social interactions on functional disability prevention for older adults: Propensity score matching and instrumental variable analyses, JAGES Taketoyo study. *Journal of Epidemiology and Community Health, 69*(9), 905–910. doi:10.1136/jech-2014-205345

Leonard, S. D., & Karlamangla, A. (2015). Dose-dependent sedating and stimulating effects of mirtazapine. *Proceedings of UCLA Healthcare, 19,* 1–2. Retrieved from https://proceedings.med.ucla.edu/wp-content/uploads/2016/11/Dose-Dependent-Sedating-and-Stimulating-Effects-of-Mirtazapine.pdf

Levitt, A., & O'Neil, J. (2018). Older adults with unintended weight loss: The role of appetite stimulants. *Home Healthcare Now, 36*(5), 312–318. doi:10.1097/NHH.0000000000000692

Softic, A., Beganlic, A., Pranjic, N., & Sulejmanovic, S. (2013). The influence of the use of benzodiazepines in the frequency falls in the elderly. *Medical Archives, 67*(4), 256–259. doi:10.5455/medarh.2013.67.256-259

Tannenbaum, C. (2015). Inappropriate benzodiazepine use in elderly patients and its reduction. *Journal of Psychiatry & Neuroscience, 40*(3), E27–E28. doi:10.1503/jpn.140355

Wedgeworth, M., LaRocca, M. A., Chaplin, W. F., & Scogin, F. (2017). The role of interpersonal sensitivity, social support, and quality of life in rural older adults. *Geriatric Nursing, 38*(1), 22–26. doi:10.1016/j.gerinurse.2016.07.001

REFERENCES

American Geriatrics Society. (2011). *A guide to the management of psychotic disorders and neuropsychiatric symptoms of dementia in older adults.* Retrieved from https://pdfs.semanticscholar.org/1557/84a956733eedc5ed069224050388d871e0e9.pdf

Albert, S., Roth, T., Toscani, M., Vitiello, M. V., & Zee, P. (2017). Sleep health and appropriate use of OTC sleep aids in older adults. *Gerontologist, 57*(2), 163–170. doi:10.1093/geront/gnv139

American Psychiatric Association. (2013). *Diagnostic and statistical manual of mental disorders* (5th ed.). Arlington, VA: American Psychiatric Publishingdoi:10.1176/appi.books.9780890425596

American Sleep Association. (n.d.). *Sleep disorders.* Retrieved from https://www.sleepassociation.org/sleep-disorders

Baldwin, D. (2018). Generalized anxiety disorder in adults: Epidemiology, pathogenesis, clinical manifestations, course, assessment, and diagnosis. In M. B. Stein & R. Hermann (Eds.), *UpToDate.* Retrieved from https://www.uptodate.com/contents/generalized-anxiety-disorder-in-adults-epidemiology-pathogenesis-clinical-manifestations-course-assessment-and-diagnosis

Blackburn, P., Wilkins-Ho, M., & Wiese, B. (2017). Depression in older adults: Diagnosis & management. *British Columbia Medical Journal, 59*(3), 171–177. Retrieved from http://www.bcmj.org/articles/depression-older-adults-diagnosis-and-management

Centers for Disease Control and Prevention and National Association of Chronic Disease Directors. (2008). The state of mental health & aging in America: Issue Brief #1: What do the data tell us? Atlanta, GA: National Association of Chronic Disease Directors. Retrieved from https://www.cdc.gov/aging/pdf/mental_health.pdf

Centers for Disease Control and Prevention and National Association of Chronic Disease Directors. (2009). The state of mental health & aging in America: Issue Brief #2: Addressing depression in older adults: Selected evidence-based programs. Atlanta, GA: National Association of Chronic Disease Directors. Retrieved from https://www.cdc.gov/aging/pdf/mental_health_brief_2.pdf

Comella, C. L. (2014). Treatment of restless legs syndrome. *Neurotherapeutics, 11*(1), 177–187. doi:10.1007/s13311-013-0247-9

Craske, M., & Bystritsky, A. (2019). Approach to treating generalized anxiety disorder in adults. In M. B. Stein & R. Hermann (Eds.), *UpToDate*. Retrieved from https://www.uptodate.com/contents/approach-to-treating-generalized-anxiety-disorder-in-adults

Epocrates. (2019a). Buspirone. Epocrates Essentials [Mobile application software]. Retrieved from http://www.epocrates.com/mobile

Epocrates. (2019b). Pregabalin. Epocrates Essentials [Mobile application software]. Retrieved from http://www.epocrates.com/mobile

Espinoza, R. T., & Unützer, J. (2017). Diagnosis and management of late-life unipolar depression. In P. P. Roy-Byrne, K. E. Schmader, & D. Solomon (Eds.), *UpToDate*. Retrieved from https://www.uptodate.com/contents/diagnosis-and-management-of-late-life-unipolar-depression

Hauk, L. (2018). Deprescribing antipsychotics for behavioral & psychological symptoms of dementia & insomnia. *American Family Physician, 98*(6), 394–395. Retrieved from https://www.aafp.org/afp/2018/0915/p394.html

Kuerbis, A., Sacco, P., Blazer, D. G., & Moore, A. A. (2014). Substance abuse among older adults. *Clinical Geriatric Medicine, 30*(3), 629–654. doi:10.1016/j.cger.2014.04.008

Lloyd, S. L., & Striley, C. W. (2018). Marijuana use among adults 50 years or older in the 21st century. *Gerontology & Geriatric Medicine, 4*. doi:10.1177/2333721418781668

Matheson, E., & Hainer, B. L. (2017). Insomnia: Pharmacologic therapy. *American Family Physician, 96*(1), 29–35. Retrieved from https://www.aafp.org/afp/2017/0701/p29.html

Mental Health America. (n.d.). *Mental health in older adults: Anxiety in older adults*. Retrieved from https://www.mentalhealthamerica.net/anxiety-older-adults

National Institute of Mental Health. (2018). Anxiety disorders. Retrieved from https://www.nimh.nih.gov/health/topics/anxiety-disorders/index.shtml

National Sleep Foundation. (n.d.). Periodic limb movements disorder. Retrieved from https://www.sleepfoundation.org/articles/periodic-limb-movements-disorder

Substance Abuse and Mental Health Services Administration-Health Resources and Services Administration Center for Integrated Health Solutions. (n.d.). SBIRT: Screening, brief intervention, and referral to treatment. Retrieved from https://www.integration.samhsa.gov/clinical-practice/sbirt

Singh, J., & Mims, N. (2015). Screening tools for the obstructive sleep apnea for the cardiovascular clinician. Retrieved from https://www.acc.org/latest-in-cardiology/articles/2015/07/14/11/04/screeing-tools-for-the-obstructive-sleep-apnea-for-the-cardiovascular-clinician

Valiengo, L. C. L., Stella, F., & Forlenza, O. V. (2016). Mood disorders in the elderly: Prevalence, functional impact, and management challenges. *Neuropsychiatric Disease & Treatment, 12*, 2105–2114. doi:10.2147/ndt.s94643

World Health Organization. (2017). Mental health of older adults. Retrieved from https://www.who.int/news-room/fact-sheets/detail/mental-health-of-older-adults

Xiong, G. L. (2019). Geriatric sleep disorder. In A. Ategan (Ed.), *Medscape*. Retrieved from https://emedicine.medscape.com/article/292498-overview

22 Musculoskeletal Disorders

Amanda M. Bellile

OBJECTIVES
1. Identify risk factors for the development of osteoporosis and fractures
2. Review screening tools for identifying osteoporosis
3. Select appropriate treatment options for osteoporosis
4. Recognize adverse effects associated with treatment options for osteoarthritis

INTRODUCTION
A significant component to body aging is a progressive decrease in muscle mass, which can then lead to a variety of complications and disorders. Restricted mobilization is a major player in the development of this muscular atrophy. Additionally, geriatric patients have a higher likelihood of developing fractures due to a decline in bone mass and a decrease in bone minerals. Being able to recognize these changes can help us to prevent and treat symptoms from these common disorders in the older patient population.

PATHOPHYSIOLOGY
Starting around age 30, bone density begins to diminish in adults. This process accelerates in women once they have hit menopause. This loss of bone density leads to bone disorders such as osteoporosis and possible fractures. Osteoporosis is acknowledged as the most prevalent bone disorder in the world. Joints are also affected by aging due to progressive changes in cartilage and connective tissue. Cartilage inside of the joints becomes thinner, which makes joints less resilient and more susceptible to damage. This may lead to osteoarthritis in aging adults. Range of motion may additionally be limited as connective tissue within ligaments and tendons becomes more rigid and brittle. Additionally, loss of muscle starts to occur around age 30 and progresses through aging. Gradually decreasing size and number of muscle fibers and tissue correlates to the loss of muscle mass and strength. This can put more pressure on already weaker joints and lead to injury. Loss of muscle mass and strength can be partially overcome or delayed by maintaining regular exercise.

MUSCULOSKELETAL DISORDERS
Osteoporosis and Fractures
Definitions
A "bone fracture" is defined as the continuity of the bone being broken. The main reasons for fractures in elderly patients are falls and osteoporosis (Cheong, Peh, &

Guglielmi, 2008). "Osteoporosis" is defined as "a [silent] skeletal disorder characterized by compromised bone strength predisposing to an increased risk of fracture. Bone strength reflects the integration of two main features: bone density and bone quality" (National Institutes of Health Consensus Development Panel on Osteoporosis Prevention, Diagnosis, and Therapy, 2001). A patient is diagnosed with osteoporosis when he or she has a T-score of −2.5 standard deviations below the bone mineral density of a healthy younger person of the same sex. Osteopenia is diagnosed when the standard deviations are −1 to −2.5 below normal (World Health Organization, 1994).

Prevalence

Osteoporosis is often underdiagnosed and undertreated, especially in adults over 75 years old (Ensrud et al., 1997). For women, osteoporosis prevalence is approximately 50% at age 85. This prevalence is lower in men at about 20% at age 85 (Woolf & Pfleger, 2003). Changing population demographics estimates a doubling of the number of people with osteoporosis in the next 20 years (Coughlan & Dockery, 2014).

Risk Factors

Gender and ethnicity can play a major role in the development of osteoporosis and fractures. It is estimated that 80% of patients suffering from osteoporosis are women (Athanatou, 2007). Ethnic differences can play a major role in osteoporosis as mineral density is higher in Black women and lower in Asian women (Barrett-Connor et al., 2005). Additional risk factors for the development of osteoporosis include age 65 years and over, family history of osteoporosis or fractures, smoking, early menopause, and an excessive alcohol intake of three or more drinks daily (Camacho et al., 2016). Despite prevalent risk factors, fewer than one in four women aged greater than 67 with an osteoporosis-related fracture undergoes bone density measurement or begins osteoporosis treatment (Kanis, Melton, Christiansen, Johnston, & Khaltaev, 1994). Additionally, there is a wide variety of risk factors that can predispose elderly patients to falls and fractures, which include, but are not limited to, neurologic disorders, impaired vision, impaired hearing, frailty and deconditioning, proximal myopathy, sarcopenia, medications, and environmental factors.

Screening Tools and Diagnosis

The bone mineral density is most widely measured using dual-energy x-ray absorptiometry (DXA; Coughlan & Dockery, 2014). T-score changes have been traditionally used in clinical trials to assess efficacy of the medications used to treat osteoporosis. There are several fracture risk predictor tools that have been derived using data from large cohort and population studies. The Fracture Risk Assessment Tool (FRAX) has been endorsed by several institutions including the National Institute for Health and Care Excellence (NICE), the American Association of Clinical Endocrinologists (AACE), and the American College of Endocrinology (ACE; Rabar, Lau, O'Flynn, Li, & Barry, 2012). FRAX predicts the 10-year probability of hip fracture and major osteoporotic fracture (hip, clinical spine, humerus, or forearm) by assessing risk factors of age, sex, body mass index, smoking, alcohol use, prior fracture, parenteral history of hip fracture, use of glucocorticoids, rheumatoid arthritis, secondary osteoporosis, and femoral neck bone mineral density (Lewiecki et al., 2011). It is important to note that FRAX underestimates future fracture risk as it reports risk only for hip and major fractures and it underestimates risk in patients with multiple osteoporosis-related fractures (Lewiecki et al., 2011).

Guidelines for Prevention and Treatment

Guidelines for the diagnosis and treatment of osteoporosis have been established by AACE and ACE. The guidelines recommend evaluating all postmenopausal women aged 50 or more years for osteoporosis risk through a detailed history, exam, and utilizing FRAX. They recommend measuring bone mineral density based on the clinical fracture risk profile. Additionally, when osteoporosis is diagnosed, patients should be evaluated for causes of secondary osteoporosis and for vertebral fractures (Camacho et al., 2016).

The guidelines recommend monitoring vitamin D levels and replacing when insufficient. General counseling on diet, exercise, and reducing fall risk is recommended as well. The guidelines suggest pharmacologic treatment for patients with osteopenia and a history of fragility fracture of the hip or spine, patients with a T-score of −2.5 or lower, and patients with a T-score between −1.0 and −2.5 if the FRAX 10-year probability for major osteoporotic fracture is ≥20% or the 10-year probability of hip fracture is ≥3%. The AACE considers successful osteoporosis treatment as stable or increasing bone mineral density with no evidence of new fractures or fracture progression. They recommend a "bisphosphonate holiday" after 5 years of stability in moderate-risk patients or after 6 to 10 years of stability in higher risk patients. The ending of the "holiday" for bisphosphonate treatment should be based on individual patient circumstances, including fracture risk and change in bone mineral density (Camacho et al., 2016).

Preventive Measures

There are several lifestyle modifications and supplements that may help to improve musculoskeletal integrity and balance, preserve bone strength, and prevent future fractures from occurring. Vitamin D is a major player in calcium absorption and bone health as well as muscle performance, balance, and improving fall risk (Camacho et al., 2016). Additionally, vitamin D may help to enhance the response to bisphosphonate therapy, increase bone mineral density, and prevent fractures (Holick et al., 2011). Vitamin D levels should be regularly monitored and corrected if levels of 25-hydroxy-D fall below 30 ng/mL (Camacho et al., 2016).

Ensuring adequate calcium intake is an essential aspect of osteoporosis prevention and treatment. For adults aged 50 and older, the recommended calcium intake (including diet) is 1,200 mg/day (Ross et al., 2011). The average dietary calcium intake among American adults is approximately 600 mg/day; so many adults are in need of additional calcium supplementation. There are two forms of calcium available over the counter: calcium carbonate and calcium citrate. Calcium carbonate is a cheaper option but may result in more gastrointestinal upset than calcium citrate. Data is inconclusive regarding magnesium intake.

Multiple studies have found that there are several nonpharmacologic lifestyle modifications that can play a major role in preventing osteoporosis. Patients should be advised to limit caffeine intake to less than one to two servings per day as there is an association between caffeinated beverage consumption and fractures (Hallström, Wolk, Glynn, & Michaëlsson, 2006). Excessive alcohol intake and smoking cigarettes have also both been linked with increased fracture risk and should be avoided (Giampietro et al., 2010; Kanis, 2005). Additional nonpharmacologic measures include regular weight-bearing exercise (e.g., walking 30–40 min per session, plus back and posture exercises for a few minutes, 3–4 days per week), fall prevention techniques (anchor rugs, minimize clutter, install handrails, etc.), hip protectors, and physical therapy (Camacho et al., 2016).

Medications for Treatment

There are many pharmacologic agents approved by the U.S. Food and Drug Administration (FDA) for prevention and/or treatment of postmenopausal osteoporosis (see Table 22.1). There are four medications (alendronate, risedronate, zoledronic acid, and denosumab) that have evidence for "broad spectrum" antifracture efficacy

TABLE 22.1 Medications Approved by the FDA for Treatment of Postmenopausal Osteoporosis

Generic Drug (Trade Name)	Dose	Fracture Risk Reduction			Common Adverse Effects
		Vertebral	Nonvertebral	Hip	
Alendronate (Fosamax)	Prophylaxis: 5 mg once daily or 35 mg once weekly Treatment: 10 mg once daily or 70 mg once weekly	Yes	Yes	Yes	GI upset, musculoskeletal pain, transient decreased serum calcium
Calcitonin (Miacalcin, Fortical)	Intranasal: 200 units (1 spray) in one nostril daily	Yes	No effect demonstrated	No effect demonstrated	Rhinitis, back pain, nausea
Denosumab (Prolia)	60 mg subcutaneously every 6 months	Yes	Yes	Yes	Headache, dermatitis, peripheral edema, arthralgia, upper respiratory infection
Ibandronate (Boniva)	150 mg orally once monthly or 3 mg IV every 3 months	Yes	No effect demonstrated	No effect demonstrated	Dyspepsia, back pain, upper respiratory tract infection
Raloxifene (Evista)	60 mg orally once daily	Yes	No effect demonstrated	No effect demonstrated	Peripheral edema, hot flash, infection, arthralgia, flu-like symptoms
Risedronate (Actonel, Atelvia)	Immediate release: 5 mg orally once daily or 35 mg once weekly Delayed release: 35 mg orally once weekly	Yes	Yes	Yes	Hypertension, headache, skin rash, GI disease, UTI, arthralgia, back pain

Teriparatide (Forteo)	20 mcg subcutaneously once daily	Yes	Yes	No effect demonstrated	Hypercalcemia, orthostatic hypotension, dizziness, headache, nausea, arthralgia
Zoledronic acid (Reclast)	5 mg IV once a year	Yes	Yes	Yes	Lower extremity edema, headache, insomnia, depression, dermatitis, nausea, UTI, anemia, dyspnea, back pain, fever

FDA, Food and Drug Administration; GI gastrointestinal; IV, intravenous; UTI urinary tract infection.

Sources: Data from Camacho, P. M., Petak, S. M., Binkley, N., Clarke, B. L., Harris, S. T., Hurley, D. L., . . . Watts, N. B. (2016). American Association of Clinical Endocrinologists and American College of Endocrinology clinical practice guidelines for the diagnosis and treatment of postmenopausal osteoporosis — 2016. *Endocrine Practice, 22*(Suppl. 4), 1–42. doi:10.4158/ep161435.gl; Lexicomp. (2018). Lexicomp Online. Retrieved from https://online.lexi.com/lco/action/home

including spine, hip, and nonvertebral fracture risk reduction and should generally be considered initial options (Camacho et al., 2016). Patients who have a low or moderate fracture risk can be started on oral therapy, reserving injectable agents (teriparatide, denosumab, or zoledronic acid) for those with the highest fracture risk or unable to tolerate the oral medications due to gastrointestinal problems. For patients at risk for spine fractures but not hip or nonvertebral fractures, ibandronate or raloxifene may be appropriate (Camacho et al., 2016).

Bisphosphonates

Bisphosphonates (alendronate, ibandronate, risedronate, and zoledronic acid) are the most widely utilized medications for osteoporosis and work by binding to hydroxyapatite in bone to reduce the activity of osteoclasts. Bisphosphonates should be taken in the morning with a full glass of water and the patient should remain upright for 30 to 60 minutes after taking to promote absorption and avoid gastrointestinal adverse effects (Camacho et al., 2016). Safety concerns associated with bisphosphonates include acute-phase reactions, osteonecrosis of the jaw, and atypical femur fractures (Camacho et al., 2016).

Additional Agents

Denosumab is a monoclonal antibody that prevents receptor activator of nuclear factor kappa-B ligand (RANKL) from binding to its receptor and thereby reducing differentiation of precursor cells into mature osteoclasts and decreasing function and survival of activated osteoclasts. This medication is a 60-mg subcutaneous injection that the patient receives once every 6 months. A "drug holiday" is not recommended with denosumab (Cummings et al., 2009). Raloxifene is approved for the treatment of postmenopausal osteoporosis as well as the reduction of risk of breast cancer (Evista Package Insert, 2011). Raloxifene has not been shown to reduce hip or nonvertebral fracture and is associated with approximately a threefold increase in the occurrence of thromboembolic diseases (similar to estrogen) and a high rate of menopausal symptoms (Barrett-Connor et al., 2006). Intranasal calcitonin, estrogen, teriparatide, and strontium are utilized less frequently for the treatment of osteoporosis.

Bone mineral testing can be done prior to initiating treatment as well as to monitor the response to treatment. For patients on treatment, bone mineral density monitoring is recommended every 1 to 2 years (Camacho et al., 2016). Length of therapy is determined by weighing the risks or benefits. Due to bisphosphonates accumulating and residing in the bone, "bisphosphonate holidays" are often utilized to reduce the risk of developing adverse reactions such as osteonecrosis of the jaw. The optimal duration of the "bisphosphonate holiday" has not been established and frequent monitoring during these breaks is important (Camacho et al., 2016). It is important to convey risks associated with therapy to patients and allow shared decision-making so that patients play an active role in their osteoporosis management.

Osteoarthritis

Definitions

Osteoarthritis can be defined as a group of distinct, but overlapping diseases, which may have different etiologies, but similar biological, morphological, and clinical outcomes affecting the articular cartilage, subchondral bone, ligaments, joint capsule, synovial membrane, and periarticular muscles (Salter, 2002). The most common symptom of osteoarthritis is joint pain. The pain tends to worsen with activity, especially following a period of rest (Sinusas, 2012). The joints most commonly affected by osteoarthritis are hands, knees, hips, and spine, but almost any joint can be involved. Symptoms of osteoarthritis often result in loss of function due to pain and stiffness (Sinusas, 2012).

Prevalence and Risk Factors

Osteoarthritis is the most common joint disease in individuals who are aged 65 years or older with radiographic prevalence as high as approximately 90% of women and 80% of men (Zhang et al., 2002). Risk factors for osteoarthritis include genetics, female sex, past trauma, advancing age, and obesity (Sinusas, 2012).

Screening Tools and Diagnosis

The diagnosis of osteoarthritis is often made by physical examination. Plain radiographs can help confirm the diagnosis as well as grade the severity of the osteoarthritis. The features that show osteoarthritis on radiographic imaging are focal/nonuniform narrowing of the joint space in the areas subjected to the most pressure, subchondral cysts, subchondral sclerosis, and osteophytes (Braun & Gold, 2012).

Guidelines for Diagnosis and Treatment

The American College of Rheumatology (ACR) came out with recommendations on the nonpharmacologic and pharmacologic treatment of osteoarthritis of the hand, hip, and knee. Updates to these guidelines are expected to be released in 2019. Additionally, the American Academy of Family Physicians released guidance on the diagnosis and treatment of osteoarthritis in 2012. Treatment recommendations are similar across both sets of guidelines focusing on exercise, weight loss, and nonopioid analgesics for pain management (Hochberg, 2012; Sinusas, 2012).

The ACR recommendations for pharmacologic treatment vary based on which joints are affected by osteoarthritis. For the hand joints, ACR recommends topical capsaicin, topical nonsteroidal anti-inflammatory drugs (NSAIDs), oral NSAIDs, and tramadol. They recommend not using intra-articular therapies or opioid analgesics for the hand and do not recommend oral NSAIDs for patients over the age of 75 years. For osteoarthritis of the knee, the guidelines recommend acetaminophen, oral and topical NSAIDs, tramadol, and intra-articular corticosteroid injections. They recommend against the use of chondroitin sulfate, glucosamine, and topical capsaicin and have no recommendations regarding the use of intra-articular hyaluronates, duloxetine, and opioid analgesics. The recommendations for hip osteoarthritis from ACR are acetaminophen, oral NSAIDs, tramadol, and intra-articular corticosteroid injections. They recommend against chondroitin sulfate and glucosamine and have no recommendations for topical NSAIDs, intra-articular hyaluronate injections, duloxetine, and opioid analgesics (Hochberg, 2012).

Nonpharmacologic Measures

Nonpharmacologic treatment for osteoarthritis often begins with exercise particularly for knee and hip osteoarthritis. The guidelines strongly recommend cardiovascular and/or resistance land-based exercise as well as aquatic exercise and weight loss for individuals who are overweight (Hochberg, 2012). Several Cochrane reviews have been conducted that have found both land-based and aquatic exercises result in short-term reduction of pain and improvement in physical function (Bartels et al., 2016; Fransen & McConnell, 2008). For patients with osteoarthritis in weight-bearing joints, swimming, elliptical training, and cycling are all good exercise options. Additionally, obesity is a major risk factor in the development of osteoarthritis and one meta-analysis found that weight loss of 5% from baselines was sufficient to reduce disability in knee osteoarthritis (Christensen, 2007).

Bracing and splinting may be an option for some patients in order to help support painful or unstable joints. The ACR guidelines recommend hand splints for patients with trapeziometacarpal osteoarthritis and medially directed patellar taping for knee osteoarthritis. There are also nonpharmacologic measures that the ACR guidelines conditionally recommend for knee osteoarthritis including psychosocial interventions, insoles for lateral and medial compartment osteoarthritis, thermal agents, walking aids if needed, tai chi, Chinese acupuncture, and transcutaneous electrical nerve stimulation (TENS); see Hochberg (2012). If a cane is utilized to reduce weight load in patients with hip or knee osteoarthritis, it needs to be properly fitted and used on the side contralateral to the affected joint (Manek & Lane, 2000).

Medications

See Table 22.2 for an overview of osteoarthritis medications.

Acetaminophen

Acetaminophen is considered the mainstay of treatment for osteoarthritis due to its effectiveness, safety, and low cost. A 2006 Cochrane review found that acetaminophen was better than placebo in treating mild osteoarthritis and equal to NSAIDs with fewer gastrointestinal-related adverse effects (Towheed et al., 2006). The U.S. FDA recommends no more than 4,000 mg of acetaminophen per day from all sources to avoid liver toxicity (FDA, 2011). For patients who do not have an adequate response to maximum doses of acetaminophen, the next step is topical and oral NSAIDs.

Nonsteroidal Anti-Inflammatory Drugs

NSAIDs can be very effective for the treatment of osteoarthritis, but patients should be cautioned about potential adverse effects including gastrointestinal bleeding, renal dysfunction, and blood pressure elevation (Towheed et al., 2006). The ACR guidelines recommend utilizing topical NSAIDs over oral in patients who are above 75 years of age. They also recommend utilizing either a cyclooxygenase 2 (COX 2) selective NSAID or a nonselective NSAID in combination with a proton-pump inhibitor (PPI) in patients with a history of a symptomatic or complicated upper gastrointestinal ulcer (Hochberg, 2012).

Intra-Articular Steroid Injections

Intra-articular injections of corticosteroids provide primarily short-term relief of osteoarthritis lasting from 4 to 8 weeks (Sinusas, 2012). The ACR guidelines recommend intra-articular steroid injections for knee and hip osteoarthritis, but not hand (Hochberg, 2012). This is due to studies that have found greater efficacy for steroid injections in the knee and hip than in areas such as the hand and shoulder (American Academy of Orthopedic Surgeons, 2009; Arroll & Goodyear-Smith, 2004; Meenagh, Patton, Kynes, & Wright, 2004). Providers often inject a corticosteroid along with a local anesthetic. Patients should be educated that they may experience a potential flare-up of symptoms within the first 24 hours, followed by an improvement from baseline at 48 hours. Many providers limit corticosteroid injections to four annually in the same joint (American Academy of Orthopedic Surgeons, 2009).

Other Medication Options

Due to their abuse potential, opioids should be avoided unless there are contraindications to first-line treatment options. If they are utilized, they should be started at low doses and monitored closely. The available guidelines do not have any recommendations on the use of duloxetine for pain in osteoarthritis; however, they mention that it may be an option if patients fail other treatment options (Hochberg, 2012). Intra-articular hyaluronate, chondroitin sulfate, and glucosamine are not recommended in guidelines due to their lack of efficacy in clinical trials.

SUMMARY

Musculoskeletal disorders are extremely prevalent in older adults. It is imperative that healthcare professionals recognize risk factors for the development of osteoporosis

Musculoskeletal Disorders | 205

TABLE 22.2 Pharmacology and Dosing of Osteoarthritis Medications

Generic Drug (Trade Name)	Time to Peak	Serum Half-Life	Typical Dosage for Osteoarthritis	Maximum Dose	Common Adverse Effects (Frequency >5%)
Acetaminophen* (Tylenol)	10–60 min	2–3 hours	1,000 mg TID	4,000 mg/day	No common adverse effects
Celecoxib (Celebrex)	~3 hours	~11 hours	200 mg daily or 100 mg BID	400 mg/day	Diarrhea, dyspepsia, upper respiratory tract infection
Diclofenac sodium (Cambia, Voltaren)	Immediate release: ~1 hour, delayed release: ~2 hours, extended release: ~5 hours	~2 hours	Immediate release: 50 mg 2–3 times daily, delayed release: 50 mg 2–3 times daily or 75 mg BID, extended release: 100 mg daily	150 mg/day	Edema, headache, dizziness, pruritus, gastrointestinal upset, anemia, increased liver enzymes
Topical diclofenac sodium (Voltaren Gel)	10–14 hours	N/A	Lower extremities: 4 g four times daily; Upper extremities: 2 g four times daily	32 g/day	Pruritus, application site rash, dermatitis, xeroderma, application site pain
Ibuprofen* (Advil)	1–2 hours	~2 hours	400 to 800 mg 3–4 times daily	3,200 mg/day	Decreased hemoglobin, increased liver enzymes
Meloxicam (Mobic)	Capsule: within 2 hours, tablet: 4–5 hours	~15–22 hours	5–15 mg once daily	15 mg/day	Edema, abdominal pain, dyspepsia, urinary tract infection
Naproxen* (Aleve)	~2 hours	~12–17 hours	500–1,000 mg/day in two divided doses	1,000 mg/day	Edema, dizziness, pruritus, headache, fluid retention, gastrointestinal upset, hemolysis, dyspnea

*Available over the counter.
BID, two times per day; TID, three times per day.
Source: Data from Lexicomp. (2018). Lexicomp Online. Retrieved from https://online.lexi.com/lco/action/home

and help to prevent a disabling fracture. Additionally, osteoarthritis is a common reason for loss of function and pain in older adults. The effective management of these disease states can keep older adults active and functional.

MUSCULOSKELETAL INTERPROFESSIONAL CASE STUDY
Megan Hebdon
Patient Presentation

Betty is a 92-year-old woman who presents to your clinic with her daughter-in-law for evaluation of chronic back pain, which she has had for almost 50 years, and bilateral knee pain which she has had for 10 years. She reports that this pain affects her sleep, eating patterns, and social activities. She has been told that she has arthritis in her knees, but she has never had a clear diagnosis for her lower back pain. When asked where her back hurts, she states "everywhere," and "everything makes it worse." It is painful when she sits, stands, or lies down.

She has been on multiple prior medications for the pain including hydrocodone with acetaminophen, oxycodone with acetaminophen, NSAIDs, acetaminophen alone, and tramadol. She is currently on a 25-mcg fentanyl patch, but her daughter-in-law is concerned due to daytime sleepiness. She states that sometimes her mother-in-law will fall asleep mid conversation. Betty lives in a retirement community, but she is widowed. Her daughter-in-law is worried about her safety in her home. Her daughter-in-law also states that she thinks Betty is using too much ibuprofen and acetaminophen for the breakthrough pain.

Betty has had physical therapy and lumbar epidural steroid injections for the pain. She has never had surgery nor is she currently interested in anything invasive.

History

Betty is a widow, has not been sexually active for 20 years, has three children, and lives alone in a retirement community. Her only chronic health conditions are her arthritis and her lower back pain. She has seen multiple providers over the past 3 years for her pain. She denies use of alcohol, tobacco, or illicit drugs. She eats dinner with friends in the retirement community and reports no current leisure activities due to the pain. She is a retired preschool teacher.

Medications

Fentanyl 25 mcg (change the patch every 48 hours), acetaminophen 500 mg as needed, and ibuprofen 600 mg as needed.

Physical Exam

Vital signs are: Blood pressure: 108/64 mmHg; Pulse: 72 beats per minute; Respirations: 18 breaths per minute; Oxygen saturation: 96%.

She is alert, oriented, and cooperative. During the exam, she holds her lower back with her left hand and leans slightly forward. Her cardiac, pulmonary, and neurologic exams are unremarkable. Her musculoskeletal exam demonstrates pain with flexion and extension, tenderness to palpation of the lumbar spine and paraspinal muscle tension. Her toe and heel walking are intact. Her knee flexion and extension are limited by her pain. She has no edema to her knee and mild pain to palpation along the joint line. There is no knee joint laxity bilaterally.

Diagnostic Testing

You review her prior bilateral knee x-rays, which demonstrate moderate joint space narrowing in both knees. Her lumbar MRI is reviewed from 2 years ago, because her pain has not changed. This shows mild spinal stenosis, disc bulging at L3 and L4, facet joint arthropathy at multiple levels, and disc degeneration at L5 and S1.

You perform a urine drug screening at the appointment, with initial results demonstrating appropriate medication use by the patient.

You administer the back pain functional scale (BPFS) and the Geriatric Depression Scale (GDS). She scores low on the functional scale and screens positive for depressive symptoms. She denies suicidal or homicidal ideation.

You also check a complete blood count (CBC) and comprehensive metabolic panel (CMP) to evaluate fatigue and medication side effects. All values are within normal limits for her age.

Plan of Care

Betty has long-standing chronic pain related to arthritis, vertebral disc disease, and spinal stenosis. She is not interested in invasive measures, and her age might preclude this. Her current pain medications are neither effective for her pain nor safe for independent living. You discuss these issues with the patient and her daughter-in-law. You also discuss the medication safety concerns related to ibuprofen and renal, gastrointestinal, and cardiac side effects. You suggest a topical alternative: diclofenac gel 4 grams to both knees twice daily. You offer two alternatives to her current fentanyl treatment: reduce to 12.5 mcg/hour or switch to a buprenorphine patch 7.5 mcg/hour. You discuss the risks and benefits of both, including decreased pain control, withdrawal symptoms, or improvement or worsening of side effects. You discuss a plan for the buprenorphine switch, including use of over-the-counter acetaminophen or short-term hydrocodone/acetaminophen 2.5/325 for breakthrough pain. You also offer a lidocaine patch for her lower back pain along with nonpharmacologic treatment approaches: use of heat/cold therapy (not over medication patches), deep breathing exercises, chiropractic care, and referral for counseling and physical therapy. Finally, you ensure she has a current prescription for naloxone, and provide training regarding administration of the medication.

Interprofessional Collaboration

There is in-house physical therapy and a tai chi class at the retirement community. You refer Betty for physical therapy and strongly suggest that she do tai chi one to two times per week. As part of the physical therapy referral, you request evaluation for a TENS unit. Additionally, you refer Betty for cognitive behavioral therapy to help with the pain and with her depressive symptoms. You are concerned about her depressive symptoms but are reluctant to add another medication at this time. With Betty and her daughter-in-law, you discuss your hope for improvement in pain and depressive symptoms using these pharmacologic and nonpharmacologic approaches.

Case Study References

Centers for Disease Control and Prevention. (n.d.). *Calculating total daily dose of opioids for safer dosage*. Retrieved from https://www.cdc.gov/drugoverdose/pdf/calculating_total_daily_dose-a.pdf

Centers for Disease Control and Prevention Guideline for Prescribing Opioids for Chronic Pain. (2016). Recommendations and reports. *65*(1), 1–49. Retrieved from http://www.cdc.gov/mmwr/volumes/65/rr/rr6501e1.htm

Galicia-Castillo, M. C., & Weiner, D. K. (2019). Treatment of persistent pain in older adults. In K. E. Schmader, S. Fishman, & M. Crowley (Eds.), *UpToDate*. Retrieved from https://www.uptodate.com/contents/treatment-of-persistent-pain-in-older-adults

Purdue Pharma. (n.d.). Butrans®: Use the dose conversion tool. Retrieved from https://butrans.com/resources/opioid-conversion-tool.html

RxFiles. (n.d.). *Opioid tapering template*. Retrieved from https://www.rxfiles.ca/rxfiles/uploads/documents/opioid-taper-template.pdf

Shirley Ryan AbilityLab. (2013). Back pain functional scale. Retrieved from https://www.sralab.org/rehabilitation-measures/back-pain-functional-scale

Wu, A. (2018). Special considerations for opioid use in elderly patients with chronic pain. *US Pharmacist, 43*(3), 26–30. Retrieved from https://www.uspharmacist.com/article/special-considerations-for-opioid-use-in-elderly-patients-with-chronic-pain

REFERENCES

American Academy of Orthopedic Surgeons. (2009). *The treatment of glenohumeral joint osteoarthritis: Guidelines and evidence report*. Rosemont, IL: Author. Retrieved from http://www.aaos.org/research/guidelines/gloguideline.pdf

Arroll, B., & Goodyear-Smith, F. (2004). Corticosteroid injections for osteoarthritis of the knee: Meta-analysis. *British Medical Journal, 328*(7444), 869. doi:10.1136/bmj.38039.573970.7c

Athanatou, E. (2007). *Medical and Surgical Clinic Nursing* (7th ed.). Athens: The Tavitha.

Barrett-Connor, E., Mosca, L., Collins, P., Geiger, M. J., Grady, D., Kornitzer, M., . . . Wenger, N. K. (2006). Effects of raloxifene on cardiovascular events and breast cancer in postmenopausal women. *New England Journal of Medicine, 355*(2), 125–137. doi:10.1056/nejmoa062462

Barrett-Connor, E., Siris, E. S., Wehren, L. E., Miller, P. D., Abbott, T. A., Berger, M. L., . . . Sherwood, L. M. (2005). Osteoporosis and fracture risk in women of different ethnic groups. *Journal of Bone and Mineral Research, 20*(2), 185–194. doi:10.1359/jbmr.041007

Bartels, E. M., Juhl, C. B., Christensen, R., Hagen, K. B., Danneskiold-Samsøe, B., Dagfinrud, H., & Lund, H. (2016). Aquatic exercise for the treatment of knee and hip osteoarthritis. *Cochrane Database of Systematic Reviews*. doi:10.1002/14651858.cd005523.pub3

Camacho, P. M., Petak, S. M., Binkley, N., Clarke, B. L., Harris, S. T., Hurley, D. L., . . . Watts, N. B. (2016). American Association of Clinical Endocrinologists and American College of Endocrinology Clinical Practice guidelines for the diagnosis and treatment of postmenopausal osteoporosis—2016. *Endocrine Practice, 22*(Suppl. 4), 1–42. doi:10.4158/ep161435.gl

Cheong, H. W., Peh, W. C. G., & Guglielmi, G. (2008). Imaging of diseases of the axial and peripheral skeleton. *Radiologic Clinics of North America, 46*(4), 703–733. doi:10.1016/j.rcl.2008.04.007

Christensen, R., Bartels, E. M., Astrup, A., & Bliddal, H. (2007). Effect of weight reduction in obese patients diagnosed with knee osteoarthritis: A systematic review

and meta-analysis. *Annals of the Rheumatic Diseases, 66*(4), 433–439. doi:10.1136/ard.2006.065904
Coughlan, T., & Dockery, F. (2014). Osteoporosis and fracture risk in older people. *Clinical Medicine, 14*(2), 187–191. doi:10.7861/clinmedicine.14-2-187
Cummings, S. R., Martin, J. S., McClung, M. R., Siris, E. S., Eastell, R., Reid, I. R., . . . Christiansen, C. (2009). Denosumab for prevention of fractures in postmenopausal women with osteoporosis. *New England Journal of Medicine, 361*(8), 756–765. doi:10.1056/nejmoa0809493
Ensrud, K. E., Black, D. M., Palermo, L., Bauer, D. C., Barrett-Connor, E., Quandt, S. A., . . . Karpf, D. B. (1997). Treatment with alendronate prevents fractures in women at highest risk: Results from the Fracture Intervention Trial. *Archives of Internal Medicine, 155*, 2617–2624. doi:10.1001/archinte.1997.00440430099012
Evista (raloxifene hydrochloride). (2011). *Tablet for Oral Use* [package insert]. Indianapolis, IN: Eli Lilly and Company.
Fransen, M., & McConnell, S. (2008). Exercise for osteoarthritis of the knee. *Cochrane Database of Systematic Reviews,* (4), CD004376. doi:10.1002/14651858.CD004376.pub2
Giampietro, P. F., McCarty, C., Mukesh, B., McKiernan, F., Wilson, D., Shuldiner, A., . . . Ghebranious, N. (2010). The role of cigarette smoking and statins in the development of postmenopausal osteoporosis: A pilot study utilizing the Marshfield Clinic Personalized Medicine Cohort. *Osteoporosis International, 21*(3), 467–477. doi:10.1007/s00198-009-0981-3
Braun, H. J., Gold, G. E. (2012). Diagnosis of osteoarthritis: imaging. *Bone, 51*(2), 278–288. doi: 10.1016/j.bone.2011.11.019
Hallström, H., Wolk, A., Glynn, A., & Michaëlsson, K. (2006). Coffee, tea and caffeine consumption in relation to osteoporotic fracture risk in a cohort of Swedish women. *Osteoporosis International, 17*(7), 1055–1064. doi:10.1007/s00198-006-0109-y
Hochberg, M. C., Altman, R. D., April, K. T., Benkhalti, M., Guyatt, G., McGowan, J., . . . Tugwell, P. (2012). American College of Rheumatology 2012 recommendations for the use of nonpharmacologic and pharmacologic therapies in osteoarthritis of the hand, hip, and knee. *Arthritis Care & Research, 64*(4), 465–474. doi:10.1002/acr.21596
Holick, M. F., Binkley, N. C., Bischoff-Ferrari, H. A., Gordon, C. M., Hanley, D. A., Heaney, R. P., . . . Weaver, C. M. (2011). Evaluation, treatment, and prevention of Vitamin D deficiency: An endocrine society clinical practice guideline. *The Journal of Clinical Endocrinology & Metabolism, 96*(7), 1911–1930. doi:10.1210/jc.2011-0385
Kanis, J. A., Johansson, H., Johnell, O., Oden, A., De Laet, C., Eisman, J. A., . . . Tenenhouse, A. (2005). Alcohol intake as a risk factor for fracture. *Osteoporosis International, 16*(7), 737–742. doi:10.1007/s00198-004-1734-y
Kanis, J. A., Melton, L. J. 3rd., Christiansen, C., Johnston, C. C., & Khaltaev, N. (1994). The diagnosis of osteoporosis. *Journal of Bone and Mineral Research, 9*, 1137–1141. doi:10.1002/jbmr.5650090802
Lewiecki, E. M., Compston, J. E., Miller, P. D., Adachi, J. D., Adams, J. E., Leslie, W. D., & Kanis, J. A. (2011). FRAX® Bone Mineral Density Task Force of the 2010 Joint International Society for Clinical Densitometry & International Osteoporosis Foundation Position Development Conference. *Journal of Clinical Densitometry, 14*, 223–225. doi:10.1016/j.jocd.2011.05.018
Manek, N. J., & Lane, N. E. (2000). Osteoarthritis: current concepts in diagnosis and management. *American Family Physician, 61*(6), 1795–1804. Retrieved from https://www.aafp.org/afp/2000/0315/p1795.html
Meenagh, G. K., Patton, J., Kynes, C., & Wright, G. D. (2004). A randomised controlled trial of intra-articular corticosteroid injection of the carpometacarpal joint of the thumb in osteoarthritis. *Annals of the Rheumatic Diseases, 63*(10), 1260–1263. doi:10.1136/ard.2003.015438
National Institutes of Health Consensus Development Panel on Osteoporosis Prevention, Diagnosis, and Therapy. (2001). Osteoporosis prevention, diagnosis, and therapy. *The Journal of the American Medical Association, 285*(6), 785–795. doi:10.1001/jama.285.6.785

Rabar, S., Lau, R., O'Flynn, N., Li, L., & Barry, P. (2012). Risk assessment of fragility fractures: Summary of NICE guidance. *British Medical Journal, 345*, e3698–e3698. doi:10.1136/bmj.e3698

Ross, A. C., Manson, J. E., Abrams, S. A., Aloia, J. F., Brannon, P. M., Clinton, S. K., . . . Shapses, S. A. (2011). The 2011 report on dietary reference intakes for calcium and vitamin D from the Institute of Medicine: What clinicians need to know. *The Journal of Clinical Endocrinology & Metabolism, 96*(1), 53–58. doi:10.1210/jc.2010-2704

Salter, D. M. (2002). Degenerative joint disease. *Current Diagnostic Pathology, 8*(1), 11–18. doi:10.1054/cdip.2001.0090

Sinusas, K. (2012). Osteoarthritis: Diagnosis and treatment. *American Family Physician, 85*(1), 49–56. Retrieved from https://www.aafp.org/afp/2012/0101/p49.html

Towheed, T., Maxwell, L., Judd, M., Catton, M., Hochberg, M. C., & Wells, G. A. (2006). Acetaminophen for osteoarthritis. *Cochrane Database of Systematic Reviews*, (1), CD004257. doi:10.1002/14651858.cd004257.pub2

U.S. Food and Drug Administration. (2011). FDA drug safety communication: Prescription acetaminophen products to be limited to 325 mg per dosage unit; Boxed warning will highlight potential for severe liver failure. Retrieved from https://www.fda.gov/drugs/drug-safety-and-availability/fda-drug-safety-communication-prescription-acetaminophen-products-be-limited-325-mg-dosage-unit

Woolf, A. D., & Pfleger, B. (2003). Burden of major musculoskeletal conditions. *Bulletin of World Health Organization, 81*, 646–656. Retrieved from https://apps.who.int/iris/bitstream/handle/10665/269026/PMC2572542.pdf?sequence=1&isAllowed=y

World Health Organization Study Group. (1994). Assessment of fracture risk and its application to screening for postmenopausal osteoporosis. *World Health Organization Technical Report Series, 843*, 1–129. Retrieved from https://apps.who.int/iris/bitstream/handle/10665/39142/WHO_TRS_843_eng.pdf?sequence=1&isAllowed=y

Zhang, Y., Niu, J., Kelly-Hayes, M., Chaisson, C. E., Aliabadi, P., & Felson, D. T. (2002). Prevalence of symptomatic hand osteoarthritis and its impact on functional status among the elderly: The Framingham Study. *American Journal of Epidemiology, 156*(11), 1021–1027. doi:10.1093/aje/kwf141

23 Pain Management

Amanda M. Bellile

OBJECTIVES

1. Assess pain characteristics and intensity in older adults
2. Develop a treatment plan for older adults to manage chronic and acute pain
3. Monitor for common adverse effects associated with analgesics
4. Describe educational points for patients who are initiated on treatment with opiates

INTRODUCTION

"Pain" is described as an "unpleasant sensory or emotional experience associated with actual or potential tissue damage or described in terms of such damage" (Merskey & Bogduk, 1994). Geriatric patients are often untreated or undertreated for pain due to a variety of reasons, including challenges in assessing their pain, misconceptions surrounding tolerance and addiction to opioids, uncertainty regarding changing pharmacokinetics and pharmacodynamics in aging patients, as well as a desire to avoid adding more medications, particularly those with higher rates of possible adverse effects. Undertreating pain in elderly patients can have a negative impact on quality of life and can result in depression, anxiety, social isolation, cognitive impairment, immobility, and sleep disturbances (Cavalieri, 2002). As the number of people over the age of 65 continues to rise, chronic diseases associated with symptoms of pain are likely to increase as well. Between 25% and 50% of community-dwelling older adults experience chronic pain (Abdulla et al., 2013). There are even higher rates of geriatric patients with pain in nursing homes estimated to be between 83% and 93% (Abdulla et al., 2013).

Pain can be classified as being nociceptive and neuropathic in origin or a combination of both. Nociceptive pain is caused by damage to body tissue, and the pain can be either visceral or somatic. It is often described as sharp, aching, or stabbing pain (Nicholson, 2006). Neuropathic pain occurs when there is nerve damage and is described as shooting, tingling, numbness, or burning (Nicholson, 2006). Oftentimes, pain can be categorized as being cancer-associated pain or noncancer pain. The most common sources for noncancer pain in geriatric patients are arthritis and postherpetic neuralgia (Pergolizzi et al., 2008).

Assessment of pain in geriatric patients can be challenging, especially when there is any cognitive impairment. Self-reporting of pain may be less evident, and it is more important to examine function and physical appearance. Older patients may not self-report pain because they may view pain as expected with old age or they are fearful of the stigma associated with it (American Geriatrics Society, 2009). In patients with dementia, agitation, changes in functional status, altered gait, and social isolation may all be signs of pain (Sansome & Schmitt, 2004). A visual analog scale, numerical scale, pain thermometer scale, and pain faces scale can all be helpful pain assessment tools in geriatric patients (American Geriatrics Society, 2009). After initiating pain management therapy, pain should be reassessed on a regular basis in order to modify current therapy for the best response. These reassessments should include evaluation of compliance as well as the presence of any adverse drug effects (Ferrell, 2001).

PHARMACOLOGICAL THERAPY

Acetaminophen

Acetaminophen is a first-line agent for the treatment of mild to moderate pain in the geriatric population (Makris, Abrams, Gurland, & Reid, 2014). This is due to the fact that it has a low side-effect profile and is safe and effective when used appropriately. The American Geriatric Society's 2009 guidelines recommend acetaminophen over other agents for mild pain, and it is often utilized for osteoarthritis of the knee and hip as well as low back pain (Marcum, Duncan, & Makris, 2016). Acetaminophen works by selectively inhibiting prostaglandin in the central nervous system (CNS; Borsheski & Johnson, 2014). It is rapidly absorbed from the gastrointestinal (GI) tract, and trials have found that the rate and extent of absorption do not appear to be age-dependent. Acetaminophen is metabolized by phase II hepatic conjugative metabolism, and advanced age is not thought to affect clearance (O'Neil, Hanlon, & Marcum, 2012).

The maximum daily recommended dose is 4 grams; this includes "hidden sources" as acetaminophen is an ingredient in more than 600 over-the-counter and prescription drugs (Horgas, 2017; Kaye, Baluch, & Scott, 2010). This often requires extensive patient education as exceeding the maximum recommended dose can result in hepatotoxicity. In patients with preexisting hepatic insufficiency, cirrhosis, and/or active alcohol use, it is recommended not to exceed 2 grams/day for short-term use (Bosilkovska, Walder, Besson, Daali, & Desmeules, 2012).

Nonsteroidal Anti-Inflammatory Drugs (NSAIDs)

NSAIDs are often the most effective agents for pain caused by inflammation (e.g., rheumatologic diseases; Horgas, 2017). For this reason, NSAIDs are widely prescribed for musculoskeletal pain and are also readily accessible over the counter. Nonselective NSAIDs (e.g., ibuprofen, naproxen) work by reversibly inhibiting cyclooxygenase 1 and 2 (COX 1 and 2) enzymes, which results in decreased formation of prostaglandin precursors. This allows them to have antipyretic, analgesic, and anti-inflammatory properties (Ibuprofen prescribing information, 2017). COX 2 selective inhibitors (e.g., celecoxib) do not inhibit COX 1 and may therefore have fewer GI-related adverse effects (Celecoxib prescribing information, 2018).

Despite efficacy in musculoskeletal conditions, NSAIDs should be used with extreme caution in elderly patients due to the high risk of potentially serious adverse effects (Abdulla et al., 2013). These adverse effects include GI, renal, and cardiovascular effects that can be seen with all types of NSAIDs (Abdulla et al., 2013). NSAID use causes an estimated 41,000 hospitalizations and 3,300 deaths each year among older adults (Griffin, 1998). Elderly patients are at increased risk of adverse effects from NSAIDs, especially GI toxicity (Boers, Tangelder, van Ingen, Fort, & Goldstein, 2007). GI toxicity includes peptic ulcers and bleeding and may be dose-related as well as time-dependent (American Geriatric Society, 2009). The risk of GI-related adverse effects increases when an NSAID is coadministered with a low-dose aspirin, which is often used for cardiovascular protection. NSAIDs should be avoided in patients on medications for anticoagulation. GI adverse effects may be reduced by prescribing misoprostol or a proton-pump inhibitor (PPI) such as omeprazole or pantoprazole together with an NSAID (Abdulla et al., 2013). Both of these agents are effective, but misoprostol is often not well tolerated in older adults (Greenberger, 1996).

Renal vasoconstriction and increased tubular sodium reabsorption may cause fluid retention. NSAIDs can contribute to worsening of chronic renal failure, particularly in patients prescribed diuretics or angiotensin-converting enzyme inhibitors (Nikolaus & Zeyfang, 2004). For this reason, NSAIDs should be avoided in older adults with chronic kidney disease (CKD; creatinine clearance <30 mL/min; American Geriatrics Society, 2015).

The U.S. Food and Drug Administration (FDA) issued a warning in 2005 that NSAID use could cause heart attacks and strokes that could lead to death. They then strengthened this warning in 2015 based on a comprehensive review of safety information and stated that all prescription NSAID labels must contain information on the risk of heart attack and stroke (FDA, 2015). Selective COX 2 inhibitors are contraindicated in patients with established ischemic heart disease and cerebrovascular disease. They should be used with caution in patients with risk factors for cardiovascular disease including hypertension, hyperlipidemia, smoking, and diabetes mellitus (Abdulla et al, 2013). It is recommended that when NSAIDs are used in elderly patients, it is for the shortest time necessary where benefits outweigh the associated risks.

Opioids

When pain increases, persists, or causes functional impairment, opioids may be an appropriate option for geriatric pain management (Makris et al., 2014). Prescribers are often hesitant to start geriatric patients on opioids due to concerns for adverse effects, including respiratory depression and falls. However, opioids can be a viable option for moderate to severe pain when started at low doses and monitored closely. Studies have demonstrated that opiate requirements decline with age (Fine, 2001). Slow titration is often necessary to find the optimal dose for geriatric patients while avoiding unwanted adverse effects. Patients who are opioid-naïve should start with short-acting opioid analgesics. If pain is persistent, it may require an extended release opioid to provide around-the-clock pain relief. Short-acting opioids should be given with long-acting opioids for breakthrough pain (Horgas, 2017). Nonopioid analgesics should be continued along with opioids to limit the number of opioids needed. However, it should be noted that some opioids come in combination with acetaminophen or NSAIDs, and maximum daily doses of these products should be carefully monitored.

Common adverse effects associated with opioids include sedation, dizziness, pruritus, nausea and vomiting, urinary retention, and constipation (Podichetty, Mazanec, & Biscup, 2003). We expect most adverse effects to resolve after 2 or 3 days of therapy; however, constipation will not resolve and often requires patients to be on a stimulant laxative while taking opioids (Abdulla et al., 2013). Opioid therapy for chronic, noncancer pain in elderly adults has been associated with increased risk of falls, fall-related injuries, hospitalization, and all-cause mortality (O'Neil et al., 2012).

Opioids work by binding to μ, κ, and δ opioid receptors found in varying locations throughout the body (Borsheski & Johnson, 2014). Tolerance to opioids may occur over time via receptor upregulation, meaning higher doses of opioids will be required over time to provide the same level of efficacy (Borsheski & Johnson, 2014). Opioid absorption and distribution are generally not altered in older adults despite age-related changes in body composition (Naples, Gellad, & Hanlon, 2016). An exception to this is morphine, which has greater absorption in older patients than younger patients (Fine, 2001). However, age-related changes in metabolism are more apparent. All opioids are metabolized by the liver. Table 23.1 specifies which opioids undergo phase I and phase II metabolism. Decreased systemic clearance and therefore increased elimination half-life may occur due to age-related decreases in CYP3A4

TABLE 23.1 Pharmacology and Dosing of Opioid Medications for Pain Management

Generic Drug	Serum Half-Life	Metabolism	Active Metabolite	Excretion
Codeine	~3 hours	Phase I, CYP2D6	Morphine	Urine (~90%, ~10% unchanged drug); feces
Hydrocodone/APAP	~4 hours	Phase I, CYP2D6	Hydromorphone	Urine (~12% unchanged drug, ~88% as metabolites)
Oxycodone	3.2–4 hours (immediate release)	Phase I, CYP3A4	Oxymorphone and noroxycodone	Urine (~19% as parent drug, >64% as metabolites)
Morphine	2–4 hours (immediate release)	Phase II, UGT	Morphine-3-glucuronide and morphine-6-glucuronide	Urine (~2%–12% excreted unchanged); feces (~7%–10%)
Hydromorphone	2–3 hours (immediate release)	Phase II, UGT	Hydromorphone-3-glucuronide	Urine (primarily as glucuronide conjugates, ~7% unchanged)
Fentanyl	20–27 hours (transdermal patch)	Phase I, CYP3A4	None	Urine 75% (primarily as metabolites, ~7%–10% unchanged drug)
Methadone	8–59 hours	Phase I, CYP3A4	None	Urine (<10% as unchanged drug), increased with urine pH <6
Buprenorphine	~37 hours (sublingual tablet), ~26 hours (transdermal patch)	Phase I, CYP3A4	None	Feces (~70%, 33% as unchanged drug); urine (~27%, 1% as unchanged drug)
Oxymorphone	~7–9 hours (immediate release)	Phase II, UGT	6 hydroxy-oxymorphone	Urine (<1% as unchanged drug); feces
Tapentadol	~4 hours (immediate release)	Phase II, UGT	Tapentadol O-glucuronide	Urine (99%: 70% metabolites, 3% unchanged drug)

CYP, cytochrome P450; UGT, uridine 5'-diphospho-glucuronosyltransferase.

Source: Data from Naples, J. G., Gellad, W. F., & Hanlon, J. T. (2016). The role of opioid analgesics in geriatric pain management. *Clinics in Geriatric Medicine, 32*(4), 725–735. doi:10.1016/j.cger.2016.06.006; Lexicomp. (2018). Lexicomp Online. Retrieved from https://online.lexi.com/lco/action/home

(FDA, 2015). All opioids are eliminated by the kidneys, and renal function is often reduced with age. Decline in renal function may lead to opioid toxicity due to the accumulation of active metabolic by-products (Naples et al., 2016). This is especially true for meperidine, which should be avoided in geriatric patients.

Patients should be educated on responsible medication use when prescribed opioids. They should be encouraged to store opioids in a locked box to minimize risk for diversion. A history of substance abuse should be taken into consideration prior to prescribing opioids as this is a strong predictor of opioid misuse (Ives et al., 2006). Urine drug screens, pain agreements, and distribution of naloxone kits should be utilized on a regular basis for safety and monitoring while patients are prescribed opioids. Additionally, patients should be educated not to drive or operate machinery after taking opioids. If goals are not met by opioids, patients experience intolerable adverse effects, or if misuse occurs, patients should be assisted with a slow taper off opioids.

Adjuvants

"Adjuvant" pain medications are medications that can be added to pain regimens or be used alone for their unique mechanisms of action that may provide analgesic benefit. Adjuvants are often utilized to target neuropathic pain from a wide variety of etiologies (e.g., diabetic peripheral neuropathy, postherpetic neuralgia, central poststroke pain, phantom limb pain) or other refractory, persistent pain (Kaye, Baluch, & Scott, 2010). The most common medication classes utilized for adjuvant therapy are antidepressants, anticonvulsants, and muscle relaxants.

As many older adults with chronic pain may experience comorbid depression, antidepressants may be used for their synergistic effects on pain as well as depression (Makris et al., 2014). The exact mechanism for antidepressant use in pain is not fully known, but antidepressants are thought to exert their therapeutic effects by inhibition of neurotransmitters (e.g., serotonin and norepinephrine) as well as by acting on histamine receptors and sodium channels (Gallagher, 2006). The antidepressants that are most efficacious for the management of chronic neuropathic pain are tricyclic antidepressants (TCAs) and serotonin and norepinephrine reuptake inhibitors (SNRIs). TCAs should generally be avoided in geriatric patients due to the increased risk of adverse effects such as anticholinergic effects and cognitive impairment (American Geriatrics Society, 2015). SNRIs are generally well tolerated by older adults and have fewer adverse effects than TCAs (Marcum et al., 2016). Venlafaxine is associated with increased blood pressure; therefore, duloxetine is preferred in patients with a history of hypertension (Marcum et al., 2016).

Anticonvulsants such as gabapentin and pregabalin were initially indicated for seizures, but have been shown effective in treating neuropathic pain (Jensen, 2002). Gabapentin and pregabalin work by binding to the alpha-2-delta subunit of the calcium channels in the CNS (Marcum et al., 2016). Gabapentin and pregabalin have been shown to have similar efficacy in pain reduction (Ziegler & Fonseca, 2015). Common adverse effects include dizziness, drowsiness, fatigue, weight gain, and peripheral edema. Both agents are excreted primarily renally and should be monitored and dose adjusted in patients with renal impairment (American Geriatrics Society, 2015).

Skeletal muscle relaxants can fall into one of two categories: antispasticity agents and antispasmodics (Witenko et al., 2014). The use of these agents is associated with sedation and confusion, which can lead to an increase in falls (Spence, Shin, Lee, & Gibbs, 2013). For this reason, the 2015 Beers Criteria considered muscle relaxants (including cyclobenzaprine, carisoprodol, methocarbamol, and metaxalone) high-risk medications in older adults (American Geriatrics Society, 2015). Baclofen is one centrally acting muscle relaxant not included in the Beers criteria because it has a decreased occurrence of CNS depression and is generally better tolerated than other muscle relaxants (Marcum et al., 2016). Additionally, tizanidine is a centrally acting alpha-2-adrenergic agonist that increases the inhibition of presynaptic motor neurons (Marcum et al., 2016). The use of tizanidine is limited in older adults due to adverse effects and the possibility of prolonged QT intervals (Marcum et al., 2016).

Table 23.2 outlines the pharmacology and dosing of various nonopioid medications for pain management in older adults.

Topicals

Topical agents can be a safe and effective option for pain in localized areas. The topical route of administration is advantageous in the geriatric population as it decreases the likelihood of adverse effects, drug–drug interactions, and overall pill burden (Kaestli, Wasilewski-Rasca, Bonnabry, & Vogt-Ferrier, 2008). However, absorption of transdermal medications can be affected in elderly patients due to decreased skin hydration, tissue thickness, and surface lipids on the skin (Kaestli et al., 2008). Commonly used topical pain medications include menthol, capsaicin, lidocaine, and diclofenac.

Menthol/methyl salicylate is available in a variety of creams, gels, patches, and so on over the counter. Menthol can provide pain relief by causing a cooling sensation and counterirritant effects (Topp, Brosky, & Pieschel, 2013). Capsaicin is derived from hot peppers and is available over the counter as a cream or by prescription as a patch. Capsaicin works to reduce pain by decreasing substance P and desensitizing epidermal nociceptive nerves (Argoff & Viscusi, 2014). Patients may initially experience burning but if tolerated, they should apply it consistently 3 to 4 times daily, and the burning should subside within 1 to 2 weeks (Argoff & Viscusi, 2014). Capsaicin has been shown effective in postherpetic neuralgia, diabetic neuropathy, and osteoarthritis (Rains & Bryson, 1995).

Lidocaine is available in various topical formulations and decreases pain by blocking sodium ion channels and stopping afferent pain signals (Argoff & Viscusi, 2014). The lidocaine patch should be applied for 12 hours and removed for 12 hours for the greatest efficacy. The American Geriatrics Society recommends utilizing lidocaine for neuropathic pain (American Geriatrics Society, 2009). The final topical option is diclofenac gel, which is the first topical NSAID approved by the U.S. FDA. Diclofenac gel is often utilized for musculoskeletal pain or inflammatory arthritis (Zacher et al., 2008). A systemic review showed that topical NSAIDs are almost as effective as oral NSAIDs and carry a lower risk of severe adverse effects including GI toxicity (Makris, Kohler, & Fraenkel, 2010). With all topical medications, patients should be educated not to apply the medication to open skin as this may increase systemic absorption (Marcum et al., 2016).

Table 23.3 provides an overview of common topical agents.

NONPHARMACOLOGICAL THERAPY

Nonpharmacologic options are increasingly popular for managing pain in geriatric patients in order to avoid polypharmacy, adverse effects, and drug–drug interactions (Makris et al., 2014). The long-term efficacy of nonpharmacologic interventions in elderly patients as well as their ability to sustain their use is not well-known. However, there is often little risk involved with trialing these techniques, and they may offer significant benefit to patients. Some of the commonly used nonpharmacologic interventions for pain include physical therapy, osteopathic manipulation, massage therapy, transcutaneous electrical nerve stimulation (TENS) unit, acupuncture, biofeedback, cognitive behavioral therapy, and psychotherapy (Borsheski & Johnson, 2014). These techniques may be used alone or in combination with medications to help with pain management. The success of these interventions often depends on the type of pain that the patient has as well as the patient's capabilities.

Pain Management | 217

TABLE 23.2 Pharmacology and Dosing of Nonopioid Medications for Pain Management

Generic Drug (Trade Name)	Serum Half-Life	Protein Binding	Metabolism	Dosing	Renal Dosing Adjustment	Hepatic Dosing Adjustment
Acetaminophen (Tylenol)	2–3 hours	10%–25%	Hepatic conjugation	≤4,000 mg/day	GFR 10–50: administer every 6 hours; GFR <10: administer every 8 hours	Use with caution; most experts recommend avoiding when possible and if used, limiting it to short-term use at doses ≤2 g/day
Ibuprofen (Advil)	~2 hours	>99%	Oxidation	1,200 to 2,400 mg/day (maximum of 3,200 mg/day)	eGFR 30–59: avoid use in patients with intercurrent disease, which increases risk of AKI; eGFR <30: avoid use	No dosage adjustments
Celecoxib (Celebrex)	~11 hours	~97%	CYP2C9	100 to 200 mg twice daily	Use not recommended in severe impairment or with advanced renal disease	Moderate impairment: reduce dose by 50%, severe impairment or abnormal liver function tests: use is not recommended
Amitriptyline (Elavil)	~13–36 hours	>90%	Rapid hepatic metabolism to demethylation to nortriptyline	Start 10 mg/day, titrate as tolerated	Use with caution due to renal elimination	Use with caution due to hepatic metabolism

(continued)

TABLE 23.2 Pharmacology and Dosing of Nonopioid Medications for Pain Management (*continued*)

Generic Drug (Trade Name)	Serum Half-Life	Protein Binding	Metabolism	Dosing	Renal Dosing Adjustment	Hepatic Dosing Adjustment
Duloxetine (Cymbalta)	~12 hours	>90%	CYP1A2, CYP2D6	Start at 30–60 mg/day, titrate to 60–120 mg/day	Avoid use if CrCl <30 mL/min	Avoid use in hepatic impairment
Gabapentin (Neurontin)	~5–7 hours	<3%	Not metabolized	Start at 300 mg/day TID, titrate to 1,800–3,600 mg/day TID	CrCl >30–59: 200–700 mg BID CrCl >15–29: 200–700 mg once daily CrCl 15: 100 to 300 mg once daily CrCl <15: reduce daily dose in proportion to CrCl	No dosag adjustments
Pregabalin (Lyrica)	6.3 hours	0%	Negligible	Start at 150 mg/day BID, titrate to 150–300 mg/day BID to TID	CrCl 30–60: 75–300 mg/day CrCl 15–30: 25–150 mg/day CrCl <15: 25–75 mg/day	No dosage adjustments

Baclofen	3.75 ± 0.96 hours	30%	Hepatic (15% of dose)	5 mg 2–3 times/day (maximum of 80 mg/day)	CrCl 50–80: start at 5 mg Q12H CrCl 30–49: start at 2.5 mg Q8H CrCl <30: start at 2.5 mg Q12H	No dosage adjustments
Tizanidine	~2.5 hours	~30%	CYP1A2	Start at 2 mg <3 times/day, titrate as tolerated (maximum of 36 mg/day)	CrCl <25: use reduced doses and with caution	Avoid use in hepatic impairment; if used, reduce doses

AKI, acute kidney injury; BID, two times per day; CrCl, creatinine clearance; CYP, cytochrome P450; eGFR, estimated glomerular filtration rate; GFR, glomerular filtration rate; TID, three times per day.

Source: Data from Marcum, Z. A., Duncan, N. A., & Makris, U. E. (2016). Pharmacotherapies in geriatric chronic pain management. *Clinics in Geriatric Medicine, 32*(4), 705–724. doi:10.1016/j.cger.2016.06.007; Bosilkovska, M., Walder, B., Besson, M., Daali, Y., & Desmeules, J. (2012). Analgesics in Patients with Hepatic Impairment. *Drugs, 72*(12), 1645–1669. doi:10.2165/11635500-000000000-00000; Lexicomp. (2018). Lexicomp Online. Retrieved from https://online.lexi.com/lco/action/home

TABLE 23.3 Topical Agents for Pain Management

Generic Name (Trade Name)	Preparation Strength	Formulations	Application Instructions	Absorption
Menthol/M-salicylate topical (Icy Hot, BenGay, Salonpas Arthritis Pain)	Methyl salicylate 10% Menthol 1.5%–3%	Cream, foam, patch, spray, balm, stick	Apply 3–4 times daily, leave patch in place for no more than 8 hours	Relatively low systemic exposure
Capsaicin (Zostrix, Salonpas Gel Patch, Qutenza)	0.025%–8%	Cream, gel, lotion, patch	Apply 3 to 4 times daily, leave patch in place for no more than 8 hours	Transient and low (<5 ng/mL)
Lidocaine topical (Lidoderm, Xylocaine)	2%–5%	Cream, gel, jelly, lotion, ointment, patch	Apply to skin 3–4 times daily, apply patch for 12 hours on and 12 hours off	3% ± 2% following application of 3 patches
Diclofenac topical (Voltaren, Flector, Pennsaid)	1%–3%	Cream, gel, solution, patch	Apply to affected area 4 times daily (lower extremities: 4 g with max of 16 g per joint per day, upper extremities: 2 g with max of 8 g per joint per day)	3% gel absorbs 6% to 10%

Source: Data from Marcum, Z. A., Duncan, N. A., & Makris, U. E. (2016). Pharmacotherapies in geriatric chronic pain management. *Clinics in Geriatric Medicine, 32*(4), 705–724. doi:10.1016/j.cger.2016.06.007; Lexicomp. (2018). Lexicomp Online. Retrieved from https://online.lexi.com/lco/action/home

Psychological factors play a major role in how patients interpret, respond to, and cope with pain. This is why pharmacological therapy may not be completely effective in managing all types of pain (Abdulla et al., 2013). Depression is common in geriatric patients, and it is important to acknowledge the association between chronic pain and depression (Abdulla et al., 2013). Cognitive behavioral therapy aims to modify the patient's beliefs and attitudes and increase the patient's control over pain and how he or she manages it (Eccleston, Williams, & Morley, 2009). The limited and weak evidence available that examined the effects of mindfulness and meditation in older adults with chronic back pain found that they experienced less pain, better sleep, and improved quality of life (Green, Hadjistavropoulos, & Sharpe, 2008). Additionally, guided imagery and biofeedback may be helpful for providing relaxation, but there is limited evidence for their efficacy.

Remaining physically active and participating in exercise are important factors in managing persistent pain in older adults. Reduced levels of fitness and function can lead to increased levels of disability (Abdulla et al., 2013). There is a wide variety of beneficial exercises that can be done including walking, resistance exercise, hydrotherapy, tai chi, and yoga. Acupuncture has shown positive benefits in a few small randomized controlled trials; however, the duration of effect may be short term (Williamson, Wyatt, Yein, & Melton, 2007). Some evidence suggests age-related changes may limit the use of TENS units in older populations, and they should therefore be utilized in combination with other therapies if trialed (Miller, Hickman, & Lemasters, 1992). Additionally, gentle massage has been found to help with pain and anxiety in older patients with chronic pain living at long-term care facilities (Sansome & Schmitt, 2004).

SUMMARY

Chronic and acute pain can have a major impact on function and quality of life in older adults. Assessing pain can be a barrier to appropriate treatment in this patient population. Finding the right pain management treatment option involves closely assessing patients when initiating therapy, titrating doses slowly, and monitoring for adverse effects. Sometimes the best treatment may be encouraging movement and nonpharmacologic therapy options.

PAIN INTERPROFESSIONAL CASE STUDY

Phyllis Brown Whitehead

Patient Presentation

Paul is a 77-year-old Caucasian male who has been receiving home healthcare for the previous 5 weeks. His daughter, Nancy, contacts you regarding his symptoms of increased confusion and fall. You instruct his daughter to take Paul to the ED for further evaluation. This will be his third ED visit in 3 weeks. During intake, his daughter, Nancy, reports Paul has been more confused, eating and drinking less. She also states that the falling and pain have increased. According to Nancy, Paul has been having more difficulty sleeping and has been complaining of severe right hip pain.

History

His past medical history includes early-stage dementia (diagnosed in 2013), hypertension, CKD stage 3 (glomerular filtration rate [GFR] 30–59 mL/min), coronary artery heart disease, chronic diastolic heart failure, diabetes, and osteoarthritis.

Medications

Paul's medications include amlodipine, metoprolol, lisinopril, metformin, naproxen as needed for pain, and hydrocodone as needed for severe pain.

Physical Exam

ED exam: His review of systems revealed no fevers, chest pain, or shortness of breath. On physical exam, he is confused and restless. Paul complains of severe pain and weakness. His heart rhythm and rate are regular and radial pulses are intact with no pulse deficit. His pedal pulses are difficult to palpate due to the 1+ edema. Paul is not able to quantify his pain on the 1–10 pain intensity scale but is able to state it is moderate to severe in his right hip and bilateral feet. Contusions are noted on his right hip and thigh.

Diagnostic Testing

During the ED evaluation, a complete blood count (CBC), comprehensive metabolic panel (CMP), vitamin D, magnesium, phosphorus, and A1C are obtained. His creatinine shows an increasing trend with a calculated GFR of 16 mL/min/1.73 m^2, A1C is 7, and his vitamin D, magnesium, calcium, and phosphorus are stable. A right hip x-ray is ordered to rule out fracture and/or dysplasia. The findings are unremarkable.

Plan of Care

Inpatient plan of care: Paul is admitted to the progressive care unit (PCU) for confusion, dehydration, hip pain, and deconditioning. The hospitalist team is concerned that Paul has been taking too high a dose of hydrocodone, which has been contributing to his imbalance, falling, and confusion. They also consider a diagnosis of diabetic peripheral neuropathy, which is contributing to his insomnia and pain. They assess him using behavioral pain assessment tools such as the Pain Assessment in Advanced Dementia Scale (PAINAD). Cognitive changes, including delirium, are evaluated using tools such as the Mini-Mental State Exam (MMSE), the Short Portable Mental Status Questionnaire (SPMSQ), the Delirium Observation Screening Scale, and the Confusion Assessment Method (CAM). While hospitalized, Paul has fluctuating delirium, which worsens at nighttime and with the use of opioids.

Interprofessional Collaboration

Paul has one living daughter, Nancy, who has been caring for her father for the past 12 years, first at Paul's home and then at her home. She shares that the patient has been living with her for the past 5 years. His wife and siblings are deceased. Nancy is married with two adult children and four adult grandchildren. She is solely responsible for Paul's care and shares that her husband has expressed frustration that she is spending all of her time with Paul. She is considering nursing home placement because she can no longer care for him. A social worker is contacted to assist Nancy in disposition planning.

While Paul is hospitalized, interprofessional rounds with the attending physician, the pain clinical nurse specialist, bedside nurse, social worker, and pharmacist occur to better integrate Paul's care. They find that his pain is better controlled with bed rest although he continues to be restless and groans when repositioned. The pharmacist expresses concern about the use of an NSAID even short term and recommends stopping it. The pharmacist also suggests a low dose of gabapentin at bedtime to help with the diabetic peripheral neuropathy and insomnia. The clinical nurse specialist suggests adding scheduled vitamin D, magnesium, and Tylenol and the use of non-pharmacological interventions such as heat and cold therapies and massage for the patient's hip pain. The clinical nurse specialist suggests minimizing the use of opioids and lowering the dose to 2.5 mg due to the patient's delirium. On discharge, she provides a pain management plan with the medication changes and instructions for assessing Paul's function and cognition using the

Clinically Aligned Pain Assessment (CAPA) tool, Minimum Data Set 2 (MDS-2), or the Functional Assessment Staging Tool (FAST). You plan to follow her recommendations to continue to optimize functioning and pain management.

When you see him in the outpatient setting for hospital follow-up, you discuss multiple strategies to help Paul and his daughter cope with cognitive changes. The hospital social worker was able to locate an assisted living facility with therapy services in-house. In addition to the changed living circumstances, he was referred to a local center for healthy aging to optimize management of his dementia and functionality.

You discuss physical therapy for gait training, strengthening, and pain management. The physical therapist suggests a TENS unit for Paul's hip pain. With improved pain management, Paul makes good progress in gait training with the use of a walker, and he is less confused. With improved pain management, Paul's appetite also increases.

As you follow up with Paul regularly, you initiate end-of-life discussions with Paul and his daughter. His daughter is his power of attorney, and he signed a do-not-resuscitate (DNR) order several years ago. In addition to these decisions, you describe the care options available, such as palliative care and hospice, for continued quality of life and a smooth transition to end-of-life care.

Case Study References

American Geriatric Society Panel. (2009). Pharmacological management of persistent pain in older persons. *Journal of the American Geriatrics Society*, 57(8), 1331–1346. doi:10.1111/j.1532-5415.2009.02376.x

Chang, A., Bijur, P. E., Esses, D., Barnaby, D. P., & Baer, J. (2017) Effect of a single dose of oral opioid and non-opioid analgesics on acute extremity pain in the ED. *Journal of the American Medical Association*, 318(17), 1661–1667. doi:10.1001/jama.2017.16190

Donaldson, G., & Chapman, C.R. (2013). *Pain management is more than just a number*. Salt Lake City: University of Utah Health/Department of Anesthesiology.

Dowell, D., Haegerich, T. M., & Chou, R. (2016). CDC guideline for prescribing opioids for chronic pain. *Morbidity and Mortality Weekly Report:Recommendations and Reports*, 65(1), 1–49. doi:http://dx.doi.org/10.15585/mmwr.rr6501e1

Gloth, FM, III., Scheve, A. A., Stober, C. V., Chow, S., & Prosser, J. (2002). The *Functional Pain Scale*: Reliability, validity, and responsiveness in an elderly population. *Journal of the American Medical Directors Association*, 3(2 Suppl.), S71–S75. doi:10.1016/S1525-8610(04)70443-0

Ives, T., Chelminski, P., Hammet-Stabler, C., Malone, R., Perhac, J., Potisek, N., . . . Pignone, M. (2006). Predictors of opioid misuse in patients with chronic pain: A prospective cohort study. *BMC Health Services Research*, 6(1). doi:10.1186/1472-6963-6-46

Malec, M., & Shega, J. (2015). Pain management in the elderly. *Medical Clinics of North America*, 99, 337–350. doi:10.1016/j.mcna.2014.11.007

National Alliance of Advocates for Buprenorphine Treatment. (2008). The Words We Use Matter. Reducing Stigma through Language. Retrieved from https://www.naabt.org/documents/NAABT_Language.pdf

National Institute on Drug Abuse. (2014). NIDA Quick Screen V1.0. Retrieved from https://www.drugabuse.gov/sites/default/files/files/QuickScreen_Updated_2013%281%29.pdf

Project Know. (2017). Addiction glossary of terms, phrases, and definitions. Retrieved from http://projectknow.com/research/addiction-glossary-of-terms-and-phrases

Topham, D., & Drew, D. (2017). Quality improvement project: Replacing the numeric rating scale with a CAPA tool. *Pain Management Nursing, 18*(6), 363–371. doi:10.1016/j.pmn.2017.07.001

REFERENCES

Abdulla, A., Adams, N., Bone, M., Elliott, A. M., Gaffin, J., Jones, D., . . . British Geriatric Society. (2013). Guidance on the management of pain in older people. *Age and Ageing, 42*(Suppl. 1), i1–i57. doi:10.1093/ageing/afs200

American Geriatrics Society Beers Criteria Update Expert Panel. (2015). American Geriatrics Society 2015 updated Beers Criteria for potentially inappropriate medication use in older adults. *Journal of the American Geriatrics Society, 63*(11), 2227–2246. doi:10.1111/jgs.13702

American Geriatrics Society Panel on Pharmacological Management of Persistent Pain in Older Persons. (2009). Pharmacological management of persistent pain in older persons. *Journal of the American Geriatrics Society, 57*(8), 1331–1346. doi:10.1111/j.1532-5415.2009.02376.x

Argoff, C. E., & Viscusi, E. R. (2014). The use of opioid analgesics for chronic pain: Minimizing the risk for harm. *The American Journal of Gastroenterology Supplements, 2*(1), 3–8. doi:10.1038/ajgsup.2014.3

Boers, M., Tangelder, M. J. D., van Ingen, H., Fort, J. G., & Goldstein, J. L. (2007). The rate of NSAID-induced endoscopic ulcers increases linearly but not exponentially with age: A pooled analysis of 12 randomised trials. *Annals of the Rheumatic Diseases, 66*(3), 417–418. doi:10.1136/ard.2006.055012

Borsheski, R., & Johnson, Q. L. (2014). Pain management in the geriatric population. *Missouri Medicine, 111*(6): 508–511. Retrieved from https://www.ncbi.nlm.nih.gov/pmc/articles/PMC6173536

Bosilkovska, M., Walder, B., Besson, M., Daali, Y., & Desmeules, J. (2012). Analgesics in patients with hepatic impairment. *Drugs, 72*(12), 1645–1669. doi:10.2165/11635500-000000000-00000

Cavalieri, T. A. (2002). Pain management in the elderly. *The Journal of the American Osteopathic Association, 102*, 481–485. Retrieved from https://jaoa.org/article.aspx?articleid=2092643

Eccleston, C., Williams, A. C., & Morley, S. (2009). Psychological therapies for the management of chronic pain (excluding headache) in adults. *Cochrane Database of Systematic Reviews*, (4), CD007407. doi:10.1002/14651858.CD007407.pub2

Ferrell, B. A. (Ed). (2001). Pain management in the elderly. *Clinics in Geriatric Medicine, 17*, 417–615.

Fine, P. G. (2001). Opioid analgesic drugs in older people. *Clinics in Geriatric Medicine, 17*(3), 479–487. doi:10.1016/s0749-0690(05)70081-1

Gallagher, R. M. (2006). Management of neuropathic pain. *The Clinical Journal of Pain, 22*(Suppl.), S2–S8. doi:10.1097/01.ajp.0000193827.07453.d6

Green, S. M., Hadjistavropoulos, T., & Sharpe, D. (2008). Client personality characteristics predict satisfaction with cognitive behavior therapy. *Journal of Clinical Psychology, 64*(1), 40–51. doi:10.1002/jclp.20429

Greenberger, N. J. (1996). Update in gastroenterology. *Annals of Internal Medicine, 12*, 489–500.

G.D. Searle LLC Division of Pzifer Inc. (2018). Celebrex (celecoxib): Highlights of prescribing information. Retrieved from https://www.accessdata.fda.gov/drugsatfda_docs/label/2018/020998s050lbl.pdf#page=21

Griffin, M. R. (1998). Epidemiology of nonsteroidal antiinflammatory drug–associated gastrointestinal injury. *The American Journal of Medicine, 104*(3 Suppl. 1), 23S–29S. doi:10.1016/s0002-9343(97)00207-6

Horgas, A. L. (2017). Pain management in older adults. *Nursing Clinics of North America, 52*(4), e1–e7. doi:10.1016/j.cnur.2017.08.001

Ives, T. J., Chelminski, P. R., Hammett-Stabler, C. A., Malone, R. M., Perhac, J. S., Potisek, N. M., ... Pignone, M. P. (2006). Predictors of opioid misuse in patients with chronic pain: A prospective cohort study. *BMC Health Services Research, 6*(1). doi:10.1186/1472-6963-6-46. Retrieved from https://bmchealthservres.biomedcentral.com/articles/10.1186/1472-6963-6-46

Jensen, T. S. (2002). Anticonvulsants in neuropathic pain: Rationale and clinical evidence. *European Journal of Pain, 6*(Suppl. A), 61–68. doi:10.1053/eujp.2001.0324

Kaestli, L.-Z., Wasilewski-Rasca, A.-F., Bonnabry, P., & Vogt-Ferrier, N. (2008). Use of transdermal drug formulations in the elderly. *Drugs & Aging, 25*(4), 269–280. doi:10.2165/00002512-200825040-00001

Kaye, A. D., Baluch, A., & Scott, J. T. (2010). Pain management in the elderly population: A review. *Ochsner Journal, 10*(3), 179–187. Retrieved from http://www.ochsnerjournal.org/content/10/3/179

Makris, U. E., Abrams, R. C., Gurland, B., & Reid, M. C. (2014). Management of persistent pain in the older patient: A clinical review. *Journal of the American Medical Association, 312*(8), 825–836. doi:10.1001/jama.2014.9405

Makris, U. E., Kohler, M. J., & Fraenkel, L. (2010). Adverse effects of topical nonsteroidal antiinflammatory drugs in older adults with osteoarthritis: A systematic literature review. *The Journal of Rheumatology, 37*(6), 1236–1243. doi:10.3899/jrheum.090935

Marcum, Z. A., Duncan, N. A., & Makris, U. E. (2016). Pharmacotherapies in geriatric chronic pain management. *Clinics in Geriatric Medicine, 32*(4), 705–724. doi:10.1016/j.cger.2016.06.007

Merskey, H., & Bogduk, N. (1994). *Taxonomy of pain terms & definitions.* Seattle, WA: International Association for the Study of Pain Press.

Miller, A. C., Hickman, L. C., & Lemasters, G. K. (1992). A distraction technique for control of burn pain. *Journal of Burn Care & Rehabilitation, 13*(5), 276–280. doi:10.1097/00004630-199209000-00012

Naples, J. G., Gellad, W. F., & Hanlon, J. T. (2016). The role of opioid analgesics in geriatric pain management. *Clinics in Geriatric Medicine, 32*(4), 725–735. doi:10.1016/j.cger.2016.06.006

Nicholson, B. (2006). Differential diagnosis: Nociceptive and neuropathic pain. *American Journal of Managed Care, 12*(9 Suppl.), S256–S262. Retrieved from https://www.ajmc.com/journals/supplement/2006/2006-06-vol12-n9suppl/jun06-2326ps256-s262

Nikolaus, T., & Zeyfang, A. (2004). Pharmacological treatments for persistent non-malignant pain in older persons. *Drugs & Aging, 21*(1), 19–41. doi:10.2165/00002512-200421010-00003

O'Neil, C. K., Hanlon, J. T., & Marcum, Z. A. (2012). Adverse effects of analgesics commonly used by older adults with osteoarthritis: Focus on non-opioid and opioid analgesics. *The American Journal of Geriatric Pharmacotherapy, 10*(6), 331–342. doi:10.1016/j.amjopharm.2012.09.004

Pergolizzi, J., Böger, R. H., Budd, K., Dahan, A., Erdine, S., Hans, G., ... Sacerdote, P. (2008). Opioids and the management of chronic severe pain in the elderly: Consensus statement of an international expert panel with focus on the six clinically most often used World Health Organization step III opioids (Buprenorphine, Fentanyl, Hydromorphone, Methadone, Morphine, Oxycodone). *Pain Practice, 8*(4), 287–313. doi:10.1111/j.1533-2500.2008.00204.x

Pharmacia & Upjohn Company: Division of Pfizer Inc.. (2007). Motrin- Ibuprofen Tablets, USP Medication Guide. Retrieved from http://www.accessdata.fda.gov/drugsatfda_docs/label/2007/017463s105lbl.pdf

Podichetty, V. K., Mazanec, D. J., & Biscup, R. S. (2003). Chronic non-malignant musculoskeletal pain in older adults: Clinical issues and opioid intervention. *Postgraduate Medical Journal, 79*(937), 627–633. doi:10.1136/pmj.79.937.627

Rains, C., & Bryson, H. M. (1995). Topical capsaicin. *Drugs & Aging, 7*(4), 317–328. doi:10.2165/00002512-199507040-00007

Sansome, P., & Schmitt, L. (2004). Providing tender touch massage to elderly nursing home residents: A demonstration project. *Geriatric Nursing Midwifery, 10*, 209–216. doi:10.1067/mgn.2000.108261

Spence, M. M., Shin, P. J., Lee, E. A., & Gibbs, N. E. (2013). Risk of injury associated with skeletal muscle relaxant use in older adults. *Annals of Pharmacotherapy, 47*(7–8), 993–998. doi:10.1345/aph.1r735

Topp, R., Brosky, J. A., & Pieschel, D. (2013). The effect of either topical menthol or a placebo on functioning and knee pain among patients with knee OA. *Journal of Geriatric Physical Therapy, 36*(2), 92–99. doi:10.1519/jpt.0b013e318268dde1

U.S. Food and Drug Administration. (2015). FDA strengthens warning that non-aspirin nonsteroidal anti-inflammatory drugs (NSAIDs) can cause heart attacks or strokes. Retrieved from http://www.fda.gov/Drugs/DrugSafety/ucm451800.htm

Williamson, L., Wyatt, M. R., Yein, K., & Melton, J. T. K. (2007). Severe knee osteoarthritis: A randomized controlled trial of acupuncture, physiotherapy (supervised exercise) and standard management for patients awaiting knee replacement. *Rheumatology, 46*(9), 1445–1449. doi:10.1093/rheumatology/kem119

Witenko, C., Moorman-li, R., Motycka, C., Duane, K., Hincapie-Castillo, J., Leonard, P., & Valaer, C. (2014). Considerations for the appropriate use of skeletal muscle relaxants for the management of acute low back pain. *P & T, 39*(6), 427–435. Retrieved from https://www.ncbi.nlm.nih.gov/pmc/articles/PMC4103716

Lexicomp. (2018). Lexicomp Online. Retrieved from https://online.lexi.com/lco/action/home

Zacher, J., Altman, R., Bellamy, N., Brühlmann, P., Da Silva, J., Huskisson, E., & Taylor, R. S. (2008). Topical diclofenac and its role in pain and inflammation: An evidence-based review. *Current Medical Research and Opinion, 24*(4), 925–950. doi:10.1185/030079908x273066

Ziegler, D., & Fonseca, V. (2015). From guideline to patient: A review of recent recommendations for pharmacotherapy of painful diabetic neuropathy. *Journal of Diabetes and Its Complications, 29*(1), 146–156. doi:10.1016/j.jdiacomp.2014.08.008

24 Renal Impairments

Abimbola Farinde and Megan Hebdon

OBJECTIVES
1. Discuss the anatomy of the renal system
2. Review what constitutes renal impairment and adjustments that need to be made in older adults
3. List and analyze drugs that require adjustment with renal impairment

INTRODUCTION
Renal function often declines with aging, and this may worsen due to chronic diseases such as hypertension and diabetes. In older adults, chronic kidney disease (CKD) with decreased renal function is an important factor for nurse practitioners to address medically and pharmacologically. Nurse practitioners must also consider renal excretion of drugs when prescribing medications and make appropriate dose adjustments for decreased renal function. This chapter provides an overview of prescribing considerations in renal disease.

RENAL ANATOMY
In order to fully understand the importance of dosing, it is vital to recognize the importance of the anatomy of the kidneys and how this can play a role in drug dosing and drug administration, especially in the geriatric population. The kidneys are viewed as paired retroperitoneal structures that are located between the transverse processes of T12–L3 vertebrae. The bean-shaped kidneys, about 4.5 inches long and 2.5 inches wide, are about the size of a closed fist (Schmidler, 2019). Even though the kidneys are small, they serve several important roles, which include filtration and excretion of metabolic wastes, the regulation of fluids, electrolytes, and acid–base balance, and the promotion of red blood cell production (Chalouhy, 2017). In addition, the kidney can serve to regulate an individual's blood pressure through the renin–angiotensin–aldosterone system and serve to control the reabsorption of water and aids with the maintenance of intravascular volume (Chalouhy, 2017). In general, the renal system is composed of the kidneys, ureters, urinary bladder, and urethra (Schmidler, 2019). All of these play an important role in the functionality of this organ.

RENAL IMPAIRMENT IN GERIATRIC POPULATION
With advancing age in various societies and the incidence of CKD is increasing consistently as well, the accurate monitoring of kidney function in this population

is of great clinical interest, especially to determine those who may be at risk for developing CKD (Fliser, 2008). After the age of 30, the glomerular filtration rate (GFR) begins to decline at a rate of 8 mL/min/1.73m² per decade, and the significance of age-related decline in kidney function has been thought to contribute to the effects of hypertension, atherosclerosis, and cardiovascular disease (Coresh, Astor, Greene, Eknoyan, & Levey, 2003). Additionally, research suggests that very elderly individuals (>80 years of age) with modest reductions in estimated GFR can have a higher prevalence of CKD-related complications (Phoon, 2012). With time, as estimated GFR gradually declines with less than 60 mL/min/1.73 m², there can also be an associated increase in the development of cardiovascular events and mortality.

RENAL IMPAIRMENT CATEGORIES

In most elderly people with CKD, the symptoms may not be apparent, but proper screening can include urinary albumin, serum estimated GFR, creatinine ratio, and blood pressure assessment (Phoon, 2012). There are currently five stages of CKD and GFR for each stage. In stage 1, an individual can present with normal or high GFR (>90 mL/min); in stage 2, there is mild CKD (GFR 60–89 mL/min); in stage 3A, there is moderate CKD (GFR 45–59 mL/min); in stage 3B, there is moderate CKD (GFR 30–44 mL/min); in stage 4, there is severe CKD (GFR 15–29 mL/min); and finally, stage 5 is regarded as end-stage CKD (GFR <15 mL/min).

RENAL DISORDERS

The use of the serum creatinine is considered to be an unreliable indication of the GFR in the elderly population, especially for those who may be sick or malnourished, which is why more reliable indicators such as timed creatinine clearance, serum creatinine–based equations such as Modification Diet in Renal Disease Formula, and serum cystatin C are utilized (Fliser, 2008).

While kidney disease may not have any specific symptoms, the two main risk factors for the development of CKD, which are known to contribute to two-thirds of the cases of this disease, are diabetes and high blood pressure. The presence of uncontrolled diabetes and blood pressure can contribute to kidney damage not only in the elderly population but in the general population (National Kidney Foundation, n.d.). Other diseases that have the ability to damage the kidneys include autoimmune disorders (e.g., systemic lupus erythematosus, scleroderma) or birth defects of the kidneys, injury to the kidney, or problems with the arteries that feed the kidneys (Silberberg, 2015).

RENALLY ADJUSTED DRUGS

There are a number of drugs that require renal adjustments based on the stage and severity of an individual's renal impairment, and this is even more important in the elderly population. The most notable physiological change that can occur in elderly individuals is with renal function. The kidneys can experience changes with blood flow, glomerular filtration, and nephron function decrease (Moini, 2013). As a result of a reduction in cardiac output and blood flow in the circulatory system, the kidneys can be impacted. By the age of 70, the blood flow to the kidneys can be reduced as much as 40% (Moini, 2013). Due to kidney dysfunction, the effectiveness of a particular drug dose can be reduced; or if a number of drugs are being administered, this can increase the effect of these drugs in an elderly individual; or if the renal system is decreased, the half-life of a drug can be extended resulting in drug toxicity (Moini, 2013). The drugs or drug classes in Table 24.1 require renal adjustment based on renal function (creatinine clearance value) or additional special considerations when given to elderly individuals.

RENIN–ANGIOTENSIN SYSTEM DRUGS

Renin–angiotensin system drugs such as angiotensin-converting enzyme inhibitors (ACE inhibitors) and angiotensin receptor blockers (ARBs) are widely acknowledged as renal protective drugs and are often the first-line hypertension treatment

TABLE 24.1 Drugs and Drug Classes Requiring Renal Adjustment Based on Creatinine Clearance

Drug/Drug Classes	Adjustment Based on CrCl
Aminoglycosides (gentamicin, tobramycin, amikacin)	Aminoglycosides Gentamicin: CrCl 10–50: give q12–48h; CrCl <10: give q48–72h; HD: give 1–1.7 mg/kg after dialysis Tobramycin: (conventional interval dosing) CrCl 50–70: give q8–24h; CrCl 10–50: give q24–48h; CrCl <10: give q48–72h; HD: give 50% usual dose after dialysis; PD: give supplement (extended interval dosing) CrCl 40–59: give q36h; CrCl 20–39: give q48h; CrCl <20: give 5–7 mg/kg ×1, then adjust dose based on serum levels Amikacin: CrCl 50–80: give q12–24h; CrCl 10–50: give q24–48h; CrCl <10: give q48–72h; HD: give supplement
Vancomycin	CrCl 50–90: 15 mg/kg ×1, then usual dose q12–24h; CrCl 10–50: 15 mg/kg ×1, then usual dose q24–96h; CrCl <10: 15 mg/kg ×1, then usual dose q4–7 days; HD: give supplement only if high-flux dialyzer used; PD: no supplement
Cephalosporins	Example: cephalexin CrCl 50–90: give q6–8h; CrCl 10–50: give q8–12h; CrCl <10: give q12–24h; HD: give dose after dialysis, no supplement; PD: no supplement
Penicillins	Example: nafcillin Consider decreasing dose if concomitant hepatic impairment; HD/PD: no supplement
Imipenem/Cilastatin	CrCl <70: see package insert; HD: give q12h after dialysis; PD: no supplement

(*continued*)

TABLE 24.1 Drugs and Drug Classes Requiring Renal Adjustment Based on Creatinine Clearance (*continued*)

Drug/Drug Classes	Adjustment Based on CrCl
Nonsteroidal anti-inflammatory agents	Example: aspirin CrCl <10: avoid use; HD: give dose after dialysis, no supplement; PD: no supplement
Chemotherapeutic agents	Example: mitomycin Stomach cancer, refractory (20 mg/m^2 IV ×1 on day 1 of 42- or 56-day cycle) Info: part of multidrug chemo regimen Pancreatic cancer, refractory (20 mg/m^2 IV ×1 on day 1 of 42- or 56-day cycle) Info: part of multidrug chemo regimen Cr >1.7: contraindicated
ACE inhibitors	Example: lisinopril (HTN) CrCl 10–30: start 5 mg QD, max 40 mg/day; CrCl <10: start 2.5 mg QD, max 40 mg/day; HD/PD: no supplement (CHF) CrCl <30: start 2.5 mg QD, max 40 mg/day; HD/PD: no supplement (MI) CrCl <30: start 2.5 mg QD, max 40 mg/day; HD/PD: no supplement
Fluoroquinolones (ciprofloxacin, levofloxacin,)	Ciprofloxacin: (PO route) CrCl 30–50: 250–500 mg q12h; CrCl 5–29: 250–500 mg q18h; CrCl <5: not defined; HD/PD: 250–500 mg q24h after dialysis, no supplement (IV route) CrCl 5–29: 200–400 mg q18–24h; CrCl <5: not defined; HD/PD: 200 mg q12h after dialysis, no supplement Levofloxacin: (if usual dose 750 mg QD) CrCl 20–49: 750 mg q48h; CrCl 10–19: 750 mg ×1, then 500 mg q48h; CrCl <10: not defined; HD/PD: no supplement (if usual dose 500 mg QD) CrCl 20–49: 500 mg ×1, then 250 mg q24h; CrCl 10–19: 500 mg ×1, then 250 mg q48h; CrCl <10: not defined; HD/PD: no supplement (if usual dose 250 mg QD) CrCl 10–19: 250 mg q48h; CrCl <10: not defined; HD/PD: not defined; info: no dose adjustment for uncomplicated UTI
Sulfamethoxazole/Trimethoprim	CrCl 15–30: decrease dose 50%; CrCl <15: avoid use; HD: give supplement; PD: no supplement

(*continued*)

Renal Impairments

TABLE 24.1 Drugs and Drug Classes Requiring Renal Adjustment Based on Creatinine Clearance (*continued*)

Drug/Drug Classes	Adjustment Based on CrCl
Nitrofurantoin: note, used in elderly females receiving long-term prophylaxis for recurrent UTIs	100 mg po q12h × 5–7 days CrCl <60: contraindicated
Azoles: fluconazole (<50 mL/min/), voriconazole (<50 mL/min)	Fluconazole: CrCl <50: give usual loading dose ×1, then decrease dose 50%; HD: give usual dose after dialysis, no supplement, decrease usual dose 50% on nondialysis days; PD: decrease dose 50%, no supplement Voriconazole: (IV route) CrCl <50: avoid use, PO route preferred due to accumulation of toxic IV vehicle; HD/PD: no supplement
Acyclovir	(PO route) CrCl <25: see package insert; HD: give supplement; PD: no supplement (IV route) CrCl 25–50: give q12h; CrCl 10–24: give q24h; CrCl <10: decrease dose 50%, give q24h; HD: give supplement; PD: no supplement
Ribavirin	(Peginterferon alfa-2a combo tx) CrCl 30–50: 200 mg tab QOD alternate w/ 400 mg tab QOD; CrCl <30: 200 mg tab QD (all other combo tx) CrCl <50: contraindicate
Glyburide	CrCl <50: avoid use
Metformin	eGFR 30–45: avoid use; eGFR <30: contraindicated
Saxagliptin/Sitagliptin	Saxagliptin CrCl <50: 2.5 mg QD; HD: give dose after dialysis, no supplement; PD: not defined Sitagliptin CrCl 30–49: 50 mg QD; CrCl <30: 25 mg QD; HD/PD: no supplement
Exenatide	CrCl 30–50: caution advised; CrCl <30: avoid use
Metoclopramide	CrCl 41–50: decrease dose 25%; CrCl 10–40: decrease dose 50%; CrCl <10: decrease dose 75%; HD/PD: no supplement
Levetiracetam	(Adjust dose amount, frequency) CrCl 50–80: 500–1,000 mg q12h; CrCl 30–50: 250–750 mg q12h; CrCl <30: 250–500 mg q12h; HD: 500–1,000 mg q24h, then give 250–500 mg as supplement; PD: 500–1,000 mg q24h, no supplement

(*continued*)

TABLE 24.1 Drugs and Drug Classes Requiring Renal Adjustment Based on Creatinine Clearance (*continued*)

Drug/Drug Classes	Adjustment Based on CrCl
Hydrochlorothiazide	Severe impairment: caution advised; anuria: contraindicated
Potassium-sparing diuretics (amiloride, spironolactone)	Amiloride: renal impairment/creatinine >1.5: contraindicated Spironolactone: CrCl <10, anuria, or acute renal impairment: contraindicated
Topiramate	(Immediate release form) CrCl 10–70: decrease dose 50%; CrCl <10: decrease dose 75%; HD: give supplement (Extended-release form) CrCl <70: decrease dose 50%; HD: give supplement
Pregabalin/Gabapentin	Pregabalin: CrCl 30–60: 75–300 mg/day divided BID-TID; CrCl 15–30: 25–150 mg/day divided QD-BID; CrCl <15: 25–75 mg QD; HD: give 25–50 mg as supplement if on 25 mg/day; 50–75 mg if on 25–50 mg/day; 75–100 mg if on 50–75 mg/day; 100–150 mg if on 75 mg/day Gabapentin: CrCl 30–60: 200–700 mg BID; CrCl 16–29: 200–700 mg QD; CrCl 15: 100–300 mg QD; CrCl <15: decrease dose proportionately to CrCl; HD: give 125–350 mg as supplement; PD: no supplement
Atenolol	CrCl 10–50: decrease dose 50%, give q48h, max 50 mg/day; CrCl <10: decrease dose 50%–70%, give q96h, max 25 mg/day; HD: give dose after dialysis, no supplement; PD: no supplement
Digoxin	Renal impairment: see package insert; HD/PD: no supplement
Enoxaparin	(DVT prophylaxis) CrCl <30: 30 mg SC QD; HD/PD: no supplement (DVT tx, unstable angina, NQWMI) CrCl <30: 1 mg/kg SC QD; HD/PD: no supplement (STEMI, <75 yo) CrCl <30: 30 mg IV plus 1 mg/kg SC ×1, then 1 mg/kg SC QD; HD/PD: no supplement (STEMI, 75 yo and older) CrCl <30: 1 mg/kg SC QD; HD/PD: no supplement
Dabigatran	(Thromboembolism/stroke prophylaxis) CrCl 15–30: 75 mg BID; CrCl <15: not defined; HD: not defined (DVT/PE prophylaxis, recurrent) CrCl <30: not defined; HD: not defined (DVT/PE prophylaxis, hip replacement)

(*continued*)

TABLE 24.1 Drugs and Drug Classes Requiring Renal Adjustment Based on Creatinine Clearance (*continued*)

Drug/Drug Classes	Adjustment Based on CrCl
	CrCl <30: not defined; HD: not defined (DVT/PE tx) CrCl <30: not defined; HD: not defined
Zoledronate	(Hypercalcemia, malignant) Severe renal impairment: weigh risk/benefit (all other indications) CrCl <60: avoid use; info: dose adjustment not possible w/ ready-to-use bag
Ranitidine/Famotidine	(PO route) CrCl <50: 150 mg QD; CrCl <10: 75–150 mg QD; HD: give dose after dialysis, no supplement; PD: no supplement; info: dose may be cautiously increased to q12h if required (IV route) CrCl <50: 50 mg q18–24h; HD: give dose after dialysis, no supplement; PD: no supplement; info: dose may be cautiously increased to q12h if required
Venlafaxine	CrCl 10–70: decrease dose 25%–50%; CrCl <10: decrease dose 50%; HD/PD: no supplement
Sotalol	(PO route) CrCl 30–59: give q24h; CrCl 10–29: give q36–48h; CrCl <10: individualize dose; HD: caution advised; info: may increase dose after 5–6 doses (IV route) CrCl 40–60: give q24h; CrCl <40: contraindicated
Risperidone	CrCl <30: start 0.5 mg BID, may increase by up to 0.5 mg BID to 1.5 mg BID, then increase dose no more frequently than QWK; HD: not defined
Paliperidone	CrCl 50–79: start 3 mg qam, max 6 mg/day; CrCl 10–49: start 1.5 mg qam, max 3 mg/day; CrCl <10
Lithium	CrCl 10–50: decrease dose 25%–50%; CrCl <10: decrease dose 50%–75%; HD: give dose after dialysis, no supplement; PD: no supplement; info: ER form cannot be cut, consider IR form for dose adjustments
Amantadine	CrCl 30–50: 200 mg ×1, then 100 mg QD; CrCl 15–29: 200 mg ×1, then 100 mg q48h; CrCl <15: 200 mg q7 days; HD/PD: no supplement

ACE, angiotensin-converting enzyme; BID, two times per day; CHF, congestive heart failure; CrCl, creatinine clearance; DVT, deep vein thrombosis; eGFR, estimated glomerular filtration rate; ER, extended release; HD, hemodialysis; HTN, hypertension; IV, intravenous; IR, immediate release; MI, myocardial infarction; NQWMI, non-Q wave myocardial infarction; PD, peritoneal dialysis; PE, pulmonary embolism; QD, one time per day; QOD, every other day; QWK, every week; SC, subcutaneous; STEMI, ST-elevation myocardial infarction; TID, three times per day; UTI, urinary tract infection.

for patients at risk for kidney disease. They may also be used for the treatment of microalbuminuria in diabetic patients. The beneficial effects of these medications include lower intraglomerular pressure, lower blood pressure, slowed progression of kidney disease, proteinuria reduction, and cardiovascular disease risk reduction (Kidney Disease: Improving Global Outcomes [KDIGO] Blood Pressure Work Group, 2012). There is also evidence suggesting lower mortality risk with the use of these agents in CKD (Molnar et al., 2014).

Common side effects of these medications such as hyperkalemia, early rise in GFR, and hypotension can often be managed without completely discontinuing the medication. These medications are contraindicated in the presence of moderate or severe aortic stenosis and bilateral renal artery stenosis (KDIGO Blood Pressure Work Group, 2012; Workeneh, Agraharker, & Gupta, 2018).

There is risk of acute kidney injury with the use of ACE inhibitors and ARBs in select patients. Risk for this increases in volume depleted states, some heart failure patients, stenosis of a dominant or single kidney, or for those with bilateral renal artery stenosis (Schoolwerth, Sica, Ballerman, & Wilcox, 2001; Workeneh et al., 2018). If a patient develops new azotemia or worsening renal function after short-term or long-term ACE inhibitor or ARB use, it is recommended that diagnostic studies to rule out renal artery stenosis be performed (Spinowitz & Rodriguez, 2018).

CHEMOTHERAPEUTIC AGENTS

Many chemotherapeutic agents are eliminated through the renal system; so dosage adjustments are often required in patients with renal impairment to avoid renal injury, electrolyte disorders, or increased drug toxicity (Merchan & Jhaveri, 2016). Some agents are nephrotoxic even in the absence of renal insufficiency, requiring close monitoring of kidney function. Potential kidney injury mechanisms include damage to the renal vasculature through capillary leak syndrome or thrombotic microangiopathy; damage to the glomeruli through sclerosis or minimal change disease; or damage to the tubulointerstitium due to acute tubular necrosis, tubulopathies, interstitial nephritis, or crystal nephropathy. Risk factors for kidney injury with the use of antineoplastic medications include older age, pharmacogenetics, immune response genes, tumor-related kidney effects such as renal infiltration or myeloma-related kidney injury, volume depletion, concomitant use of other nephrotoxic drugs, urinary tract obstruction, and intrinsic renal disease (Merchan & Jhaveri, 2018; Perazella, 2012).

In order to make dosage modifications, the optimal approach is to use the estimated GFR using serum creatinine concentration and estimation equations (Cockcroft–Gault, Modification of Diet in Renal Disease, and Chronic Kidney Disease Epidemiology Collaboration). Table 24.2 provides an overview of commonly used chemotherapeutic agents, effects on the renal system, monitoring required, and recommended dosage adjustments. In dialysis patients, dose reduction may be required, or timing of chemotherapeutic medication administration may need to be adjusted based on dialysis treatments (Merchan & Jhaveri, 2018; Perazella, 2012). It is recommended that the following medications be given after hemodialysis: fluorouracil, capecitabine, carboplatin, cisplatin, cyclophosphamide, doxorubicin, epirubicin, irinotecan, methotrexate, oxaliplatin, and vinorelbine. Docetaxel, etoposide, and paclitaxel may be given before or after hemodialysis, while it is recommended to administer gemcitabine 6 to 12 hours prior to hemodialysis (Janus, Thariat, Boulanger, Deray, & Launay-Vacher, 2010).

TABLE 24.2 Overview of Commonly Used Chemotherapeutic Agents and Their Effects on the Renal System

Drug	Renal Effects	Monitoring	Dosage Adjustments
Cisplatin	Nephrotoxicity	BUN/Creatinine, GFR	Manufacturer: do not administer until serum creatinine is <1.5 mg/100 mL and/or BUN <25 mg/100 mL Empiric guidelines suggest 25% dose reduction for CrCl of 46–60 mL/min and 50% dose reduction for CrCl of 31–45 mL/min
Carboplatin	Nephrotoxicity—less than cisplatin	BUN/Creatinine, GFR	Dosing based on AUC dose calculation (AUC × time), Calvert formula: total carboplatin dose (mg) = target AUC × (estimated CrCl +25) FDA recommends limiting max GFR to 125 mL/min For obese patients, recommend using adjusted weight (actual weight − ideal weight) × 0.40
Oxaliplatin	Cleared by kidneys, acute tubular necrosis rarely occurs in presence of immune-mediated intravascular hemolysis	BUN, creatinine, GFR	Reduce starting dose in patients with severe renal impairment (CrCL <30 mL/min)
Bendamustine	Increased frequency of grade 3 or 4 treatment-related toxicity with renal impairment	BUN, creatinine, GFR	Avoid use in patients with CrCl <40 mL/min
Cyclophosphamide	Hemorrhagic cystitis, hyponatremia due to increased effect of ADH	Sodium, BUN, creatinine, GFR	Consider dosage reduction for those with marked renal insufficiency (CrCL <30 mL/min)
Ifosfamide	Hemorrhagic cystitis and SIADH	Electrolytes, anion gap, BUN, creatinine, GFR, phosphate	Suggested dosage reductions: CrCl 46–60 mL/min: 80% dose CrCl 31–45 mL/min: 75% dose CrCl <30 mL/min: 70% dose

(continued)

TABLE 24.2 Overview of Commonly Used Chemotherapeutic Agents and Their Effects on the Renal System (*continued*)

Drug	Renal Effects	Monitoring	Dosage Adjustments
Nitrosoureas	Progressive, chronic interstitial nephritis	Creatinine, BUN, proteinuria	Dosage reduction for streptozocin and lomustine: CrCl 10–50 mL/min: 75% dose; CrCL <10 mL/min: 25%–50% dose
Melphalan	SIADH	Creatinine, BUN	50% dose reduction in patients with BUN ≥30 mg/dL
Mitomycin C	Renal failure, microangiopathic hemolytic anemia	Creatinine, BUN, CBC	Avoid use in patients with serum creatinine >1.7 mg/dL
Bleomycin	Treatment-related toxicity	Creatinine, BUN	Dose reduction for CrCl <50 mL/min
Anthracyclines	Some urinary excretion	Creatinine, BUN	Epirubicin dose adjustment with severe renal impairment (serum creatinine >5 mg/dL); Daunorubicin 50% dose reduction in patients with serum creatinine >3 mg/dL
Capecitabine	Renally excreted	Creatinine, BUN	Contraindicated in patients with severe renal impairment (CrCl <30 mL/min), initial dose reduced by 25% in patients with CrCl 30–50 mL/min
Hydroxyurea	Renally excreted	Creatinine, BUN	Dose reduction in patients with renal impairment
Methotrexate	Precipitation in renal tubules, transient decrease in GFR, SIADH	Creatinine, BUN	Dose reduction for CrCl 10–50 mL/min, avoid in patients with CrCl of <10 mL/min
Pemetrexed	Rarely associated with renal damage (acute tubular necrosis, renal tubular acidosis, and diabetes insipidus)	Creatinine, BUN	Avoid in patients with CrCL <45 mL/min. Avoid NSAIDs prior to and following each dose of pemetrexed with mild to moderate renal dysfunction (CrCl 45–79 mL/min)

Drug	Adverse Effect	Monitoring	Comments
Pralatrexate	Dose reduction suggested in renal impairment	Creatinine, BUN	Dose reduction for patients with severe renal impairment (CrCl <30 mL/min/1.73 m^2)
Pentostatin	Dose reduction suggested in renal impairment	Creatinine, BUN	Some suggest dose reduction for patients with CrCl <60 mL/min
Fludarabine and cladribine	Renally excreted	Creatinine, BUN	Dose reduction for renal impairment
Gemcitabine	Renal failure, thrombotic microangiopathy	CBC, Creatinine, BUN	Administer with caution in patients with significant renal dysfunction
Cytarabine	Dose reduction suggested in renal impairment	Creatinine, BUN	Some clinicians suggest dose reduction for patients receiving high-dose cytarabine (>2 g/m^2)
Vinca alkaloids	SIADH	Electrolytes, creatinine, BUN	Dose reduction of vinorelbine in patients with ESRD undergoing hemodialysis
Topotecan	Increased medication toxicity	Creatinine, BUN	Dosage adjustment for patients with CrCl <50 mL/min
Etoposide	Renally excreted	Creatinine, BUN	Dosage adjustment for patients with CrCl <50 mL/min
Irinotecan	Toxicity in patients with ESRD	Creatinine, BUN	Not recommended for patients on dialysis
Lenalidomide	Increased risk of toxicity in renal impairment, rarely drug-induced renal failure	Creatinine, BUN	Renal dosing specific to disease being treated
Eribulin	Potential for toxicity in renal impairment	Creatinine, BUN	Dose adjustment for CrCl 15–49 ml/min: 1.1 mg/m^2
Arsenic trioxide	Increased risk of toxicity in renal impairment	Creatinine, BUN	Caution in renal impairment, no defined dose adjustments

(continued)

TABLE 24.2 Overview of Commonly Used Chemotherapeutic Agents and Their Effects on the Renal System (*continued*)

Drug	Renal Effects	Monitoring	Dosage Adjustments
Ixazomib	Increased risk of toxicity in renal impairment	Creatinine, BUN	CrCl <30: start 3 mg
VEGF pathway inhibitors	Proteinuria, nephrotic syndrome, elevated blood pressure, drug-specific toxicity in renal impairment	Urinalysis, creatinine, BUN	VEGF ligand inhibitors: periodic assessment for proteinuria, withhold drug if protein excretion exceeds >2 g/24 hours Tyrosine kinase inhibitors: dose adjustment in renal insufficiency
EGFR pathway inhibitors	Hypomagnesemia, secondary hypocalcemia, hypokalemia, and potential for increased toxicity in renal impairment	Creatinine, BUN, magnesium, potassium, and calcium	Drug-specific monitoring and dosage modification
Imatinib	Acute/chronic kidney injury rare, SIADH in one case report	Creatinine, BUN, sodium	CrCl 40–59: max 600 mg/day; CrCl 20–39: decrease starting dose by 50%, max 400 mg/day; CrCl <20: decrease dose, amount undefined
Rituximab	Electrolyte imbalance and acute renal failure in patients with high tumor burden	Electrolytes, creatinine, BUN	Discontinue with rising creatinine or oliguria
Bosutinib	Decline in GFR	Creatinine, BUN	CrCl 30–50: 400 mg daily; CrCL <30: 300 mg daily
Crizotinib	Decline in GFR	Creatinine, BUN	CrCl <30: starting dose at 250 mg daily
Brentuximab	Severe adverse reactions and death risk increased in severe renal impairment	Creatinine, BUN	Avoid if CrCl <30
Ibrutinib	Renal failure	Creatinine, BUN	No defined dose adjustments

Vemurafenib and dabrafenib	Decreased CrCl and acute kidney injury	Creatinine, BUN	Caution advised in severe renal impairment
Olaparib	Caution in renal impairment	Creatinine, BUN	CrCl 31–50: 300 mg twice daily; CrCl <31: dose adjustment undefined
Interleukin-2	Capillary leak syndrome (edema, volume depletion, and fall in GFR)	Creatinine, BUN	Avoid use in patients who have underlying renal failure, are on other nephrotoxic drugs, and who are older
Interferons	Proteinuria, nephropathy, and rare thrombotic microangiopathy	Periodic urinalysis, creatinine, BUN	Caution in renal impairment, dose adjustments undefined

ADH, antidiuretic hormone; AUC, area under the curve; BUN, blood urea nitrogen; CBC, complete blood count; CrCl, creatinine clearance; EGFR, epidermal growth factor receptor; ESRD, end-stage renal disease; FDA, U.S. Food and Drug Administration; GFR, glomerular filtration rate; NSAID, nonsteroidal anti-inflammatory drug; SIADH, syndrome of inappropriate antidiuretic hormone secretion; VEGF, vascular endothelial growth factor.

Sources: Data from Epocrates. (2017). Epocrates RX for Android (Version 16.11) [Mobile application software]. Retrieved from http://www.epocrates.com; Merchan, J. R., & Jhaveri, K. D. (2018). Chemotherapy-related nephrotoxicity and dose modification in patients with renal insufficiency: Conventional cytotoxic agents. In R. E. Drews, J. S. Berns, D. M. F. Savarese, & A. Q. Lam (Eds.), *UpToDate.* Retrieved from https://www.uptodate.com/contents/chemotherapy-nephrotoxicity-and-dose-modification-in-patients-with-renal-insufficiency-conventional-cytotoxic-agents

KEY POINTS

- As the population ages, the people with CKD continues to grow. Practitioners must be aware of appropriate dosing protocols and measures that must be taken to ensure optimal patient care is provided each time.
- After the age of 30 years, the GFR begins to decline at a rate of 8 mL/min/1.73m² per decade.
- There are a number of drugs that require renal adjustments based on the stage and severity of an individual's renal impairment.
- The care of an individual with advanced renal disease requires engagement of an interprofessional healthcare team to address diet, function, medication, and management of comorbidities.
- ACE inhibitors and ARBs are widely acknowledged as renal protective drugs in individuals with diabetes and hypertension. They should be used with caution in those with aortic stenosis or bilateral renal artery stenosis. Kidney function should be routinely monitored with these medications. If an individual has an abrupt decline in kidney function following initiation of these medications, they should be worked up for renal artery stenosis.
- Many chemotherapeutic agents have renal toxicity; so careful consideration of renal function, use of other nephrotoxic drugs, and dosage adjustments should be addressed in patients with existing renal disease.

SUMMARY

Renal anatomy and drug dosing can come hand in hand, especially when an individual has a renal impairment and is an older adult. The ability to dose medications in renal, geriatric patients can sometimes be viewed as a challenge for prescribers and practitioners (Zuber, 2013). As the number of people with CKD continues to grow, practitioners must be aware of appropriate dosing protocols and measures that must be taken to ensure optimal patient care is provided each time. Prior to 1998, there was no specific requirement for testing medication in CKD patients at different levels of renal functioning, but this changed in 1998 when the Food and Drug Administration provided published guidelines requiring renal dosing for several medications, including those for CKD patients, that uses a glomerular filtration calculation for dosing adjustments (Zuber, 2013).

RENAL INTERPROFESSIONAL CASE STUDY

Megan Hebdon

Patient Presentation

Robert is a 74-year-old male patient whom you are seeing in your internal medicine practice for his multiple chronic diseases. During his follow-up appointment, he reports fatigue and increased pedal edema. He has gained 10 pounds over the past 3 months although he reports eating less due to nausea almost on a daily basis. He denies any change in his medications and states that he has been taking his medications as prescribed when his medication is reviewed. He reports that he has been sitting a lot more due to his fatigue as well as neuropathic pain in his hands and feet. He does become short of breath with exertion but denies chest pain or palpitations. He denies changes in memory but does feel as if it takes him more time to process or retrieve information.

History

Robert has a past medical history of hypertension, type 2 diabetes mellitus (T2DM), non–ST-elevation myocardial infarction (STEMI) 10 years ago, hyperlipidemia, stage 4 CKD, sleep apnea, and diabetic neuropathy. His past surgical history includes a percutaneous coronary intervention (PCI) with stent placement. He has a wife and three grown children who are fairly supportive although his wife has health problems of her own and two of his children live out of state. He has insurance through Medicare and has some healthcare covered by the Department of Veterans Affairs (VA) due to his former military service. He has told you that they rely mostly on Social Security for their income.

Medications

He is allergic to penicillin. His current medications include insulin glargine once daily, insulin lispro with meals, metoprolol tartrate, lisinopril, furosemide, rosuvastatin, gabapentin, ergocalciferol, and sevelamer.

Physical Exam

On physical exam, he is pale and his affect is flat. He has a positive depression screen using the Beck Depression Inventory. He has decreased sensation to his feet with the monofilament, and on the Mini-Mental State Exam, he has difficulty with recall and calculating serial sevens. His heart rhythm and rate are regular, and his radial pulses are intact with no pulse deficit. His pedal pulses are difficult to palpate due to the 2+ pitting edema. He has mild dyspnea and wheezing on auscultation. He has bruising to his arms but no other skin lesions. His timed get up and go test is 30 seconds.

Diagnostic Testing

For workup of his symptoms, you decide to check A1C, complete blood count (CBC), comprehensive metabolic panel (CMP), parathyroid hormone (PTH), vitamin D, magnesium, and phosphorus The results indicate that his A1C is high at 9.6, but stable, his CBC shows worsening anemia, his creatinine is increasing with a calculated GFR of 16 mL/min/1.73 m^2, and his PTH, vitamin D, magnesium, calcium, and phosphorus are stable.

Plan of Care

Due to the decline in kidney function and worsening anemia, you consult with his nephrologist regarding his symptoms and health status. His nephrologist requests to see Robert for a follow-up appointment. Following the consult with nephrology, it is determined that Robert is now a candidate for dialysis because he is both symptomatic and on the cusp of stage V CKD. Robert has been aware that dialysis and/or kidney transplantation were potential treatment options if his kidney function continued to decline. He, his family, and his nephrologist determine that hemodialysis would be the best treatment option for his current condition. He will be having an arterial–venous fistula placed in the next month, and he will be starting on additional medications including erythropoietin, vitamin C, B-complex vitamin, and folic acid. He will also be getting an iron panel checked to see if he will need iron supplementation.

Robert expresses multiple concerns regarding hemodialysis, including dietary and medication concerns. You discuss the importance of a low-protein diet and avoidance of foods high in potassium, such as oranges, bananas, prunes, and high levels of dairy intake. You also discuss the importance of eating prior to his dialysis appointments.

Interprofessional Collaboration

He is confused as to how to take his medication on dialysis days. You educate him on the importance of working with his nephrologist and dialysis team on dosing of his medications. You discuss that any medications that are removed by dialysis would need to be dosed at night, and that he will need to check his blood pressure before dialysis to determine if he should take his morning metoprolol dose. You also note that medications may be dosed lower or less frequently moving forward; so he needs to be aware of this when seeing other providers and starting on new medications.

Recognizing that Robert will require an interprofessional team to manage his care, you refer him to a dietitian for education on a renal diet. You discuss the option of a home health nurse for a short time to do weekly assessments and education while he is adjusting to medication and dialysis. Due to his decline in physical activity, you also discuss physical therapy and occupational therapy options with him through home health or an outpatient clinic to enhance his physical functioning. Social work involvement may be needed to assist Robert with medical transportation and community support services. He has a positive depression screen with no history of a manic episode. You discuss a psych referral to support Robert and his family, but he declines. You recommend starting on low-dose sertraline, and he states that he will think about it.

You review the chronic nature of his disease with him and approach the topic of palliative care and advance directives. You review the Physician Orders for Scope of Treatment (POST) form and ask if he and his family would be open to a visit from a palliative care team in his home. He reports that he is not ready but agrees to readdress palliative care at his next visit.

While Robert is experiencing a significant change in his chronic disease management with the addition of hemodialysis, he continues to have other chronic health conditions. Many patients respond well to an interprofessional nephrology clinic for patients on dialysis, but this is not available for Robert. Additional medical specialties involved in Robert's care might include cardiology due to his history of myocardial infarction (MI) and hematology for management of anemia from his end-stage renal disease. Effective communication strategies such as shared notes, letters, and phone consults with team members are essential to manage Robert's chronic health needs.

Case Study References

Arora, P. (2019). Chronic kidney disease clinical presentation. In V. Batuman (Ed.), *Medscape*. Retrieved from http://emedicine.medscape.com/article/238798-clinical#b3

Berns, J. S. (2016). Hemodialysis in the older adult. In S. J. Schwab & A. M. Sheridan (Eds.), *UpToDate*. Waltham, MA.

Centers for Disease Control & Prevention. (2015). *The timed up and go (TUG) test*. Retrieved from https://www.ons.org/sites/default/files/TUG_Test-a.pdf

Dahlin, C. (Ed.). (2013). *Clinical practice guidelines for quality palliative care* (3rd ed.). Pittsburgh, PA: National Consensus Project for Quality Palliative Care.

Davita. (n.d.). Stage 4 of chronic kidney disease. Retrieved from https://www.davita.com/kidney-disease/overview/stages-of-kidney-disease/stage-4-of-chronic-kidney-disease/e/4751

Hedayati, S. S., Yalamanchili, V., & Finkelstein, F. O. (2012). A practical approach to the treatment of depression in patients with chronic kidney disease and end-stage renal disease. *Kidney International, 81*(3), 247–255. doi:10.1038/ki.2011.358

Johansen, K. L. (2007). Exercise in the end-stage renal disease population. *Journal of the American Society of Nephrology, 18*(6), 1845–1854. doi:10.1681/ASN.2007010009

Kidney Disease: Improving Global Outcomes Blood Pressure Work Group. (2012). KDIGO clinical practice guideline for the management of blood pressure in chronic kidney disease. *Kidney International, 2*(5), 337–414. Retrieved from https://kdigo.org/wp-content/uploads/2016/10/KDIGO-2012-Blood-Pressure-Guideline-English.pdf

Lynn, R. (n.d.). 7 common drugs prescribed for dialysis patients. Retrieved from https://www.davita.com/kidney-disease/dialysis/treatment-options/common-drugs-prescribed-for-dialysis-patients/e/5271

Manitoba Renal Program. (n.d.). Guidelines for managing hospitalized hemodialysis patients. Retrieved from http://www.kidneyhealth.ca/wp/wp-content/uploads/pdfs/P&P/80.20.05.pdf

National Kidney Foundation. (2015). KDOQI clinical practice guidelines for hemodialysis adequacy: 2015 update. *American Journal of Kidney Diseases, 66*(5), 884–930. doi:10.1053/j.ajkd.2015.07.015

National Physician's Orders for Life-Sustaining Treatment Paradigm. (n.d.). POLST & advance care planning. Retrieved from http://polst.org/polst-advance-care-planning

O'Daniel, M., & Rosenstein, A. H. (2008). Professional communication and team collaboration. In R. G. Hughes (Ed.), *Patient safety and quality: An evidence-based handbook for nurses*. Rockville, MD: Agency for Healthcare Research and Quality. Retrieved from https://www.ncbi.nlm.nih.gov/books/NBK2651/?report=reader

Rosenberg, M. (2019). Overview of the management of chronic kidney disease in adults. In G. C. Curhan & S. Motwani (Eds.), *UpToDate*. Retrieved from https://www.uptodate.com/contents/overview-of-the-management-of-chronic-kidney-disease-in-adults

Saliba, W., & El-Haddad, B. (2009). Secondary hypoparathyroidism: Pathophysiology and treatment. *Journal of the American Board of Family Medicine, 22*(5), 574–581. doi:10.3122/jabfm.2009.05.090026

Smyth, B., Jones, C., & Saunders, J. (2016). Prescribing for patients on dialysis. *Australian Prescriber, 39*(1), 21–24. Retrieved from https://www.ncbi.nlm.nih.gov/pmc/articles/PMC4816865

Snively, C. S., & Gutierrez, C. (2004). Chronic kidney disease: Prevention and treatment of common complications. *American Family Physician, 70*(10), 1921–1930. Retrieved from https://www.aafp.org/afp/2004/1115/p1921.html

University of Massachusetts Lowell. (11 January 2017). *Mini-mental status exam.* Retrieved from https://pdfs.semanticscholar.org/4370/72f1421146674eaf98e11cc9079311f23fcb.pdf

REFERENCES

Chalouhy, C. E. (2017). Kidney anatomy. In T. R. Gest (Ed.), *Medscape*. Retrieved from http://emedicine.medscape.com/article/1948775-overview

Coresh, J., Astor, B. C., Greene, T., Eknoyan, G., & Levey, A. S. (2003). Prevalence of chronic kidney disease and decreased kidney function in the adult US population: Third national health and nutrition examination survey. *American Journal of Kidney Diseases, 41*(1), 1–12. doi:10.1053/ajkd.2003.50007

Epocrates. (2017). Epocrates RX for Android (Version 16.11) [Mobile application software]. Retrieved from http://www.epocrates.com

Fliser, D. (2008). Assessment of renal function in elderly patients. *Current Opinion in Nephrology and Hypertension, 17*(6), 604–608. doi:10.1097/mnh.0b013e32830f454e

Janus, N., Thariat, J., Boulanger, H., Deray, G., & Launay-Vacher, V. (2010). Proposal for dosage adjustment and timing of chemotherapy in hemodialyzed patients. *Annals of Oncology, 21*(7), 1395–1403. doi:10.1093/annonc/mdp598

Kidney Disease: Improving Global Outcomes (KDIGO) Blood Pressure Work Group. (2012). KDIGO clinical practice guideline for the management of blood pressure in chronic kidney disease. *Kidney International, 2*(5), 337–414. Retrieved from https://kdigo.org/wp-content/uploads/2016/10/KDIGO-2012-Blood-Pressure-Guideline-English.pdf

Merchan, J. R., & Jhaveri, K. D. (2018). Chemotherapy-related nephrotoxicity and dose modification in patients with renal insufficiency: Conventional cytotxic agents. In R. E. Drews, J. S. Berns, D. M. F. Savarese, A. Q. Lam (Eds.), *UpToDate*. Retrieved from https://www.uptodate.com/contents/chemotherapy-nephrotoxicity-and-dose-modification-in-patients-with-renal-insufficiency-conventional-cytotoxic-agents

Moini, J (2013). *Student workbook for focus on pharmacology: Essentials for health professionals* (2nd ed.). Boston, MA: Pearson.

Molnar, M. Z., Kalantar-Zadeh, K., Lott, E. H., Lu, J. L., Malakauskas, S. M., Ma, J. Z., . . . Kovesdy, C. P. (2014). Angiotensin-converting enzyme inhibitor, angiotensin receptor blocker use, and mortality in patients with chronic kidney disease. *Journal of the American College of Cardiology, 63*(7), 650–658. doi:10.1016/j.jacc.2013.10.050

National Kidney Foundation. (n.d.). About chronic kidney disease. Retrieved from https://www.kidney.org/kidneyDisease/aboutckd

Perazella, M. A. (2012). Onco-nephrology: Renal toxicities of chemotherapeutic agents. *Clinical Journal of the American Society of Nephrology, 7*(10), 1713–1721. doi:10.2215/CJN.02780312

Phoon, R. (2012). Chronic kidney disease in the elderly. *Assessment and Management, 41*(12), 940–944. Retrieved from https://www.racgp.org.au/download/Documents/AFP/2012/December/201212phoon.pdf

Schmidler, C. (Ed.). (2019). Kidney anatomy and function. Retrieved from http://www.healthpages.org/anatomy-function/kidney

Schoolwerth, A. C., Sica, D. A., Ballermann, B. J., & Wilcox, C. S. (2001). Renal considerations in angiotensin converting enzyme inhibitor therapy. *Circulation, 104*(16), 1985–1991. doi:10.1161/hc4101.096153

Silberberg, C. (2015). Chronic kidney disease. University of Maryland Medical Center. Retrieved from https://www.umms.org/ummc/health-services/kidney/disease

Spinowitz, B. S., & Rodriguez, J. (2018). Renal artery stenosis guidelines. In V. Batuman, F. Talavera, & E. Lederer (Eds.), *Medscape*. Retrieved from http://emedicine.medscape.com/article/245023-guidelines

Workeneh, B. T., Agraharkar, M., & Gupta, R. (2018). Acute kidney injury treatment & management. In V. Batuman & E. Lederer (Eds.), *Medscape*. Retrieved from http://emedicine.medscape.com/article/243492-treatment

Zuber, K. (2013). Renal medication dosing. Retrieved from http://www.primaryissues.org/2013/02/renal_med_dosing

25 Genitourinary Pharmacotherapy, Urinary Tract Infections, and Sexual Health

Madeline Burke

OBJECTIVES

1. Evaluate older adults for symptoms of benign prostatic hyperplasia/hypertrophy (BPH), erectile dysfunction, and sexual health and dysfunction
2. Develop a treatment plan for BPH and sexual dysfunction
3. Distinguish between urinary tract infections (UTIs) and asymptomatic bacteriuria (ASB)
4. Select appropriate antimicrobial treatment for empiric treatment of UTI

INTRODUCTION

Older adults have a high prevalence of UTIs and may have other genitourinary (GU) changes that can affect their quality of life. Sexual health is an area of health that has historically been overlooked in older adults. Clinicians should make addressing sexual health a priority in older adults as well as other aspects of GU health.

BENIGN PROSTATIC HYPERPLASIA

Definitions and Pathophysiology

BPH is a nonmalignant overgrowth of the prostate commonly seen in aging men. The prevalence of BPH is age-dependent and affects approximately 75% of men 70 years and older and 90% of men older than 85 years (Woodard, Manigault, McBurrows, Wray, & Woodard, 2016).

The prostate is a walnut-sized gland below the urinary bladder that surrounds the proximal urethra. Its main function is to secrete fluid that is a component of semen. The normal prostate weight in an adult male is between 7 and 16 grams (Woodard et al., 2016).

Enlarged prostate reduces the bladder's ability to completely empty, which may cause lower urinary tract symptoms (LUTS). LUTS related to voiding function include urinary hesitancy, poor urinary flow, reduced sensation of complete bladder emptying, weak urinary stream, postmicturition dribbling, and prolonged urination. LUTS related to storage function include urinary frequency, nocturia, urinary urgency, and urinary incontinence. LUTS are thought to be due to bladder outflow obstruction, which may chronically lead to urinary retention, renal insufficiency, recurrent UTIs, hematuria, and bladder calculi. Overall, LUTS can have a significant effect on sleep and quality of life (Woodard et al., 2016).

Guidelines

American Urological Association (AUA) guidelines for management of BPH were last revised in 2010 with an update for surgical recommendations in the treatment of LUTS released in 2018.

Assessment and Evaluation

The patient should be evaluated for other potential causes of LUTS, such as neurogenic bladder, prostatitis, bladder cancer, prostate cancer, UTI, diabetes, erectile dysfunction, cardiovascular disease (CVD), neurologic disease, and sexually transmitted diseases (STDs); see Woodard et al. (2016).

Assessment should involve complete medical history and description of urinary symptoms. Urinalysis should be completed to screen for hematuria and serum prostate-specific antigen (PSA) should be checked, particularly if digital rectal exam (DRE) is deferred. Prostate is typically considered enlarged if the size is estimated >40 mL on DRE (Woodard et al., 2016; see Table 25.1). The American Urological Association Symptom Index (AUA-SI) is recommended to assist with determination of symptom severity. AUA-SI is scored between 1 and 35, with a score <8 indicating mild symptoms. AUA recommends watchful waiting if symptoms are mild.

Treatment

Nonpharmacological Treatment

Avoid medications that may worsen BPH, such as the following:

- Any medication with high anticholinergic activity (such as antihistamines and tricyclic antidepressants) due to risk of acute urinary retention
- Decongestants, which may cause muscle contractions and incomplete bladder emptying
- Beta-agonists, which may prevent voiding by relaxation of bladder detrusor muscle
- Opioid analgesics
- Diuretics due to increased frequency of voiding
- Testosterone replacement due to risk of prostate enlargement (Woodard et al., 2016)

Behavior modifications recommended include limiting fluid intake in the evening, reducing alcohol and caffeine intake, healthy diet, smoking cessation, and exercise. Physical activity has been shown to reduce the risk of BPH or the need for surgery due to BPH (Woodard et al., 2016).

TABLE 25.1 Evaluation of PSA

Patient Age	Correlation to Prostate Volume of 40 mL
≥50 years	1.6 mcg/L
≥60 years	2.0 mcg/L
≥70 years	2.4 mcg/L

PSA, prostate-specific antigen.

Source: Data from Woodard, T., Manigault, K., McBurrows, N., Wray, T., & Woodard, L. (2016). Management of benign prostatic hyperplasia in older adults. *The Consultant Pharmacist, 31*(8), 412–424. doi:10.4140/tcp.n.2016.412

Watchful waiting or active surveillance is recommended in patients who are asymptomatic or have mild symptoms. Some patients even have improvement with this technique (Woodard et al., 2016).

Surgical procedures for the treatment of BPH can be minimally invasive, such as a transurethral needle ablation (TUNA), or an invasive procedure, such as open prostatectomy or transurethral resection of prostate (TURP).

Pharmacotherapy

Prostate cancer should be ruled out for all patients initiating treatment for BPH, as symptoms can be similar and BPH pharmacotherapy can mask further symptoms of prostate cancer (Woodard et al., 2016; Table 25.2).

TABLE 25.2 Pharmacotherapy for LUTS Associated With BPH

Generic (Brand)	Initial/Typical Dosing	Maximum Recommended Dose	Additional Considerations
ALPHA-BLOCKERS			Floppy iris syndrome during cataract surgery May cause CNS depression Risk of orthostasis/syncope, particularly with first dose or when prescribed with other agents with antihypertensive effects Rare risk of priapism
Alfuzosin (Uroxatral)	10 mg PO once daily		Functionally uroselective alpha-blocker Caution in CrCl <30 mL/min Minimal QT prolongation
Doxazosin (Cardura)	0.5 mg PO once daily, dose is doubled every 1–2 weeks if tolerated	8 mg/day	If medication is discontinued for several days, recommend resuming at starting dose and slowly titrating back to previously effective dose to prevent side effects. Decreases in WBC have been reported. Caution in heart failure, angina, or recent MI—may exacerbate underlying myocardial dysfunction.
Silodosin (Rapaflo)	8 mg PO once daily with a meal		Reduce dose to 4 mg daily for CrCl 30–50 mL/min and avoid use if <30 mL/min.

(continued)

TABLE 25.2 Pharmacotherapy for LUTS Associated With BPH (*continued*)

Generic (Brand)	Initial/Typical Dosing	Maximum Recommended Dose	Additional Considerations
Tamsulosin (Flomax)	0.4 mg PO once daily, ~30 minutes following same meal each day	0.8 mg/day	Functionally uroselective alpha-blocker Discontinue if angina occurs or worsens Rare cross-reactivity in patients with sulfa allergy
Terazosin (Hytrin)	0.5 mg PO at bedtime, increase over several weeks—most patients will require 10 mg once daily	20 mg/day	If medication discontinued for several days, recommend resuming at starting dose and slowly titrating back to previously effective dose to prevent side effects
5-ALPHA-REDUCTASE INHIBITORS			
Dutasteride (Avodart)	0.5 mg PO once daily		Monitor PSA levels periodically.
Finasteride (Proscar)	5 mg once daily		Women who are pregnant or who may be pregnant should avoid contact with these medications due to fetal risk. Avoid blood donation on this medication due to risk of female/pregnant transfusion recipient.
COMBINATION PRODUCT			
Dutasteride/ tamsulosin (Jalyn)	Fixed dose of 0.5 mg dutasteride/ 0.4 mg tamsulosin once daily ~30 minutes after same meal each day		See individual agents.
UROSELECTIVE ANTICHOLINERGICS			
Darifenacin (Enablex)	7.5 mg PO once daily	15 mg/day	Off-label in BPH Requires dose adjustment to maximum of 7.5 mg/day with potent CYP3A4 inhibitors Caution in bladder flow obstruction, GI motility or obstructive disorders, narrow-angle glaucoma, and myasthenia gravis Most common side effects: xerostomia and constipation

(*continued*)

TABLE 25.2 Pharmacotherapy for LUTS Associated With BPH (*continued*)

Generic (Brand)	Initial/Typical Dosing	Maximum Recommended Dose	Additional Considerations
Fesoterodine (Toviaz)	4 mg PO once daily	8 mg/day	Off-label in BPH Requires dose adjustment to maximum of 4 mg/day with potent CYP3A4 inhibitors and CrCl <30 mL/min Caution in bladder flow obstruction, GI motility or obstructive disorders, narrow-angle glaucoma, and myasthenia gravis Most common side effect: xerostomia
Solifenacin (Vesicare)	5 mg PO once daily	10 mg/day	Off-label in BPH Requires dose adjustment to maximum of 5 mg/day with potent CYP3A4 inhibitors and CrCl <30 mL/min Use with caution in patients with Alzheimer's disease, bladder flow obstruction, GI motility or obstructive disorders, narrow-angle glaucoma, and myasthenia gravis May prolong QT interval (dose-related) Most common side effects: xerostomia and constipation
PDE5 INHIBITORS			**Classwide Considerations:** **May cause dose-related impairment of color discrimination** **Rare reports of hearing loss (unknown mechanism) and vision loss (associated with NAION)** **Risk of priapism** **Not recommended in hypotension, uncontrolled hypertension, angina, life-threatening arrhythmias, recent stroke, or recent MI**

(*continued*)

TABLE 25.2 Pharmacotherapy for LUTS Associated With BPH (continued)

Generic (Brand)	Initial/Typical Dosing	Maximum Recommended Dose	Additional Considerations
			Avoid/separate use of these medications and nitrate medications due to risk of life-threatening hypotension.
Avanafil (Stendra)	Off-label for BPH, the following dosing is for erectile dysfunction: 100 mg PO taken 15 mg prior to sexual activity 50 mg PO as single dose if on stable, concomitant alpha-blockers	200 mg/day (if concomitant alpha-blocker or moderate CYP3A4 inhibitor, adjusted to 50 mg/day)	Avoid with strong CYP3A4 inhibitors. Not recommended in CrCl <30 mL/min. Most common side effect is headache.
Sildenafil (Viagra)	Off-label for BPH, the following dosing is for erectile dysfunction: 25 mg PO 30 min–4 hr prior to sexual activity PRN	100 mg/day	Concomitant strong CYP3A4 inhibitors require dose reduction. Avoid use with protease inhibitors. Most common side effects include flushing, headache, dyspepsia, visual disturbance, and epistaxis.
Tadalafil (Cialis)	5 mg PO once daily Initial dose of 2.5 mg PO once daily recommended for CrCl 30–50 mL/min	5 mg/day Concomitant strong CYP3A4 inhibitors, 2.5 mg/day	Not recommended for concomitant use in BPH with alpha-blockers. Not recommended in BPH for CrCl < 30 mL/min. If concomitant with finasteride to initiate BPH therapy, recommended duration is 26 weeks or less. Most common side effects include flushing, headache, nausea, myalgia, limb pain, respiratory tract infection, and nasopharyngitis.

(continued)

TABLE 25.2 Pharmacotherapy for LUTS Associated With BPH *(continued)*

Generic (Brand)	Initial/Typical Dosing	Maximum Recommended Dose	Additional Considerations
Vardenafil (Levitra)	Off-label for BPH, the following dosing is for erectile dysfunction: 5 mg PO once ~60 minutes prior to sexual activity	20 mg/day	Requires dose reduction for CYP3A4 inhibitors and slower titration if concomitant alpha-blockers. Not recommended for use in congenital QT prolongation. Most common side effects include flushing and headache.

BPH, benign prostatic hyperplasia/hypertrophy; CNS, central nervous system; CrCl, creatinine clearance; GI, gastrointestinal; LUTS, lower urinary tract symptoms; MI, myocardial infarction; NAION, nonarteritic anterior ischemic optic neuropathy; PDE5, phosphodiesterase-5; PO, by mouth; PSA, prostate-specific antigen; WBC, white blood cell.

Source: Data from Lexicomp Online, Lexi-Drugs Online. (2019, February 10). Hudson, OH: Wolters Kluwer Clinical Drug Information, Inc.

Alpha-blockers are commonly used for treatment of LUTS associated with BPH. Agents with higher prostate-selective alpha effects are preferred in older adults to prevent risk of orthostasis and falls. Alfuzosin and tamsulosin are the most prostate-selective of these agents available in the United States.

5-alpha-reductase inhibitors (5-ARIs) work to prevent a byproduct of testosterone, called "dihydrotestosterone" (DHT), which drives prostate growth. Testosterone is converted to DHT by 5-alpha-reductase. These agents work over the long term (typically about 6 months to see effect) to reduce prostate size, but prostate cancer should be screened for and ruled out before initiating these agents (Woodard et al., 2016).

Phosphodiesterase-5 (PDE5) inhibitors, particularly tadalafil, which gained the Food and Drug Administration (FDA) approval for this indication, have shown evidence of benefit for LUTS in addition to known benefit in erectile dysfunction. The mechanism is not well established, but any symptom improvement is typically seen within 1 to 2 weeks of initiation of treatment. Nonselective alpha-blockers should be avoided with PDE5 inhibitors due to increased risk of hypotension, but prostate-selective alpha-blockers with PDE5 inhibitors are a reasonable option (Woodard et al., 2016).

Anticholinergic agents are thought to increase risk of urinary retention, but when uroselective agents were studied in men with concomitant BPH and overactive bladder, improvement in LUTS was demonstrated. No agents within this class are FDA-approved. AUA does recognize the role these medications may play in select patients. The ideal candidate for these medications would be those with BPH who are stable on their alpha-blocker and have bothersome voiding symptoms and postvoid residual (PVR) less than 250 mL. Clinicians should use caution and monitor for any systemic anticholinergic effects, including confusion (Woodard et al., 2016).

URINARY TRACT INFECTIONS AND ASYMPTOMATIC BACTERIURIA

Key recommendations for collection and interpretation of urine samples from the Infectious Diseases Society of America (IDSA) are as follows:

- Urine should not sit at room temperature >30 minutes.
- Presence of three or more species of bacteria typically indicates contamination at the time of collection.
- Do not ask the laboratory to report "everything that grows" without consulting laboratory and providing reference for interpretation of less common bacteria.
- Samples should be gathered midstream, clean catch, or straight catheterization to reduce risk of contamination with skin flora. (Miller et al., 2018)

Urinary Tract Infections

Definitions

UTIs cover a spectrum of syndromes, including cystitis and pyelonephritis, and may be accompanied by or progress to sepsis. Clinical definitions may vary and typically have alternative criteria for diagnosis of catheter-associated UTI (CAUTI) for patients who have an indwelling catheter or who have had one removed within the past 48 hours. A commonly accepted definition for UTI in older adults is dysuria alone. Alternatively, an older adult could have fever with frequency, suprapubic pain, flank pain, or new or worsening urgency or incontinence. CAUTI can be defined as fever, rigors, delirium, or new costovertebral (flank) tenderness (Cortes-Penfield, Trautner, & Jump, 2017).

Prevalence

UTIs are the second most common infection in older adults and account for 30% to 40% of healthcare infections in institutionalized elderly patients (Detweiler, Mayers, & Fletcher, 2015). Overall incidence of UTI in elderly men and women is estimated to be 1 infection per 14 to 20 person-years (Cortes-Penfield et al., 2017). UTIs accounted for an estimated 5% of all ED visits in U.S. adults aged 65 and older (Rowe et al., 2014). UTI is the most common bacterial infection in community-dwelling older women, affecting about 10% of postmenopausal women each year (Arinzon, Shabat, Peisakh, & Berner, 2012).

Presentation in Older Adults

UTIs in older adults often present with atypical, generalized symptoms, which may delay diagnosis and treatment. Underdiagnosis of UTI in these patients could lead to failure to adequately treat the infection. However, overdiagnosis of UTI in older adults can increase cost, inappropriate antibiotic use, and lead to missed alternative diagnosis and preventable admissions (Caterino et al., 2018).

Primary symptoms associated with UTI in premenopausal women were primarily localized symptoms like frequency, painful urination, and burning urination. Primary symptoms associated with UTI in postmenopausal women were more generalized symptoms, such as urgency, incontinence, lower abdominal pain, lower back pain, chills, constipation, and diarrhea (Arinzon et al., 2012).

Diagnosis of UTI is further complicated by chronic urinary incontinence, as fluctuations in urinary urgency and incontinence can occur in older women, even without infection. Additionally, nonspecific symptoms of dizziness and confusion could be due to dehydration, especially as women with urinary urgency are often told to restrict fluids (Mody & Juthani-Mehta, 2014).

For older adults, altered mental status has poor sensitivity but high specificity for infections, and absence of urinary symptoms is not always sufficient to rule out a UTI (Caterino et al., 2018).

The most common causative organisms of UTI in community-dwelling older adults are as follows:

- *Escherichia coli*
- *Enterococcus sp.*
- *Proteus mirabilis*
- *Klebsiella pneumoniae*
- *Staphylococcus saprophyticus* (Marques et al., 2012)

See Figures 25.1 and 25.2 for examples of decision tools for empiric treatment of suspected UTIs.

Risk Factors

Increased age, functional and organic changes of urinary tract, vaginitis, hormonal changes, and history of UTI are associated with a higher risk of UTI (Marques et al., 2012).

Reduced functional status is associated with a higher risk of UTI, such as the following:

- Reduced cognitive function
- Difficulty walking
- Urinary and fecal incontinence
- Malnutrition
- Delirium within the past month
- Dementia
- Vertebral fractures (Eriksson, Gustafson, Fagerström, & Olofsson, 2010; Marques et al., 2012)

Catheter use is associated with an increased risk of UTIs (Mody et al., 2017). Additionally, bacteremia from urinary sources is 3 to 39 times more common in catheter patients than noncatheterized patients (Detweiler et al., 2015).

Diabetes, BPH, and iron deficiency anemia have also been associated with an increased risk of UTI (Detweiler et al., 2015).

A strong negative predictive value was associated with the absence of pyuria, or white blood cells on urinalysis, for the presence of UTI (Detweiler et al., 2015).

Guidelines

IDSA has produced and revised guidelines for uncomplicated cystitis and pyelonephritis, which were last updated in 2011; the guideline is under review currently for update release planned for 2022. IDSA produced a separate guideline for CAUTI, which was last released in 2010 (Hooton et al., 2010).

Nonpharmacological Changes and Prevention

Recommendations for prevention of CAUTI are as follows:

- Catheter removal
- Aseptic insertion
- Use regular assessment
- Training for catheter care
- Incontinence care planning (Mody et al., 2017)

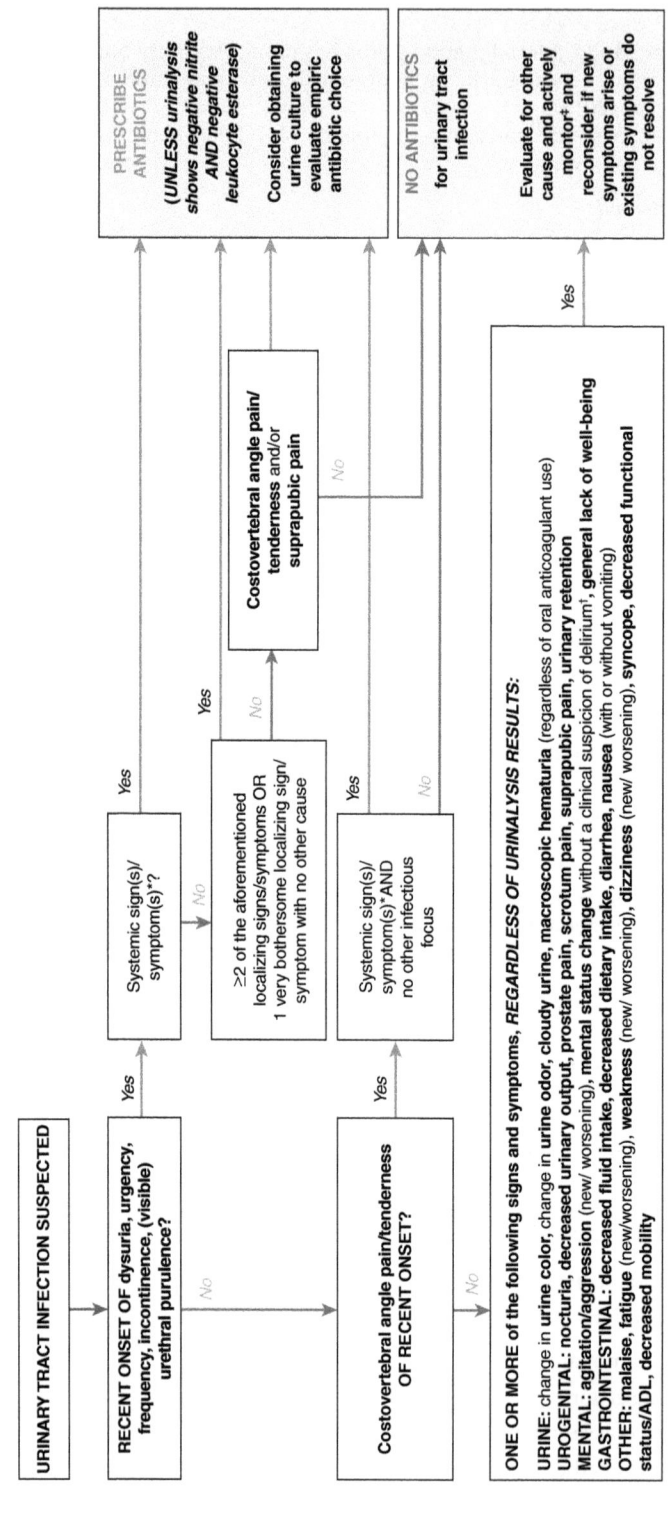

FIGURE 25.1 Decision tool for empiric treatment of suspected UTI in frail older adults without indwelling catheter.

ADL, activity of daily living; *DSM-5, Diagnostic and Statistical Manual of Mental Disorders, 5th edition*; UTI, urinary tract infection.

*Presence of at least fever (i.e., a single oral temperature >37.8°C or repeated oral temperatures >37.2°C or rectal temperatures >37.5°C or a 1.1°C increase over the baseline temperature), rigors/shaking chills and/or clear-cut delirium

†Definition of delirium according to *DSM-5*: (a) Disturbance in attention (i.e., reduced ability to direct, focus, sustain, and shift attention) and awareness (reduced orientation to the environment). (b) The disturbance develops over a short period of time (usually hours to a few days), represents an acute change from baseline attention and awareness, and tends to fluctuate in severity during the course of the day. (c) An additional disturbance in cognition (e.g., memory deficit, disorientation, language, visuospatial ability, or perception). (d) The disturbance in Criteria A and C are not better explained by a preexisting, established, or evolving neurocognitive disorder and do not occur in the context of a severely reduced level of arousal such as coma. (e) There is evidence from the history, physical examination, or laboratory findings that the disturbance is a direct physiological consequence of another medical condition, substance intoxication or withdrawal (i.e., due to a drug of abuse or to a medication), or exposure to a toxin, or is due to multiple ethiologies.

‡e.g., monitoring vital signs, paying attention to hydration status, and repeated physical assessments by nursing home staff.

Source: From van Buul, L., Vreeken, H., Bradley, S., Cnrich, C., Drinka, P., Geerlings, S., . . . Hertogh, C. M. P. M. (2018). The development of a decision tool for the empiric treatment of suspected urinary tract infection in frail older adults: A Delphi consensus procedure. *Journal of the American Medical Directors Association, 19*(9), 757–764. doi:10.1016/j.jamda.2018.05.001

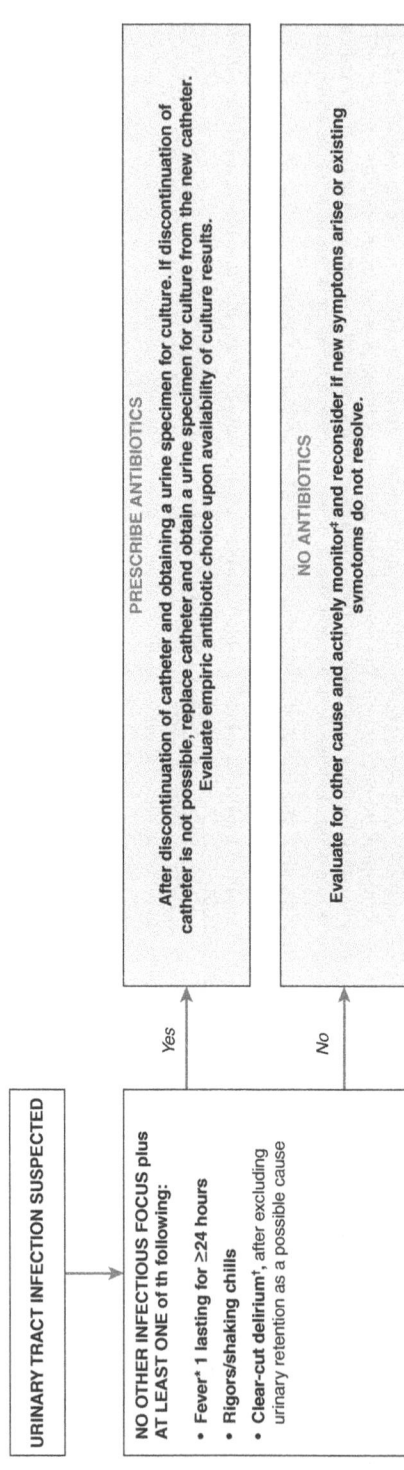

FIGURE 25.2 Decision tool for empiric treatment of suspected UTI in frail older adults with indwelling catheter.

DSM-5, Diagnostic and Statistical Manual of Mental Disorders, 5th edition; UTI, urinary tract infection.

*Defined as a single oral temperature >37.8°C OR repeated oral temperatures >37.2°C OR rectal temperature >37.5°C OR a 1.1°C increase over the baseline temperature.

†Definition of delirium according to *DSM-5*: (a) Disturbance in attention (i.e., reduced ability to direct, focus, sustain, and shift attention) and awareness (reduced orientation to the environment). (b) The disturbance develops over a short period of time (usually hours to a few days), represents an acute change from baseline attention and awareness, and tends to fluctuate in severity during the course of a day. (c) An additional disturbance in cognition (e.g., memory deficit, disorientation, language, visuospatial ability, or perception). (d) The disturbance in Criteria A and C are not better explained by a preexisting, established, or evolving neurocognitive disorder and do not occur in the context of a severely reduced level of arousal such as coma. (e) There is evidence from the history, physical examination, or laboratory findings that the disturbance is a direct physiological consequence of another medical condition, substance intoxication or withdrawal (i.e., due to a drug of abuse or to a medication), or exposure to a toxin, or is due to multiple etiologies.

‡e.g., monitoring vital signs, paying attention to hydration status and repeated physical assessments by nursing home staff.

Source: From van Buul, L., Vreeken, H., Bradley, S., Crnich, C., Drinka, P., Geerlings, S., . . . Hertogh, C. M. P. M. (2018). The development of a decision tool for the empiric treatment of suspected urinary tract infection in frail older adults: A Delphi consensus procedure. *Journal of the American Medical Directors Association, 19*(9), 757–764. doi:10.1016/j.jamda.2018.05.001

Recommendations for prevention of recurrent UTI are as follows:
- Low-dose prophylactic antibiotics
- Topical estrogen
- Increased fluid intake, >1 L/day
- Frequent voiding, at least every 3 to 4 hours (Marques et al., 2012)
- Intermittent condom catheter
- Cranberry products
- Likely not beneficial: oral estrogen and antibiotic-impregnated catheters (Detweiler et al., 2015)

Medications

See Table 25.3 for an overview of the most common medications for the treatment of UTIs.

Empiric therapy should be reassessed 48 to 72 hours after initiation (Marques et al., 2012). A high risk of antimicrobial resistance and additional adverse effects has been associated with the treatment of patients with recurrent UTI. In one study of older adults with three or more UTIs per year, there was a high rate of antimicrobial resistance and one-third of participants had nitrofurantoin as their last remaining outpatient UTI treatment option (Malik, Wu, Christie, Alhalabi, & Zimmern, 2018).

Asymptomatic Bacteriuria

Definition

ASB is the presence of one or more species of bacteria growing in the urine at >105 colony-forming units (CFU)/mL, irrespective of the presence of pyuria, in the absence of signs or symptoms attributable to UTI (Nicolle et al., 2019).

Prevalence

Urine samples are often cultured for any abnormality on a urinalysis, which may result in a positive culture. This leads to an expectation or hesitancy to not treat, whether the patient had symptoms suggestive of UTI or not. Many experts feel that too many urine cultures in older adults are not justified (Gavazzi et al., 2013).

The absence of pyuria has a strong negative predictive value for ASB and for UTI. Pyuria is present in 45% of incontinent adults and 90% of institutionalized adults regardless of infection or colonization status (Detweiler et al., 2015).

Urinalysis showing hematuria without bacteria indicates a patient's urinary symptoms are not due to infection (Mody & Juthani-Mehta, 2014).

Table 25.4 presents a summary of prevalence rates of ASB by population.

Risk Factors

Catheters are a most strongly associated risk factor for ASB, but all other risk factors for UTI listed earlier are likely relevant factors for ASB.

The most common bacteria are as follows:

- *Escherichia coli*
- *Klebsiella* spp
- *Proteus mirabilis*
- *Enterococcus* spp (Matthews & Lancaster, 2011)

TABLE 25.3 Most Common Medications for Treatment of UTI

Antibiotic	Dosing for Normal Renal Function	Renal Adjustment Required?	Additional Considerations
Amoxicillin/clavulanate	500 mg PO BID ×5–7 days for cystitis 875 mg PO BID ×10–14 days for pyelonephritis	CrCl <30 mL/min: 250 mg–500 mg PO once daily	Higher incidence of diarrhea than amoxicillin alone. Available as an oral suspension for those with difficulty swallowing. Consider local resistance patterns and/or facility antibiogram.
Cefdinir	300 mg BID ×5–7 days for cystitis 300 mg BID ×10–14 days for pyelonephritis	CrCl < 30 mL/min: 300 mg once daily	Use with caution in patients with a history of colitis. May cause reddish stools with concomitant use of iron supplements. Do not use if enterococcus is suspected.
Cephalexin	500 mg PO BID ×5–7 days for cystitis	CrCl 15–29 mL/min: 250 mg BID CrCl 5–14 mL/min: 250 mg daily CrCl 1–4 mL/min: 250 mg QOD ESRD on HD or PD: 250 mg–500 mg every 12–24 hours	Available as an oral suspension for those with difficulty swallowing. Consider local resistance patterns and/or facility antibiogram. No strong evidence to support treatment of pyelonephritis. Do not use if enterococcus is suspected.

Ciprofloxacin (immediate release)	250 mg PO BID ×3 days for cystitis 500 mg PO BID ×5–7 days for pyelonephritis	CrCl 30–50 mL/min: 250 mg–500 mg PO BID CrCl 5–29 mL/min: 250–500 mg every 18 hours ESRD on HD or PD: 250 mg–500 mg once daily	Black box warning: due to risk of serious adverse effects, reserve for use in patients with no alternative treatment options for cystitis. Risk of tendonitis, peripheral neuropathy, CNS effects (including delirium), and hypoglycemia with fluoroquinolones, particularly in elderly patients. Consider local resistance patterns and/or facility antibiogram. Risk of QT prolongation, crystalluria, aortic aneurysm and dissection, and photosensitivity.
Ertapenem	1 g IM or IV once followed by appropriate PO therapy ×5–14 days		Consider use for initial, empiric coverage in patients with history of ESBLs.
Fosfomycin	3 g PO once as a single dose for cystitis in women Off-label use in males without systemic symptoms: 3 g every 2–3 days for 3 total doses		Most common side effects include headache, diarrhea, vaginitis, and rhinitis. Comes as a flavored powder in a packet for reconstitution with 3–4 oz of cool water.
Levofloxacin	750 mg daily ×5 days	CrCl 20–49 mL/min: 750 mg every 48 hours CrCl 10–19 mL/min: 750 mg initial dose, then 500 mg every 48 hours	Black box warning: due to risk of serious adverse effects, reserve for use in patients with no alternative treatment options for cystitis.

(continued)

TABLE 25.3 Most Common Medications for Treatment of UTI (continued)

Antibiotic	Dosing for Normal Renal Function	Renal Adjustment Required?	Additional Considerations
Levofloxacin (cont.)		ESRD on HD or CAPD: 750 mg initial dose, then 500 mg every 48 hours	Risk of tendonitis, peripheral neuropathy, CNS effects (including delirium), and hypoglycemia with fluoroquinolones, particularly in elderly patients. Consider local resistance patterns and/or facility antibiogram. Risk of QT prolongation, crystalluria, aortic aneurysm and dissection, and photosensitivity.
Nitrofurantoin monohydrate macrocrystals (Macrobid)	100 mg PO BID ×5 days for females, ×7 days for males	Limited data suggests urine concentrations are adequate for treatment of cystitis even with eGFR or CrCl 30–60 mL/min	Avoid for treatment of pyelonephritis or in patients with CrCl <30 mL/min. Rare but serious hepatic reactions, optic neuritis, peripheral neuropathy, and pulmonary toxicity have been reported.

Sulfamethoxazole 800 mg/trimethoprim 160 mg (Bactrim DS)	1 tablet PO BID ×3 days for cystitis 1 tablet PO BID ×14 days for pyelonephritis (some experts will treat ×7–10 days if rapid response)	CrCl 15–30 mL/min: administer 50% of recommended dose Alternative dose reduction for GFR 10–50 mL/min is 1 tablet once, then single-strength tablet BID for remainder of therapy	Avoid in CrCl < 15 mL/min. Take with at least 8 oz of water to help prevent crystalluria. Associated with rare but life-threatening reports of Stevens–Johnson syndrome, aplastic anemia, and hepatic necrosis. May cause hyperkalemia, hypoglycemia, hyponatremia, and thrombocytopenia. Use with caution in patients with allergies, asthma, renal impairment, or thyroid dysfunction. Use with caution in older adults due to greater risk for more severe adverse reactions, including hyperkalemia, especially with concomitant medications that may also increase serum potassium. Use with caution in folate deficiency or those with potential folate deficiency.

BID, two times per day; CAPD, continuous ambulatory peritoneal dialysis; CNS, central nervous system; CrCl, creatine clearance; eGFR, estimated glomerular filtration rate; ESBL, extended-spectrum beta-lactamase; ESRD, end-stage renal disease; GFR, glomerular filtration rate; HD, hemodialysis; IM, intramuscular; IV, intravenous; PD, peritoneal dialysis; PO, by mouth; QOD, every other day; UTI, urinary tract infection.

Source: Data from Lexicomp Online, Lexi-Drugs Online. (2019, February 10). Hudson, OH: Wolters Kluwer Clinical Drug Information, Inc.

TABLE 25.4 Prevalence of ASB

Population	Prevalence, %
Healthy, premenopausal women	1–5
Healthy, pregnant women	1.9–9.5
Healthy, postmenopausal women (50–70 years)	2.8–8.6
Women with diabetes	10.8–16
Men with diabetes	0.7–11
Elderly women (70 and older) in community	10.8–16
Elderly men (70 and older) in community	3.6–19
Elderly women in long-term care facility	25–50
Elderly men in long-term care facility	15–50
Patients with short-term indwelling catheter use	3–5 (per day of catheter use)
Patients with long-term catheter use	100

ASB, asymptomatic bacteriuria.
Source: Data from Nicolle, L., Gupta, K., Bradley, S., Colgan, R., DeMuri, G., Drekonja, D., . . . Siemieniuk, R. (2019). Clinical practice guideline for the management of asymptomatic bacteriuria: 2019 Update by the Infectious Diseases Society of America. *Clinical Infectious Diseases, 68*(10), e83–e110. doi:10.1093/cid/ciy1121

Guidelines

The IDSA released an update to its ASB guideline in March 2019. Major changes to this updated guideline included highlighting the need to assess for other potential causes of delirium in older adults (see Chapter 20, Central Nervous System Impairments) with nonspecific symptoms (Nicolle et al., 2019). Assessment for other causes and careful observation without antimicrobial agents is recommended for the following:

- Older adults with functional and/or cognitive impairment with bacteriuria and delirium (acute mental status change, confusion) and without local GU symptoms or other systemic signs of infection
- Older adults with functional and/or cognitive impairment with bacteriuria and without local GU symptoms or other systemic signs of infection who experience a fall (Nicolle et al., 2019)

Updated guidelines recommend against screening and treatment of ASB in the following populations:

- Healthy, nonpregnant women (pre- or postmenopausal)
- Functionally impaired older adults residing in the community
- Older residents of long-term care facilities
- Patients with diabetes
- Renal transplant patients (<1 month postsurgery)
- Nonrenal solid organ transplant patients

- Individuals with impaired voiding following spinal cord injury
- Patients with short-term indwelling urethral catheter (<30 days)
- Patients with long-term indwelling catheters
- Elective nonurologic surgery (Nicolle et al., 2019)

Guidelines suggest against screening and treatment of ASB in patients planning to undergo surgery for artificial sphincter or penile implant or those living with implanted urologic devices (Nicolle et al., 2019).

Treatment
Antimicrobial treatment of ASB is not often recommended. Delirious inpatient older adults treated for ASB were associated with worse functional recovery (Dasgupta, Brymer, & Elsayed, 2017).

If a patient is undergoing a urologic procedure for which mucosal bleeding is expected, such as TURP, treatment of ASB is recommended. Urine culture and sensitivities should be gathered to guide tailored antimicrobial therapy prior to the procedure (Nicolle et al., 2019).

SEXUAL FUNCTION IN OLDER ADULTS
Erectile Dysfunction
Definition and Epidemiology
Erectile dysfunction is defined as the inability to achieve a full erection or inability to maintain an erection adequate for sexual intimacy. It is the most common form of sexual dysfunction in men, affecting an estimated 70% of men 70 years and older (Mobley, Khera, & Baum, 2017).

Medications or Conditions That May Worsen
Medications known to worsen erectile dysfunction include beta-blockers, thiazide diuretics, and selective serotonin reuptake inhibitors (SSRIs). Smoking, alcohol, and illicit drug use may also worsen erectile dysfunction (Mobley et al., 2017).

Psychogenic conditions that may worsen erectile dysfunction include relationship stressors, performance anxiety, trauma, and the patient's overall mental health. Obesity is associated with reduced libido. Diabetes mellitus (DM) has been associated with erectile dysfunction due to changes in the vessels and/or nerves. Prostate disease is associated with erectile dysfunction. CVD and hypertension (HTN) have strong correlation to erectile dysfunction by narrowing and hardening of arteries leading to reduced blood flow to corporal bodies (Mobley et al., 2017).

Risk Factors Associated With Erectile Dysfunction
Risk factors that have been associated with erectile dysfunction include:

- Hypertension
- Dyslipidemia
- Diabetes mellitus
- Atherosclerotic heart disease
- Age (Gokce & Yaman, 2017)
- Depression (Bella, Lee, Carrier, Bénard, & Brock, 2015)

Physical activity is associated with lower rates of erectile dysfunction in men (Bella et al., 2015).

Physiological Changes Associated With Erectile Dysfunction

Erectile dysfunction has been associated with reduced testosterone production in Leydig cells of testicles and reduced blood supply, causing erections that are less frequent or less rigid (Mobley et al., 2017).

Endothelium

Significant overlap has been demonstrated between erectile dysfunction and CVD due to changes in endothelial functioning. Proper vascular endothelial functioning is necessary for maintaining erections. Risk factors for endothelial dysfunction are common in an aging male, such as HTN, atherosclerosis, hyperlipidemia, and DM. Endothelial dysfunction then leads to reduced blood flow, which is the primary underlying mechanism in both erectile dysfunction and coronary artery disease (Bella et al., 2015).

Erection occurs with the release of nitric oxide from vascular endothelial cells. Reduced endothelial cell production of nitric oxide leads to smooth muscle inhibition in corporal bodies, which reduces smooth muscle relaxation, reduces blood supply, and ultimately leads to erectile dysfunction (Mobley et al., 2017).

Testosterone

Changes in testosterone availability in older adults lead to impaired nitric oxide synthase release, altered PDE5 expression and activity, and impaired cavernosal nerve function; contribute to veno-occlusive disease in penis; and impact function on smooth musculature within corpus spongiosum (Mobley et al., 2017).

Older adults typically have reduced testosterone production, which has been shown to increase the risk of CVD, muscle wasting, reduced bone density, and reduced libido. Testosterone replacement therapy may be considered as adjuvant to increase efficacy of PDE5 inhibitors for erectile dysfunction (Mobley et al., 2017). Use of testosterone replacement therapy is suggested in symptomatic hypogonadal elderly men with erectile dysfunction but must consider androgen-dependency risk of prostate cancer (Bella et al., 2015).

Assessment

Physical exam and laboratory tests should be performed to rule out secondary causes or other types of sexual dysfunction. If a patient has hormonal deficiency, experts suggest the treatment of deficiency before the trial of a PDE5 inhibitor (Mobley et al., 2017). If erectile dysfunction is confirmed with no previous history of CVD, cardiovascular evaluation is recommended (Mobley et al., 2017). Erectile dysfunction may manifest as a first sign of atherosclerosis and CVD (Bella et al., 2015).

Treatment

Recommend lifestyle modification when applicable at all steps, including smoking cessation, regular physical exercise, and reduction of body weight (Bella et al., 2015). First-line pharmacotherapy includes PDE5 inhibitors, which are typically safe for CVD (Mobley et al., 2017). PDE5 inhibitors should be avoided if the patient requires restriction of physical activity due to cardiac status or if the patient is prescribed concomitant nitrate therapy (Bella et al., 2015). If nitroglycerin and a PDE5 inhibitor are concomitantly prescribed, the patient should be counseled to separate the medications by at least 24 to 48 hours (48 hours for tadalafil) when possible to avoid severe vasodilation and hypotension.

If patients cannot tolerate or have contraindication to PDE5 inhibitors, second-line treatments include intracavernosal injections, vacuum erection device, and intraurethral prostaglandin suppositories (Mobley et al., 2017). Third-line treatment involves penile implants.

For stress-related erectile dysfunction, psychosexual counseling resolves about 50% to 70% of cases and should be trialed instead of or in addition to pharmacotherapy (Mobley et al., 2017).

Testosterone replacement is not recommended in older men with normal testosterone levels, even in the presence of erectile dysfunction (Buttaro, Koeniger-Donohue, & Hawkins, 2014). Herbal medications, such as yohimbine, are advertised as a treatment for erectile dysfunction but it is not recommended due to the risk and lack of evidence (Buttaro et al., 2014).

Women's Health

Sexual health needs may change as women age. One study investigated the sexual health needs or concerns most important in women younger than 65 and in women 65 and older. They found that women under 65 were more concerned about dyspareunia, body image, "normal" sex, STDs, HIV/AIDS, thinking about sex, controlling sexual urges, and orientation and practices. Older women were more concerned about orgasm difficulty, preorgasmic sexual dysfunction, partner sexual difficulties, and different desires from their partners. Older women were less comfortable bringing up their sexual health needs if the provider was young, seemed rushed, or previously seemed dismissive of the topic. Most women preferred the provider bringing up sexual health (Nusbaum, Singh, & Pyles, 2004).

Sexual dysfunction in older women is estimated to be 68% to 86%. This issue can be multifactorial including decline in estrogen production, problems with arousal, frequent UTIs, reduced body image, and/or pain. No robust data or agents support a specific treatment for sexual dysfunction in women, particularly in older women. However, some experts recommend a trial of L-arginine 1,000 mg to 3,000 mg just before intercourse. In theory, the supplement would increase nitric oxide production, which would lead to increased blood flow to the genitals. Other treatment options include psychosexual counseling, topical estrogens, and lubrication (Buttaro et al., 2014).

Dyspareunia

Vaginal atrophy affects about 50% of postmenopausal women due to reduced estrogen levels. This is thought to contribute to dyspareunia or painful intercourse. However, fewer than half of these affected postmenopausal women have discussed this issue with their provider due to embarrassment, belief that nothing can be done, or that these symptoms are a "normal" part of aging. Treatment of dyspareunia due to vaginal atrophy includes lubricants and/or topical estrogen products. Topical estrogen products should be used with caution in women with a history of thrombotic disease or malignancy, particularly breast cancer (Seehusen, Baird, & Bode, 2014).

Sexuality in Older Adults

Sexual interest and activity are still important to many older adults. Older adults have reported their sexuality remains important, even in the last days to weeks prior to death. We now believe that sexual interest and ability are constant with age, but the frequency generally declines. Overall, elderly males are more likely to be sexually active, which is likely from testosterone's effect on libido. One survey of men >70 years old found that 27% desired more frequent sexual activity. Another survey of men 70 to 80 years old found that 50% had sex within the last year, compared to 21% of women in the same age range (Camacho & Reyes-Ortiz, 2005). Interest in sex for older adults does remain, even when not sexually active. The variables most associated with remaining sexually active in older adults include male sex, married, higher education level, self-sufficient, and satisfied with present life (Bortz, Wallace, & Wiley, 1999).

Sexual health needs and education are important because many older adults are less aware of STD risk and HIV transmission or may consider it an issue for younger people. Older sexually active adults are more likely to have unprotected sex and less likely to have regular STD checks for these reasons (Camacho & Reyes-Ortiz, 2005). One alarming public health statistic relevant to this population is the estimated 25% of new HIV cases in Florida occurred in heterosexual older adults (Nusbaum et al., 2004).

Sexuality in dementia patients is an emerging "gray area" of patient rights and safety. Studies have shown that patients with dementia are more likely than others to engage in sexual activity without feeling aroused and men with dementia are more likely than men without dementia to have sex primarily out of obligation. Over 40% of men and women aged 80 to 91 years with dementia reported being sexually active (Lindau et al., 2018).

Barriers to Expression of Sexuality

Literature is notably lacking for sexuality in older adults, particularly those who are lesbian, gay, bisexual, transgender, and queer (LGBTQ; Bauer, McAuliffe, & Nay, 2007). In fact, one study found only 57% of geriatricians take sexual history for each patient (Omole et al., 2014). Expression of sexuality may not include or may have less to do with penetration in older adults. Older adults may be more uncertain about their abilities or concerned about harmful outcomes from sex (Bauer et al., 2007). From the limited data available, it does appear that aging does not abolish the need to be sexual (McAuliffe, Bauer, & Nay, 2007) and physical health was more likely to contribute to sexual problems than aging alone (Lindau et al., 2007). Medications and comorbidities often lead to sexual dysfunction, but older adults may attribute the symptom to aging when it might be easily corrected (Camacho & Reyes-Ortiz, 2005).

Older women most commonly report arthritis (Camacho & Reyes-Ortiz, 2005), lack of interest, difficulty with lubrication, inability to climax, finding sex not pleasurable, and pain as bothersome sexual problems (Lindau et al., 2007). Older men are more likely to report psychological interference with sexuality, such as alcohol abuse and depression (Camacho & Reyes-Ortiz, 2005). Most common sexual problems in older men included difficulty achieving or maintaining an erection, lack of interest in sex, climaxing too quickly, anxiety about performance, and inability to climax (Lindau et al., 2007).

Patients may be hesitant to discuss their sexual health concerns with providers because of embarrassment or believing that there is no solution or that their problem is "part of aging." When older adults were asked to define sexuality, answers included looking nice, spending time with the opposite sex, intercourse with a long-term partner, and relieving one's frustrations with a sex worker (McAuliffe et al., 2007).

Sexuality encompasses partnership, activity, behavior, attitudes, and function. Many people, particularly older women, lose their partner with age. However, negative societal values about women's sexuality and older adult sexuality may hinder discussion of patient needs and ultimately lead to patient harm (Lindau et al., 2007). Providers should acknowledge and attempt to overcome these barriers.

How to Discuss Sexuality With Older Adults

Clinicians may overlook sexual history as patients age and have more comorbidities, but sexuality does remain an important piece of overall health for older adults (Buttaro et al., 2014). Providers may be reluctant to discuss sexuality with older adults due to fear of offending patients, lack of confidence in their ability to adequately educate, and belief in myths and stereotypes surrounding sex in older adults (McAuliffe et al., 2007). Beware of one's own prejudices and subconscious feelings, do not make assumptions, and be sensitive to patient preferences. Sexuality should be discussed with patients in a private environment as any other health discussion (Taylor & Gosney, 2011).

One model for discussion of sexuality is the "PLISSIT model," which is a pneumonic for:

- Ask permission to discuss sexuality
- Provide limited information about sexual issues that affect older adults
- Specific suggestions to improve sexual health and resolve problems
- Referral for intensive therapy (Omole et al., 2014)

Open-ended questions are preferred when gathering sexual history, using the following examples. Experts recommend integrating this into their routine interview and examination of patients and suggest leading with "As part of your physical, I will ask..." to show the patient this is a routine and important part of their overall health (Omole et al., 2014).

- "Are you experiencing any problems in your sexual life?"
- "Can you tell me how you express your sexuality?"
- "In what ways has your relationship changed with age?"
- "What concerns or questions do you have about fulfilling your sexual needs?"

Selected Educational Resources for Sexuality in Older Adults

- Safersex4seniors.org
- Healthinaging.org/agingintheknow
  - Created by American Geriatrics Society Foundation for Health in Aging and offers up-to-date information for patients on health and aging, including sexual concerns
- LGBTagingproject.org
  - Nonprofit working to increase awareness of LGBT elders and caregivers and issues that impact their lives
- nyahof.org
  - Volunteer-based education promoting education, training, and advocacy to those over 50 with a diagnosis of HIV
- NIA.NIH.gov/healthinformation/publications/sexuality.htm
  - National Institute on Aging Sexuality in Later Life
- AARP.org/relationships/love-sex
  - AARP Love & Sex Website

SUMMARY

GU diseases such as BPH, erectile dysfunction, and UTIs have a significant impact on many older adults' quality of life. Sexual health remains a major part of life in aging adults and should be addressed as a part of their healthcare.

GENITOURINARY INTERPROFESSIONAL CASE STUDY

Marjorie Young

Patient Presentation

Brenda is a 66-year-old female who presents with complaints of urinary urgency and frequency and dysuria to the urgent care center in which you work. She was referred to urgent care by her primary care provider (PCP) because her physician's office had no openings today due to flu season.

Brenda states that she has noticed that her urine is cloudy, dark, and has a strong odor for the past 2 days. Last night, she started with symptoms of urgency, frequency, and burning with urination. She denies fever, chills, and sweats. She denies respiratory or cardiac symptoms. Brenda states she is a little nauseated and has some fatigue today along with slight lower abdomen pressure. She also complains of mild dyspareunia with occasional vaginal irritation, which started about 2 years ago. She denies vaginal bleeding or discharge. Brenda states that due to her irritable bowel syndrome (IBS), she has episodic diarrhea. This past week, she states she had a particularly "bad flare." Brenda states she is frustrated and concerned as this is her third UTI in a year and had only one UTI previously in her life.

History

Brenda has a past medical history of HTN, IBS, depression, and onychomycosis. Her past surgical history includes two cesarean sections, gallbladder surgery, and a uterine ablation. Brenda has been divorced for 2 years. She is currently in a new relationship and is sexually active in this relationship. Her two adult children live locally and visit frequently with her five grandchildren. They are supportive of the new relationship. She states she does not have financial worries and has private insurance from the state along with Medicare.

Medications

Brenda is allergic to penicillin. Her current medications include lisinopril, dicyclomine, ketoconazole, and sertraline. She states she also takes a multivitamin, along with glucosamine/chondroitin daily.

Physical Exam

Patient presents well-groomed and nourished. No apparent distress. She is positive and articulate. Lungs' sounds are clear in all fields, heart with regular rate and rhythm, no murmur, or gallop bowel sounds (BS) active in all four quads, mild suprapubic tenderness, and no costovertebral angle (CVA) tenderness. The patient declines a GU exam and sexually transmitted infection (STI) testing at this time.

Diagnostic Testing

A urine specimen was obtained in triage at the urgent care clinic. Urine dipstick analysis is positive for leukocyte esterase and nitrates, consistent with a UTI. Urine is sent for culture and sensitivity.

Plan of Care

Brenda is given instructions to increase her fluid intake including cranberry juice and add a high-quality probiotic. Concerning her new relationship, you encourage Brenda to void after sexual intercourse along with standard precautions for STIs, such as the avoidance of multiple sexual partners, use of condoms, reporting any new onset vaginal discharge or pelvic symptoms, and HIV testing at least once to determine HIV status. You also offer instructions on nonhormonal over-the-counter lubricant options for her dyspareunia. With the possible splashing from her IBS diarrhea, you encourage Brenda to use toileting wet wipes for personal cleansing with reinforcement on correct wiping technique and regular voiding.

When prescribing medication to treat the UTI, you avoid Bactrim DS due to her current medications of ketoconazole, sertraline, and lisinopril. When these medications are used in combination, they can increase her risk of QT prolongations due to hyperkalemia. For a good antimicrobial coverage, you prescribe nitrofurantoin along with phenazopyridine. You instruct Brenda that her urine may look orange and to use a panty liner as the medication can permanently stain her underwear.

You send the urine sample to the lab for culture and sensitivity along with instructions to follow up with her PCP 1 week after completing the antibiotic for a repeat urinalysis. You also encourage Brenda to follow up with her gastroenterologist and gynecologist.

Interprofessional Collaboration

Considering Brenda's recurrent UTIs, new relationship, dyspareunia, and IBS flare, you consider an interprofessional approach to treatment. Along with the nursing interventions discussed in her plan of care, you consider that she is postmenopausal. You recommend that she make an appointment with her gynecologist for evaluation of urogenital structures and possible use of estrogen therapy with either a vaginal cream, tablet or ring to decrease her UTIs and improve the GU symptoms associated with GU syndrome of menopause. Depending on the assessment and evaluation from Brenda's gynecologist, an adjunctive treatment would be to involve physical therapy for pelvic floor retraining.

Also recommended is a follow-up with her gastroenterologist to manage her IBS symptoms. You counsel Brenda on the importance of follow-up with her PCP for a repeat urinalysis to evaluate effectiveness of treatment and possible use of postcoital prophylaxis.

Consultation with Brenda's local pharmacist is necessary to determine drug choice based on her current medications of dicyclomine, lisinopril, ketoconazole, and sertraline with instructions to avoid use of the standard Bactrim DS. This is based on the increased cardiac risk of possible QT prolongation due to hyperkalemia. Nitrofurantoin is prescribed as first-line therapy while an alternative could be fosfomycin. After the follow-up with her PCP, if additional antibiotics with postcoital or long-term prophylaxis are needed, collaboration with a pharmacist will be beneficial.

While what may seem like a simple diagnosis of a UTI, the holistic picture of the patient is essential for quality of life. Effective communication between specialties is important for continuity of care. Providing patient education handouts and a copy of the information of her visit from the clinic will facilitate interprofessional care of the patient. Sharing the urinalysis and urine culture results with Brenda's PCP and gynecologist will facilitate the follow-up with continuity of her care.

Case Study References

Baker, J. (2018). Challenges of treating urinary tract infections in post-menopausal women. *Urologic Nursing, 38*(1), 6–19. doi:10.7257/1053-816X.38.1.6

Bass-Ware, A., Weed, D., Johnson, T., & Spurlock, A. (2014). Evaluation of the effect of cranberry juice on symptoms associated with a urinary tract infection. *Urologic Nursing, 34*(3), 121–127. doi:10.7257/1053-816X.2014.34.3.121

Davis, D., & Rantell, A. (2017). Lower urinary tract infections in women. *British Journal of Nursing, 26*(9), 12–19. doi:10.12968/bjon.2017.26.9.S12

Epocrates Rx. (2019). Medications online. Athena Health, Retrieved from https://www.epocrates.com

Hooton, T., & Gupta, K. (2019). Recurrent simple cystitis in women. In S. B. Calderwood & A. Bloom (Eds.), *UpToDate*. Retrieved from https://www.uptodate.com/contents/recurrent-simple-cystitis-in-women

Hooton, T., & Gupta, K. (2019). Acute simpl cystitis in women. In S. B. Calderwood & A. Bloom (Eds.), *UpToDate*. Retrieved from https://www.uptodate.com/contents/acute-simple-cystitis-in-women

Hopkins, L., McCroskey, D., Reeves, G., & Tanabe, P. (2014). Implementing a urinary tract infection clinical practice guideline in an ambulatory urgent care practice. *The Nurse Practitioner, 39*(4), 50–54. doi:10.1097/01.NPR.0000444651.10142.06

IBM Micromedex. (2019). IBM Micromedex Drug Ref (version 2.1) [Mobile application software]. Retrieved from https://apps.apple.com/us/app/ibm-micromedex-drug-ref/id666520138

Lexi-Comp, Inc. (2019). Lexicomp (version 5.1.1) [Mobile application software]. Retrieved from https://apps.apple.com/us/app/lexicomp/id313401238

Love, B. (2016). Physical therapy management of lower urinary tract symptoms. *The Journal of Nurse Practitioners, 12*(5), 356–357. doi:10.1016/j.nurpra.2016.02.015

Maki, K., Kaspar, K., Khoo, C., Derrig, L., Schild, A., & Gupta, K. (2016). Consumption of a cranberry juice beverage lowered the number of clinical urinary tract infection episodes in women with a recent history of urinary tract infection. *American Journal of Clinical Nutrition, 103*(6), 1434–1442. doi:10.3945/ajcn.116.130542

Price, J., Guran, L., Gregory, T., & McDonagh, M. (2016). Nitrofurantoin vs other prophylactic agents in reducing recurrent urinary tract infections in adult women: A systematic review and meta-analysis. *American Journal of Obstetrics & Gynecology, 215*(5), 548–560. doi:10.1016/j.ajog.2016.07.040

Velez, R., Richmond, E., & Dudley-Brown, S. (2017). Antibiogram, clinical practice guidelines and treatment of urinary tract infection. *The Journal of Nurse Practitioners, 13*(9), 617–622. doi:10.1016/j.nurpra.2017.07.016

Ward, K., & Deneris, A. (2016). Genitourinary syndrome of menopause: A new name for an old condition. *The Nurse Practitioner, 41*(7), 28–33. doi:10.1097/01.NPR.0000484319.60683.db

REFERENCES

Arinzon, Z., Shabat, S., Peisakh, A., & Berner, Y. (2012). Clinical presentation of urinary tract infection (UTI) differs with aging in women. *Archives of Gerontology and Geriatrics, 55*(1), 145–147. doi:10.1016/j.archger.2011.07.012

Bauer, M., McAuliffe, L., & Nay, R. (2007). Sexuality, health care and the older person: An overview of the literature. *International Journal of Older People Nursing, 2*(1), 63–68. doi:10.1111/j.1748-3743.2007.00051.x

Bella, A., Lee, J., Carrier, S., Bénard, F., & Brock, G. (2015). 2015 CUA Practice guidelines for erectile dysfunction. *Canadian Urological Association Journal, 9*(1–2), 23–29. doi:10.5489/cuaj.2699

Bortz, W., Wallace, D., & Wiley, D. (1999). Sexual function in 1,202 aging males: Differentiating aspects. *Journals of Gerontology: Series A, 54A*(5), M237–M241. doi:10.1093/gerona/54.5.M237

Buttaro, T., Koeniger-Donohue, R., & Hawkins, J. (2014). Sexuality and quality of life in aging: Implications for practice. *The Journal For Nurse Practitioners, 10*(7), 480–485. doi:10.1016/j.nurpra.2014.04.008

Camacho, M., & Reyes-Ortiz, C. (2005). Sexual dysfunction in the elderly: Age or disease? *International Journal of Impotence Research, 17*(Suppl. 1), S52–S56. doi:10.1038/sj.ijir.3901429

Caterino, J., Kline, D., Leininger, R., Southerland, L., Carpenter, C., Baugh, C., . . . Stevenson, K. B. (2018). Nonspecific symptoms lack diagnostic accuracy for infection in older patients in the emergency department. *Journal of the American Geriatrics Society, 67*(3), 484–492. doi:10.1111/jgs.15679

Cortes-Penfield, N., Trautner, B., & Jump, R. (2017). Urinary tract infection and asymptomatic bacteriuria in older adults. *Infectious Disease Clinics of North America, 31*(4), 673–688. doi:10.1016/j.idc.2017.07.002

Dasgupta, M., Brymer, C., & Elsayed, S. (2017). Treatment of asymptomatic UTI in older delirious medical in-patients: A prospective cohort study. *Archives of Gerontology and Geriatrics, 72*, 127–134. doi:10.1016/j.archger.2017.05.010

Detweiler, K., Mayers, D., & Fletcher, S. (2015). Bacteriuria and urinary tract infections in the elderly. *Urologic Clinics of North America, 42*(4), 561–568. doi:10.1016/j.ucl.2015.07.002

Eriksson, I., Gustafson, Y., Fagerström, L., & Olofsson, B. (2010). Prevalence and factors associated with urinary tract infections (UTIs) in very old women. *Archives of Gerontology and Geriatrics, 50*(2), 132–135. doi:10.1016/j.archger.2009.02.013

Gavazzi, G., Delerce, E., Cambau, E., François, P., Corroyer, B., de Wazières, B., . . . Gaillat, J. (2013). Diagnostic criteria for urinary tract infection in hospitalized elderly patients over 75 years of age: A multicenter cross-sectional study. *Médecine Et Maladies Infectieuses, 43*(5), 189–194. doi:10.1016/j.medmal.2013.02.006

Gokce, M., & Yaman, O. (2017). Erectile dysfunction in the elderly male. *Türk Üroloji Dergisi/Turkish Journal of Urology, 43*(3), 247–251. doi:10.5152/tud.2017.70482

Hooton, T., Bradley, S., Cardenas, D., Colgan, R., Geerlings, S., Rice, J., . . . Nicolle, L. E. (2010). Diagnosis, prevention, and treatment of catheter-associated urinary tract infection in adults: 2009 International clinical practice guidelines from the Infectious Diseases Society of America. *Clinical Infectious Diseases, 50*(5), 625–663. doi:10.1086/650482

Lexicomp Online, Lexi-Drugs Online. (2019, February 10). Hudson, OH: Wolters Kluwer Clinical Drug Information, Inc.

Lindau, S., Dale, W., Feldmeth, G., Gavrilova, N., Langa, K., Makelarski, J., & Wroblewski, K. (2018). Sexuality and cognitive status: A U.S. nationally representative study of home-dwelling older adults. *Journal of the American Geriatrics Society, 66*(10), 1902–1910. doi:10.1111/jgs.15511

Lindau, S., Schumm, L., Laumann, E., Levinson, W., O'Muircheartaigh, C., & Waite, L. (2007). A study of sexuality and health among older adults in the United States. *New England Journal of Medicine, 357*(8), 762–774. doi:10.1056/nejmoa067423

Malik, R., Wu, Y., Christie, A., Alhalabi, F., & Zimmern, P. (2018). Impact of allergy and resistance on antibiotic selection for recurrent urinary tract infections in older women. *Urology, 113*, 26–33. doi:10.1016/j.urology.2017.08.070

Marques, L., Flores, J., Barros Junior, O., Rodrigues, G., Mourão, C., & Moreira, R. (2012). Epidemiological and clinical aspects of urinary tract infection in community-dwelling elderly women. *The Brazilian Journal of Infectious Diseases, 16*(5), 436–441. doi:10.1016/j.bjid.2012.06.025

Matthews, S., & Lancaster, J. (2011). Urinary tract infections in the elderly population. *The American Journal of Geriatric Pharmacotherapy, 9*(5), 286–309. doi:10.1016/j.amjopharm.2011.07.002

McAuliffe, L., Bauer, M., & Nay, R. (2007). Barriers to the expression of sexuality in the older person: The role of the health professional. *International Journal of Older People Nursing*, 2(1), 69–75. doi:10.1111/j.1748-3743.2007.00050.x

Miller, J., Binnicker, M., Campbell, S., Carroll, K., Chapin, K., Gilligan, P., . . . Yao, J. D. (2018). A guide to utilization of the microbiology laboratory for diagnosis of infectious diseases: 2018 Update by the Infectious Diseases Society of America and the American Society for Microbiology. *Clinical Infectious Diseases*, 67(6), e1–e94. doi:10.1093/cid/ciy381

Mobley, D., Khera, M., & Baum, N. (2017). Recent advances in the treatment of erectile dysfunction. *Postgraduate Medical Journal*, 93(1105), 679–685. doi:10.1136/postgradmedj-2016-134073

Mody, L., Greene, M., Meddings, J., Krein, S., McNamara, S., & Trautner, B., . . . Saint, S. (2017). A national implementation project to prevent catheter-associated urinary tract infection in nursing home residents. *Journal of the American Medical Association Internal Medicine*, 177(8), 1154. doi:10.1001/jamainternmed.2017.1689

Mody, L., & Juthani-Mehta, M. (2014). Urinary tract infections in older women. *Journal of the American Medical Association*, 311(8), 844. doi:10.1001/jama.2014.303

Nicolle, L., Gupta, K., Bradley, S., Colgan, R., DeMuri, G., Drekonja, D., . . . Siemieniuk, R. (2019). Clinical practice guideline for the management of asymptomatic bacteriuria: 2019 Update by the Infectious Diseases Society of America. *Clinical Infectious Diseases*, 68(10), e83–e110. doi:10.1093/cid/ciy1121

Nusbaum, M., Singh, A., & Pyles, A. (2004). Sexual healthcare needs of women aged 65 and older. *Journal of the American Geriatrics Society*, 52(1), 117–122. doi:10.1111/j.1532-5415.2004.52020.x

Omole, F., Fresh, E., Sow, C., Lin, J., Taiwo, B., & Nichols, M. (2014). How to discuss sex with elderly patients. *The Journal of Family Practice*, 63(4), E1–E4. Retrieved from https://mdedge-files-live.s3.us-east-2.amazonaws.com/files/s3fs-public/Document/September-2017/JFP_06304_Article1W.pdf

Rowe, T., & Juthani-Mehta, M. (2014). Diagnosis and management of urinary tract infection in older adults. *Infectious Disease Clinics of North America*, 28(1), 75–89. doi:10.1016/j.idc.2013.10.004

Seehusen, D., Baird, D., & Bode, D. (2014). Dyspareunia in women. *American Family Physician*, 90(7), 465–470. Retrieved from https://www.aafp.org/afp/2014/1001/p465.html

Taylor, A., & Gosney, M. (2011). Sexuality in older age: Essential considerations for healthcare professionals. *Age and Ageing*, 40(5), 538–543. doi:10.1093/ageing/afr049

van Buul, L., Vreeken, H., Bradley, S., Crnich, C., Drinka, P., Geerlings, S., . . . Hertogh, C. M. P. M. (2018). The development of a decision tool for the empiric treatment of suspected urinary tract infection in frail older adults: A Delphi consensus procedure. *Journal of the American Medical Directors Association*, 19(9), 757–764. doi:10.1016/j.jamda.2018.05.001

Woodard, T., Manigault, K., McBurrows, N., Wray, T., & Woodard, L. (2016). Management of benign prostatic hyperplasia in older adults. *The Consultant Pharmacist*, 31(8), 412–424. doi:10.4140/tcp.n.2016.412

IV Prescribing Considerations Unique to the Geriatric Population

26 The Beers Criteria for Inappropriate Medication Use in Older Adults

Megan Hebdon

OBJECTIVES
1. Review the implications of adverse drug events in elderly patients
2. Discuss the Beers criteria and screening tool of older people's prescriptions (STOPP)/screening tool to alert to right treatment (START) criteria to aid in prescribing decision-making
3. Describe the clinical application of prescribing criteria in older adults

INTRODUCTION
Due to the physiologic changes in the body that occur with aging, geriatric patients may be more prone to adverse drug side effects (Health in Aging Foundation, 2019b). The consequences of adverse drug events in the elderly are costly due to morbidity and mortality, and financially costly to the healthcare system in the United States. Adverse drug events or inappropriate prescribing is relatively common, with one in six older adults having experienced an adverse drug event and around 40% of older adults having exposure to a potentially inappropriate medication (Beizer & Semla, 2016). For over 20 years, the American Geriatrics Society (AGS) has disseminated the Beers Criteria for Inappropriate Drug Prescribing as a guide for clinicians in medication decision-making (Health in Aging Foundation, 2019b). These guidelines are not absolute, but they are meant to guide patient-centered care (AGS Beers Criteria Update Expert Panel, 2019). In addition to the Beers criteria, the STOPP/START criteria provide useful guidance regarding medications that should be initiated or discontinued based on the clinical picture of the patient (O'Mahony et al., 2015). In addition to prescribing decisions, both sets of guidelines are useful when conducting a medication review in inpatient and outpatient settings. Medication review is further described in the next chapter, Examples of Inappropriate Medication Prescribing.

HISTORY OF THE BEERS CRITERIA
The Beers criteria were developed and published by Dr. Beers in 1991. He used an expert panel and Delphi system to identify 30 therapeutic classes or medications where the risks of use outweighed the benefits in older adults. He then used the criteria as a process measure in a cluster randomized trial for an intervention to improve prescribing for older patients in long-term care facilities (Marcum & Hanlon, 2012). The purpose of the initial guidelines was to prevent inappropriate drug prescribing (Marcum & Hanlon, 2012). These criteria were updated in 1997, where 28 drug therapeutic classes with greater risk in the elderly in long-term care or community settings were outlined. Medicare and Medicaid Services adopted a partial list from the

1997 criteria, and this list was used as a quality indicator measure for long-term care facilities (Marcum & Hanlon, 2012). Subsequently, updates to the Beers criteria have occurred in 2003, 2012, 2015, and 2019 based on new medications and new findings regarding the effects of medications on the elderly population (AGS Beers Criteria Expert Panel, 2019; Marcum & Hanlon, 2012).

The 2019 Beers Criteria for Potentially Inappropriate Prescribing were released with aims to incorporate new evidence, grade the strength and quality of potentially inappropriate medication statements, use an interdisciplinary panel of 13 experts in geriatric care and pharmacotherapeutics for a modified Delphi panel, and to incorporate exceptions to promote individualized care across multiple settings (AGS Beers Criteria Update Expert Panel, 2019). The criteria are intended for clinicians prescribing medications to adults aged 65 years or older in all settings of care, with the exceptions of hospice and palliative care (AGS Beers Criteria Update Expert Panel, 2019). The 2019 update is intended to provide support for provider education and quality measurement, but is not intended to be used as a punitive tool for providers in the clinical setting. The panel specifically addressed the challenges related to prescribing decision-making and the difficulty of making blanket statements regarding prescribing decisions that may apply only to a subgroup of the population (AGS Beers Criteria Update Expert Panel, 2019). Additionally, some recommendations were removed from the current update because the adverse medication side effects are relevant to all populations (use of medications that lower the seizure threshold in patients at risk for seizures). Therefore, there are nuances that need to be considered regarding individual comorbidities, existing pharmacotherapy, environment, access to medications, and goals of care.

Tables 26.1 to 26.6 provide a high-level overview of the 2019 Beers Criteria Update.

In addition to the recommendations of medications to avoid or use with caution, the AGS has also provided patient information to help older adults advocate for alternative medications (Health in Aging Foundation, 2019a). They recommend saline nasal rinses, corticosteroid nasal sprays, or second-generation antihistamines to be used in place of first-generation antihistamines. As alternatives to tricyclic antidepressants, they suggest selective serotonin reuptake inhibitors (SSRIs) or bupropion. For individuals with epilepsy, lamotrigine or levetiracetam is recommended in lieu of phenobarbital. Behavioral strategies are suggested for sleep and anxiety, rather than z-drugs or benzodiazepines (Health in Aging Foundation, 2019a). In addition, buspirone and SSRIs are suggested for treatment of anxiety. Pain management alternatives for nonsteroidal anti-inflammatory drugs (NSAIDs) include acetaminophen, topical capsaicin, lidocaine patches, and serotonin–norepinephrine reuptake inhibitors (SNRIs). For pain management with opioid therapy, tramadol, morphine, and immediate-release oxycodone with acetaminophen are recommended over meperidine with the disclaimer to follow the Centers for Disease Control and Prevention guidelines for safe opioid prescribing (Health in Aging Foundation, 2019a). Finally, rather than systemic estrogen, topical estrogen creams for vaginal dryness are recommended, along with gabapentin, SNRIs, or SSRIs for hot flashes and night sweats (Health in Aging Foundation, 2019a).

HISTORY OF THE STOPP/START CRITERIA

The STOPP/START criteria were initially drafted in 2003 as a response to the gaps in prescribing for older patients in routine clinical practice (O'Mahony et al., 2010). O'Mahony et al. (2010) also described some deficiencies in the Beers criteria, including listing drugs no longer available in Europe, drugs that are not contraindicated in older adults, accounting for drug–drug interactions or drug class overlap, and

TABLE 26.1 Common Medications From 2019 Beers Criteria for Potentially Inappropriate Medication Use in Older Adults

System/Therapeutic Drug Category/Examples	Rationale	Recommendation/Quality of Evidence/Strength of Recommendation
Anticholinergics		
First generation	Reduced clearance with age, highly anticholinergic (dry mouth, confusion, constipation, etc.)	Avoid/moderate/strong
Antihistamines Examples: *meclizine, promethazine, oral diphenhydramine*	Use of diphenhydramine in acute allergic reaction may be appropriate	
Antispasmodics Examples: *atropine, dicyclomine (excluding ophthalmic), scopolamine*	Highly anticholinergic	Avoid/moderate/strong
Anti-Infective		
Nitrofurantoin	Risk of pulmonary and hepatic toxicity and peripheral neuropathy	Avoid for creatinine <30 mL/min or for long-term use/low/strong
Cardiovascular		
Peripheral alpha-1 blockers for hypertension Examples: *terazosin, doxazosin, prazosin*	Risk of orthostatic hypotension	Avoid for hypertension/moderate/strong
Central alpha-agonists Examples: *clonidine for first-line hypertension treatment, guanfacine, methyldopa*	Adverse CNS effects, bradycardia, and orthostatic hypotension	Avoid clonidine as first-line hypotensive and other alpha-agonists/low/strong

(*continued*)

TABLE 26.1 Common Medications From 2019 Beers Criteria for Potentially Inappropriate Medication Use in Older Adults (continued)

System/Therapeutic Drug Category/Examples	Rationale	Recommendation/Quality of Evidence/Strength of Recommendation
Cardiovascular (continued)		
Digoxin for first-line treatment of atrial fibrillation or heart failure	Safer alternatives for atrial fibrillation and heart failure	Avoid as first-line therapy and avoid dosages >0.125 mg/d/low/strong
Nifedipine, immediate release	Risk for hypotension and ischemia	Avoid/high/strong
Amiodarone	Greater toxicities than other antiarrhythmics	Avoid as first-line therapy for atrial fibrillation unless concomitant heart failure or left ventricular hypertrophy/high/strong
CNS		
Antidepressants Examples: TCAs (amitriptyline, imipramine, nortriptyline, doxepin >6 mg/d), paroxetine	Highly anticholinergic, risk of sedation or orthostatic hypotension	Avoid/high/strong
Antipsychotics Examples: First and second generation	Increased risk of stroke, cognitive decline, and mortality in dementia. Avoid use for behavioral issues in dementia or delirium	Avoid, except in schizophrenia, bipolar disorder, or short-term antiemetic during chemotherapy/moderate/strong
Barbiturates Examples: butalbital, phenobarbital, pentobarbital	Physical dependence, tolerance, and risk of overdose	Avoid/high/strong

Benzodiazepines Examples: *alprazolam, lorazepam, temazepam, clonazepam, diazepam*	Increased sensitivity, decreased metabolism, increased risk of cognitive impairment, delirium, falls, fractures, and motor vehicle accidents. May be used in select conditions: seizure disorders, REM sleep behavior disorder, benzodiazepine or ethanol withdrawal, severe GAD, and anesthesia	Avoid/moderate/strong
Sedative-hypnotics "z-drugs" Examples: *zaleplon, zolpidem, and eszopiclone*	Adverse effects similar to benzodiazepines	Avoid/moderate/strong
Endocrine		
Androgens Examples: *methyltestosterone, testosterone*	Risk of cardiac issues and contraindicated in prostate cancer	Avoid unless confirmed hypogonadism with symptoms/moderate/weak
Desiccated thyroid	Cardiac effects, safer alternatives	Avoid/low/strong
Estrogens with or without progestins Examples: *femara, vagifem*	Carcinogenic potential, lack of cardioprotective effect or cognitive protection in women. Vaginal estrogens are safe and effective, but should be approached in caution with a history of breast cancer	Avoid systemic estrogen/high/strong Vaginal cream or tablets are acceptable/moderate/weak

(continued)

TABLE 26.1 Common Medications From 2019 Beers Criteria for Potentially Inappropriate Medication Use in Older Adults (*continued*)

System/Therapeutic Drug Category/Examples	Rationale	Recommendation/Quality of Evidence/Strength of Recommendation
Endocrine		
Growth hormone	Associated with edema, arthralgia, carpal tunnel, gynecomastia, and impaired fasting glucose	Avoid/moderate/strong
Megestrol	Minimal weight effects and increased risk of thrombotic events	Avoid/moderate/high
Sulfonylureas, long acting Examples: *glimepiride, glyburide*	Higher risk of severe and prolonged hypoglycemia	Avoid/high/strong
Gastrointestinal		
Metoclopramide	Extrapyramidal effects	Avoid unless short term for gastroparesis/moderate/strong
Oral mineral oil	Risk of adverse effects, safer alternatives	Avoid/moderate/strong
Proton-pump inhibitors Examples: *pantoprazole, omeprazole*	Risk of *Clostridium difficile* infection, bone loss, and fractures	Avoid scheduled use for over 8 weeks unless high-risk patient/high/strong
Pain		
Meperidine	Higher risk of neurotoxicity, safer alternatives	Avoid/moderate/strong

Pain		
Nonselective oral NSAIDs Examples: *aspirin >325 mg/d, diclofenac, naproxen, ibuprofen, ketorolac, indomethacin*	Risk of gastrointestinal bleeding, peptic ulcer disease, increased blood pressure, and kidney injury. Indomethacin has greatest adverse effects	Avoid chronic use unless no other alternatives or can take gastroprotective agent/moderate/strong
Skeletal muscle relaxants Examples: *carisoprodol, cyclobenzaprine, methocarbamol*	Anticholinergic effects, sedation, risk of fracture	Avoid/moderate/strong
Urinary		
Desmopressin	Hyponatremia, safer alternative available	Avoid for nocturia/moderate/strong

CNS, central nervous system; GAD, generalized anxiety disorder; NSAIDs, nonsteroidal anti-inflammatory drugs; REM, rapid eye movement; TCAs, tricyclic antidepressants.

Source: From American Geriatrics Society Beers Criteria Update Expert Panel. (2019). American Geriatrics Society 2019 updated AGS Beers Criteria for potentially inappropriate medication use in older adults. *Journal of the American Geriatrics Society, 67*(4), 674–694. doi:10.1111/jgs.15767

TABLE 26.2 Summary of the 2019 Beers Criteria for Potentially Inappropriate Medication Use Due to Drug–Disease or Drug–Syndrome Interactions

Disease or Syndrome	Drugs	Rationale
Heart failure	Avoid: cilostazol In HFrEF: nondihydropyridine CCBs Use with caution in asymptomatic heart failure patients; avoid in patients with symptomatic heart failure: NSAIDs and COX-2 inhibitors, thiazolidinediones, dronedarone	Potential for fluid retention, exacerbation of heart failure, increased mortality in older adults
Syncope	Avoid: anticholinesterase inhibitors, nonselective peripheral alpha-1 blockers, tertiary TCAs, antipsychotics (chlorpromazine, thioridazine, olanzapine)	Bradycardia, orthostatic hypotension
Delirium	Avoid: anticholinergics, antipsychotic, benzodiazepines, corticosteroids, H2-receptor antagonists, meperidine, z-drugs	Worsening delirium, stroke risk, and mortality risk in patients with dementia
Dementia or cognitive impairment	Avoid: anticholinergics, benzodiazepines, z-drugs, chronic or as-needed antipsychotics	Adverse CNS effects, stroke risk, and mortality risk
History of falls/fractures	Avoid: antiepileptics (unless for seizures or mood disorders), antipsychotics, benzodiazepines, z-drugs, TCAs, SSRIs, SNRIs, opioids	Ataxia, impaired motor function, syncope, and additional falls. Consider reducing other CNS-active drugs if one of the drugs must be used and implement fall risk strategies
Parkinson's disease	Avoid: antiemetics (metoclopramide, prochlorperazine, promethazine), all antipsychotics (except quetiapine, clozapine, pimavanserin)	Potential to worsen parkinsonism
History of GI ulcers	Avoid unless no effective alternatives or can use gastroprotective agent: aspirin >325 mg/d, nonselective NSAIDs	Additional bleeding and ulcer risk

(continued)

TABLE 26.2 Summary of the 2019 Beers Criteria for Potentially Inappropriate Medication Use Due to Drug–Disease or Drug–Syndrome Interactions (*continued*)

Disease or Syndrome	Drugs	Rationale
Chronic kidney disease (stage 4 or higher)	Avoid: NSAIDs	Risk of acute kidney injury or further renal decline
Urinary incontinence in women	Avoid: oral and transdermal estrogen, peripheral alpha-1 blockers (doxazosin, prazosin, terazosin)	Lack of efficacy (estrogens) and aggravation of incontinence (alpha-blockers)
Lower urinary tract symptoms, benign prostatic hyperplasia	Strong anticholinergic agents, except antimuscarinics for incontinence	Decreased urine flow and cause retention

CCBs, calcium channel blockers; CNS, central nervous system; COX-2, cyclooxygenase-2; GI, gastrointestinal; HFrEF, heart failure with reduced ejection fraction; NSAIDs, nonsteroidal anti-inflammatory drugs; SSRIs, selective serotonin reuptake inhibitors; SNRIs, serotonin–norepinephrine reuptake inhibitors; TCAs, tricyclic antidepressants.

Source: From American Geriatrics Society Beers Criteria Update Expert Panel. (2019). American Geriatrics Society 2019 updated AGS Beers Criteria for potentially inappropriate medication use in older adults. *Journal of the American Geriatrics Society, 67*(4), 674–694. doi:10.1111/jgs.15767

TABLE 26.3 2019 Beers Criteria: Summary of Drugs to Be Used With Caution

Drugs	Rationale	Recommendation
Aspirin for primary prevention of cardiovascular disease	Risk of bleeding with older age	Use with caution in adults 70 years and older
Dabigatran, rivaroxaban	Increased risk of GI bleeding compared to warfarin and other direct oral anticoagulants	Use with caution for treatment of VTE or atrial fibrillation in adults 75 years and older
Prasugrel	Increased risk of bleeding	Use with caution in adults 75 years or older
Antipsychotics, carbamazepine, diuretics, mirtazapine, oxcarbazepine, SNRIs, SSRIs, TCAs, tramadol	Exacerbate SIADH or hyponatremia, monitor the sodium levels closely with initiation and change in dose	Use with caution
Dextromethorphan/ quinidine	Limited efficacy, increased risk of falls, drug interactions	Use with caution

(*continued*)

TABLE 26.3 2019 Beers Criteria: Summary of Drugs to Be Used With Caution (*continued*)

Drugs	Rationale	Recommendation
Trimethoprim/sulfamethoxazole	Risk of hyperkalemia with concurrent ACEI or ARB use with reduced creatinine clearance	Use with caution as indicated

ACEI, angiotensin-converting enzyme inhibitor; ARB, angiotensin receptor blocker; GI, gastrointestinal; SIADH, syndrome of inappropriate antidiuretic hormone; SSRIs, selective serotonin reuptake inhibitors; SNRIs, serotonin–norepinephrine reuptake inhibitors; TCAs, tricyclic antidepressants; VTE, venous thromboembolism.

Source: From American Geriatrics Society Beers Criteria Update Expert Panel. (2019). American Geriatrics Society 2019 updated AGS Beers Criteria for potentially inappropriate medication use in older adults. *Journal of the American Geriatrics Society, 67*(4), 674–694. doi:10.1111/jgs.15767

TABLE 26.4 2019 Beers Criteria Summary of Drug–Drug Interactions That Should Be Avoided

Drug and Class	Interacting Drug and Class	Rationale
RAS inhibitor (ACEIs, ARBs, aliskiren) or potassium-sparing diuretics	Another RAS inhibitor	Risk of hyperkalemia
Opioids	Benzodiazepines	Overdose
Opioids	Gabapentin, pregabalin	Sedation, respiratory depression, death
Anticholinergic	Anticholinergic	Cognitive decline
Antidepressants, antipsychotics, antiepileptics, benzodiazepines, z-drugs, and opioids	Any combination of three or more of these CNS drugs	Falls, fracture
Corticosteroids	NSAIDs	GI ulcers and bleeding
Lithium	ACEIs, loop diuretics	Lithium toxicity
Peripheral alpha-blockers	Loop diuretics	Urinary incontinence in older women
Phenytoin	Trimethoprim–sulfamethoxazole	Phenytoin toxicity
Theophylline	Cimetidine, ciprofloxacin	Theophylline toxicity

(*continued*)

TABLE 26.4 2019 Beers Criteria Summary of Drug–Drug Interactions That Should Be Avoided (*continued*)

Drug and Class	Interacting Drug and Class	Rationale
Warfarin	Ciprofloxacin, amiodarone, macrolides (excluding azithromycin), trimethoprim–sulfamethoxazole, and NSAIDs	Increased risk of bleeding

ACEI, angiotensin-converting enzyme inhibitor; ARB, angiotensin receptor blocker; CNS, central nervous system; GI, gastrointestinal; NSAIDs, nonsteroidal anti-inflammatory drugs; RAS, renin-angiotensin system.

Source: From American Geriatrics Society Beers Criteria Update Expert Panel. (2019). American Geriatrics Society 2019 updated AGS Beers Criteria for potentially inappropriate medication use in older adults. *Journal of the American Geriatrics Society, 67*(4), 674–694. doi:10.1111/jgs.15767

TABLE 26.5 2019 Beers Criteria Summary of Medications That Should Be Avoided or Dose Reduced With Reduced Kidney Function

Drug	Creatinine Clearance (mL/min) and Recommendation
Ciprofloxacin	<30 reduce dose
Trimethoprim–sulfamethoxazole	<30 reduce dose, <15 avoid
Amiloride	<30 avoid
Apixaban	<25 avoid
Dabigatran	<30 avoid, dose adjust if >30, but drug–drug interactions
Dofetilide	<60 reduce dose, <20 avoid
Edoxaban	15 to 50 reduce dose, <15 avoid
Enoxaparin	<30 reduce dose
Fondaparinux	<30 avoid
Rivaroxaban	<50 reduce dose, <15 avoid in nonvalvular atrial fibrillation, <30 avoid in VTE treatment or prophylaxis
Spironolactone	<30 avoid
Triamterene	<30 avoid
Duloxetine	<30 avoid
Gabapentin	<60 reduce dose
Levetiracetam	<80 reduce dose

(*continued*)

TABLE 26.5 2019 Beers Criteria Summary of Medications That Should Be Avoided or Dose Reduced With Reduced Kidney Function (*continued*)

Drug	Creatinine Clearance (mL/min) and Recommendation
Pregabalin	<60 reduce dose
Tramadol	<30 reduce dose, immediate release, avoid extended release
Cimetidine, famotidine, nizatidine, ranitidine	<50 reduce dose
Colchicine	<30 reduce dose
Probenecid	<30 avoid

VTE, venous thromboembolism.

Source: From American Geriatrics Society Beers Criteria Update Expert Panel. (2019). American Geriatrics Society 2019 updated AGS Beers Criteria for potentially inappropriate medication use in older adults. *Journal of the American Geriatrics Society, 67*(4), 674–694. doi:10.1111/jgs.15767

TABLE 26.6 2019 Beers Criteria Summary of Drugs With Strong Anticholinergic Properties

Class	Drug(s)
Antiarrhythmic	Disopyramide
Antidepressants	Amitriptyline Amoxapine Clomipramine Doxepin >6 mg Imipramine Nortriptyline Protriptyline Trimipramine
Antiemetics	Prochlorperazine Promethazine
Antihistamines (first generation)	Brompheniramine Carbinoxamine Chlorpheniramine Clemastine Cyproheptadine Dexbrompheniramine Dexchlorpheniramine Doxylamine Hydroxyzine Meclizine

(*continued*)

TABLE 26.6 2019 Beers Criteria Summary of Drugs With Strong Anticholinergic Properties (*continued*)

Class	Drug(s)
Anticholinergic	Dicyclomine Hyoscyamine Scopolamine
Antimuscarinics	Darifenacin Fesoterodine Flavoxate Oxybutynin Solifenacin Tolterodine Trospium
Antiparkinsonian agents	Benztropine Trihexyphenidyl
Antipsychotics	Chlorpromazine Clozapine Loxapine Olanzapine Perphenazine Thioridazine Trifluoperazine
Skeletal muscle relaxants	Cyclobenzaprine Orphenadrine

Source: From American Geriatrics Society Beers Criteria Update Expert Panel. (2019). American Geriatrics Society 2019 updated AGS Beers Criteria for potentially inappropriate medication use in older adults. *Journal of the American Geriatrics Society, 67*(4), 674–694. doi:10.1111/jgs.15767

prescribing omission errors. Due to these concerns, O'Mahony et al. (2010) developed a draft of STOPP/START criteria with the following goals as a guide: capture common and important inappropriate prescribing; organize according to physiologic systems; give attention to drugs with high fall risk and opioid use in elderly patients; duplicate drug class prescription; errors of prescribing omission; and represent consensus views of an expert panel (O'Mahony et al., 2010).

Content validity for the criteria was evaluated using a Delphi consensus model, with 65 STOPP criteria and 22 START criteria when completed (Gallagher et al., 2008). STOPP stands for **s**creening **t**ool of **o**lder **p**ersons' **p**rescriptions and START stands for **s**creening **t**ool to **a**lert to **r**ight **t**reatment. Findings from one study suggested that use of the STOPP criteria detected adverse drug events leading to hospital admission 2.8 times more than Beers criteria (O'Mahony et al., 2010). The most recent version of STOPP/START criteria was released in 2015 and is referred to as version 2 (O'Mahony et al., 2015). These criteria are outlined in Table 26.7.

TABLE 26.7 STOPP/START Version 2 Criteria Overview

STOPP	
Section A: indication of medication	No evidence-based indication
	Beyond recommended treatment duration
	Duplicate drug class prescriptions
Section B: cardiovascular system	Digoxin for HF with normal ventricular function
	Verapamil or diltiazem for Class III or IV HF
	Beta-blocker in combination with verapamil or diltiazem
	Beta-blocker with bradycardia, type II or complete heart block
	Amiodarone as first-line antiarrhythmic in supraventricular tachycardia
	Loop diuretic as first-line treatment for HTN
	Loop diuretic for dependent edema without evidence of HF, liver failure, nephrotic syndrome, or renal failure
	Thiazide diuretic with hypokalemia, hyponatremia, hypercalcemia, or history of gout
	Loop diuretic for HTN with concurrent urinary incontinence
	Centrally acting antihypertensives unless intolerant of other antihypertensives
	ACEIs or ARBs in patients with hyperkalemia
	Aldosterone antagonists with potassium conserving agents – serum potassium must be monitored
	Phosphodiesterase inhibitors in HF with hypotension or concurrent nitrate therapy
Section C: antiplatelet/ anticoagulant drugs	Long-term aspirin with doses >160 mg/d
	Aspirin with history of PUD without concurrent PPI
	Antiplatelet or antithrombotic agents in the presence of significant bleeding risk
	Aspirin plus clopidogrel for secondary stroke prevention, unless stents in the previous 12 months, concurrent acute coronary syndrome, or high-grade carotid artery stenosis
	Aspirin in combination with vitamin K antagonist, direct thrombin inhibitor, or factor Xa inhibitors in patients with chronic atrial fibrillation
	Antiplatelet agents with vitamin K antagonist, direct thrombin inhibitor, or factor Xa inhibitors with stable coronary, cerebrovascular, or peripheral arterial disease
	Ticlopidine in any circumstance
	Vitamin K antagonist, direct thrombin inhibitor, or factor Xa inhibitor for first DVT for >6 months
	Vitamin K antagonist, direct thrombin inhibitor, or factor Xa inhibitor for first pulmonary embolus >12 months
	NSAID and vitamin K antagonist, direct thrombin inhibitor, or factor Xa inhibitor in combination
	NSAID with concurrent antiplatelet agents without PPI prophylaxis

(continued)

TABLE 26.7 STOPP/START Version 2 Criteria Overview (*continued*)

STOPP	
Section D: CNS and psychotropic drugs	TCAs with dementia, narrow-angle glaucoma, cardiac conduction, abnormalities, lower urinary tract symptoms, or prior history of urinary retention TCAs as first-line antidepressant Neuroleptics with moderate antimuscarinic/anticholinergic effects (chlorpromazine, clozapine, etc.) with lower prostate disease or previous urinary retention SSRIs with current or recent hyponatremia Na+ <130 mmol/L Benzodiazepines for 4 weeks or more – withdraw gradually if taken for >4 weeks Antipsychotics in parkinsonism or Lewy Body Disease Anticholinergics/antimuscarinics to treat EPS of neuroleptic medications Anticholinergics/antimuscarinics in patients with delirium or dementia Neuroleptic antipsychotic in patients with behavioral symptoms of dementia unless severe and behavioral treatments have not worked Neuroleptics as hypnotics unless sleep disorder is due to psychosis or dementia Acetylcholinesterase inhibitors with history of bradycardia, heart block, or recurrent reduced heart rate with other medications Phenothiazines as first-line treatment – more efficacious and safe alternatives Levodopa or dopamine agonists for benign essential tremor First-generation antihistamines
Section E: renal system (potentially inappropriate with renal disease or low eGFR)	Digoxin at a dose >125 mcg/d if eGFR <30 mL/min Direct thrombin inhibitors if eGFR <30 mL/min Factor Xa inhibitors if eGFR <15 mL/min NSAIDs if eGFR <50 mL/min Colchicine if eGFR <10 mL/min Metformin if eGFR <30 mL/min
Section F: GI system	Prochlorperazine or metoclopramide with parkinsonism PPI for uncomplicated PUD or esophagitis for >8 weeks Drugs with increased risk of constipation in patients with chronic constipation Oral iron doses >200 mg/d
Section G: respiratory system	Theophylline as monotherapy for COPD Systemic rather than inhaled steroids for maintenance therapy in moderate–severe COPD Antimuscarinic bronchodilators with a history of narrow-angle glaucoma or bladder obstruction Benzodiazepines with acute or chronic respiratory failure

(*continued*)

TABLE 26.7 STOPP/START Version 2 Criteria Overview (*continued*)

STOPP	
Section H: musculoskeletal system	Nonselective NSAIDs with history of PUD or GI bleeding, unless concurrent PPI or H2 antagonist NSAID with severe hypertension or severe heart failure Long-term NSAID use for osteoarthritis where acetaminophen has not been tried Long-term corticosteroids as monotherapy for rheumatoid arthritis Corticosteroids for osteoarthritis Long-term NSAID or colchicine for gout treatment when no contraindication for xanthine oxidase inhibitor COX-2 selective NSAIDs with concurrent cardiovascular disease NSAID with concurrent corticosteroids without PPI prophylaxis Oral bisphosphonates with upper GI disease or bleeding
Section I: urogenital system	Antimuscarinic drugs with dementia, mild cognitive impairment, narrow-angle glaucoma, or prostate disease Selective alpha-1 blockers with symptomatic orthostatic hypotension or micturition syncope
Section J: endocrine system	Sulfonylureas with long duration of action in T2DM Thiazolidenediones in patients with heart failure Beta-blockers in diabetes mellitus with frequent hypoglycemia Estrogens with history of breast cancer or VTE Oral estrogens with progesterone in patients with intact uterus Androgens in the absence of primary or secondary hypogonadism
Section K: drugs that increase fall risk in older people	Benzodiazepines Neuroleptic drugs Vasodilator drugs with persistent postural hypotension Hypnotic z-drugs
Section L: analgesic drugs	Oral or transdermal opioids as first-line therapy for mild pain Use of regular opioids without concomitant laxative Long-acting opioids without short-acting opioids for breakthrough pain
Section N: antimuscarinic/ anticholinergic drug burden	Use of two or more drugs with antimuscarinic/anticholinergic properties

(*continued*)

TABLE 26.7 STOPP/START Version 2 Criteria Overview (*continued*)

START	
Section A: cardiovascular system	Vitamin K antagonists, direct thrombin inhibitors, or factor Xa inhibitors in chronic atrial fibrillation
	Aspirin (75–160 mg) in chronic atrial fibrillation where other medications are contraindicated
	Antiplatelet therapy with documented history of coronary, cerebral, or peripheral arterial disease
	Antihypertensive therapy with systolic blood pressure >160 mmHg and/or diastolic blood pressure >90 mmHg; >140 mmHg systolic and/or >90 mmHg if diabetic
	Statin therapy with history of coronary, cerebral, or peripheral vascular disease, unless at the end of life or >85 years
	ACEI with systolic HF and/or documented coronary artery disease
	Beta-blocker with ischemic HF
	Appropriate beta-blocker with stable systolic HF
Section B: respiratory system	Regular inhaled beta-2 agonist or antimuscarinic bronchodilator for mild–moderate asthma or COPD
	Regular inhaled corticosteroid for moderate–severe asthma or COPD
	Home continuous oxygen with documented hypoxemia
Section C: CNS and eyes	l-DOPA or a dopamine agonist in idiopathic Parkinson's disease with functional impairment and resultant disability
	Non-TCA antidepressant drug in the presence of persistent major depressive symptoms
	Acetylcholinesterase inhibitor for mild–moderate Alzheimer's dementia or Lewy body dementia
	Topical prostaglandin, prostamide, or beta-blocker for open-angle glaucoma
	SSRI (SNRI or pregabalin if SSRI contraindicated) for persistent severe anxiety
	Dopamine agonist for RLS, once iron deficiency and renal failure have been excluded
Section D: GI system	PPI with severe GERD or peptic stricture requiring dilation
	Fiber supplementation for diverticulosis with history of constipation
Section E: musculoskeletal system	DMARD with active, disabling RA
	Bisphosphonates, vitamin D, and calcium in patients taking long-term systemic corticosteroids
	Vitamin D and calcium supplement in patients with known osteoporosis, previous fracture, and/or BMD T-scores >−2.5 in multiple sites
	Bone antiresorptive or anabolic therapy in patients with documented osteoporosis, where no contraindication exists
	Vitamin D supplementation in homebound individuals or individuals with falls or osteopenia
	Xanthine oxidase inhibitors with recurrent episodes of gout
	Folic acid supplement in patients taking methotrexate

(*continued*)

TABLE 26.7 STOPP/START Version 2 Criteria Overview (*continued*)

START	
Section F: endocrine system	ACEI or ARB in diabetes with evidence of renal disease
Section G: urogenital system	Alpha-1 blocker with symptomatic BPH 5-Alpha reductase inhibitor with symptomatic BPH Topical vaginal estrogen for symptomatic atrophic vaginitis
Section H: analgesics	High-potency opioids in moderate–severe pain, where acetaminophen, NSAIDs, or low-potency opioids are not appropriate Laxatives in patients receiving regular opioids
Section I: vaccines	Seasonal trivalent influenza vaccine Pneumococcal vaccine after age 65 according to national guidelines

BMDT, bone mineral density test; BPH, benign prostatic hyperplasia; CNS, central nervous system; COPD, chronic obstructive pulmonary disease; COX-2, cyclooxygenase-2; DMARD, disease-modifying antirheumatic drug; DVT, deep vein thrombosis; eGFR, estimated glomerular filtration rate; EPS, extrapyramidal side effects; GERD, gastroesophageal reflux disease; GI, gastrointestinal; HF, heart failure; HTN, hypertension; l-DOPA, l-3,4-dihydroxyphenylalanine; NSAID, nonsteroidal anti-inflammatory drug; PPI, proton pump inhibitor; PUD, peptic ulcer disease; RA, rheumatoid arthritis; RLS, restless leg syndrome; SSRIs, selective serotonin reuptake inhibitors; SNRIs, serotonin–norepinephrine reuptake inhibitors; START, screening tool to alert to right treatment; STOPP, screening tool of older persons' prescriptions; T2DM, type 2 diabetes mellitus; TCA, tricyclic antidepressant.

Source: From O'Mahony, D., O'Sullivan, D., Byrne, S., O'Connor, M. N., Ryan, C., & Gallagher, P. (2015). STOPP/START criteria for potentially inappropriate prescribing in older people, version 2. *Age and Ageing, 44*(2), 213–218. doi:10.1093/ageing/afu145

CLINICAL APPLICATION

When applying the Beers or STOPP/START criteria, it is important to recognize the environments in which they were developed. The Beers criteria have been developed and updated by individuals and organizations within the United States, while the STOPP/START criteria have been developed and updated by stakeholders in Europe (Marcum & Hanlon, 2012) There are some differences between the two sets of criteria, so nurse practitioners should reconcile these differences with the best available evidence for the conditions they are treating, the insurance structures that impact the cost of treatments, patient-specific concerns (comorbidities, existing medications, safety, and medication access), and priorities of care for the healthcare team (including patient and family).

CHAPTER SUMMARY

The Beers Criteria for Potentially Inappropriate Prescribing and the STOPP/START criteria provide important guidance regarding safe prescribing practices in the aging population. A key consideration when applying these criteria is the individual patient context. Prescribing guidelines do not replace clinical judgment for nurse practitioners, but provide a framework for informed decision-making.

REFERENCES

American Geriatrics Society Beers Criteria Update Expert Panel. (2019). American Geriatrics Society 2019 updated AGS Beers Criteria for potentially inappropriate medication use in older adults. *Journal of the American Geriatrics Society, 67*(4), 674–694. doi:10.1111/jgs.15767

Beizer, J. L., & Semla, T. (2016). Beers Criteria: Navigating the challenges of geriatric care [Blog post]. Retrieved from https://www.wolterskluwercdi.com/blog/beers-criteria-navigating-challenges-geriatric-care

Gallagher, P., Ryan, C., Byrne, S., Kennedy, J., & O'Mahony, D. (2008). STOPP (screening too of older person's prescriptions) and START (screening tool to alert doctors to right treatment): Consensus validation. *International Journal of Pharmacologic Therapy, 46*(2), 72–83. doi:10.5414/cpp46072

Health in Aging Foundation. (2019a). Alternatives for medications listed in the AGS Beers Criteria® for potentially inappropriate medication use in older adults. Retrieved from https://www.healthinaging.org/tools-and-tips/alternatives-medictions-listed-ags-beers-criteriar-potentially-inappropriate

Health in Aging Foundation. (2019b). Medications that older adults should avoid or use with caution: The 2019 American Geriatrics Society updated Beers Criteria®. Retrieved from https://www.healthinaging.org/medications-older-adults/medications-older-adults-should-avoid

Marcum, Z. A., & Hanlon, J. T. (2012). Commentary on the new American Geratric Society Beers Criteria for potentially inappropriate medication use in older adults. *American Journal of Geriatric Pharmacotherapy, 10*(2), 151–159. doi:10.1016/j.amjopharm.2012.03.002

O'Mahony, D., Gallagher, P., Ryan, C., Byrne, S., Hamilton, H., Barry, P., . . . Kennedy, J. (2010). STOPP & START criteria: A new approach to detecting potential inappropriate prescribing in old age. *European Geriatric Medicine, 1*(1), 45–51. doi:10.1016/j.eurger.2010.01.007

O'Mahony, D., O'Sullivan, D., Byrne, S., O'Connor, M. N., Ryan, C., & Gallagher, P. (2015). STOPP/START criteria for potentially inappropriate prescribing in older people, version 2. *Age and Ageing, 44*(2), 213–218. doi:10.1093/ageing/afu145

27 Examples of Inappropriate Medication Prescribing

Madeline Burke

OBJECTIVES
1. Describe the types of inappropriate prescribing
2. Utilize techniques to reduce risk of adverse effects in older adults

INTRODUCTION
Older adults are particularly susceptible to adverse effects of their medications, as well as polypharmacy. This chapter attempts to categorize some examples of inappropriate prescribing and provide suggestions for preventing similar situations in your practice.

One high-yield practice is to include the indication in the comments of all prescription orders for patients, such as "lisinopril 5 mg PO (by mouth) daily for kidney protection and blood pressure." It is beneficial to the pharmacist verifying the order (in any setting) and often helpful for the patient or his or her family to understand or remember why this medication is important to take as prescribed.

In a longitudinal study of potentially inappropriate prescribing in older adults, it was found that hospital admission was independently associated with increased rate of inappropriate prescriptions. Most common types of potentially inappropriate prescribing in this study included long-term proton pump inhibitor (PPI) use without compelling indication, benzodiazepines for greater than 4 weeks, and zolpidem or other "Z-drugs" used longer than indicated (Pérez et al., 2018).

DOSE CHANGES
Many commonly prescribed medications require dose adjustment for kidney and liver dysfunction. Along these lines, some medications require dose adjustment for differing indications.

Dose Too High for Indication
Example Case 1
An 82-year-old African American male presents to your clinic with a prescription he received at discharge from a recent hospitalization and asks whether you can prescribe this as a 90-day supply for him. He was recently diagnosed with atrial fibrillation and has a CHA2DS2-VASc of 5. His serum creatinine indicated on his discharge summary is 1.2 mg/dL. He is 65 inches tall and weighs 59 kg in clinic today. His prescription is for "apixaban 5 mg BID for stroke prevention." This dose is too high for this patient per the package insert, as apixaban has dose adjustment to 2.5 mg twice

daily (BID) in patients prescribed this medication for stroke prevention secondary to atrial fibrillation. The patient must meet at least two of the following criteria for dose reduction in this indication: age ≥80 years, weight <60 kg, or serum creatinine ≥1.5 mg/dL. Therefore, this patient meets the criteria for apixaban dose reduction to 2.5 mg BID for stroke prevention to reduce the risk of bleeding on this blood thinner.

Dose Too Low for Indication
Example Case 2
Mr. Smith is a 72-year-old male with relevant history of diabetes, diabetic neuropathy, and hypertension. He comes for his routine follow-up today and states, "This pill you started me on isn't doing a thing for my nerve pain." He was prescribed gabapentin 100 mg every night at bedtime (QHS) on his primary care visit 3 months ago. His estimated creatinine clearance is 50 mL/min. In patients with normal renal function, gabapentin doses of 1,800 mg/d are considered minimal effective dose for treatment of neuropathic pain (Backonja & Glanzman, 2003). However, this medication dose requires slow titration, particularly in older adults, for tolerability of side effects including drowsiness and dizziness.

MEDICATION CHANGES
Similar Agent With More Favorable Risk–Benefit Ratio
Example Case 3
Ms. Johnson is an 87-year-old African American female who presents for her annual follow-up. She still lives at home and is independent in all activities of daily living (ADLs). Her past medical history includes hypothyroidism and hypertension. Her medications include atenolol 50 mg daily and levothyroxine 88 mcg daily. She also reports an occasional acetaminophen as needed (PRN) for headache/aches/pains. Her thyroid stimulating hormone (TSH) is within normal limits (WNL) today. In clinic, her blood pressure is 132/70 mmHg with a heart rate (HR) of 68 bpm. She reports some dizziness upon standing, but otherwise reports she has "no complaints."

Example Case 3 Discussion
First-line antihypertensives do not include beta-blockers and should not be used in hypertension without a compelling indication. This is especially true with atenolol, which has been associated with increased mortality in community-dwelling hypertensive older adults (Testa, 2014). For Ms. Johnson, you recommend a taper off of atenolol (25 mg daily for 1 week, then stop) to prevent any risk of rebound hypertension or arrhythmias. You instruct her to keep a consistent blood pressure and pulse log at home and return in 2 weeks for nurse appointment to review her blood pressure trends. At that time, you plan to start amlodipine 2.5 mg daily if her blood pressure is elevated.

MEDICATION DISCONTINUED
Treatment Contraindicated or Relatively Contraindicated
Example Case 4
Ms. Smith is an 85-year-old White female who currently resides in a senior community (assisted living facility, nursing home, and hospice on-site). Her daughter brings her for an appointment in your clinic because she is concerned about her mom's increased agitation. Ms. Smith's past medical history includes dementia (likely Alzheimer's, diagnosed 4 years ago), lower extremity edema, and diabetes mellitus type 2 (now

diet controlled). She notes that her facility has been reporting increased behavioral symptoms associated with her dementia. The nurses at the facility help to administer the patient's medications; the patient's medication administration record (MAR) indicates alprazolam 0.25 mg each morning, amlodipine 2.5 mg daily, furosemide 40 mg BID, memantine 28/donepezil 10 mg daily, omeprazole 20 mg daily, quetiapine 25 mg daily, sertraline 100 mg daily, spironolactone 25 mg daily, and cholecalciferol 1,000 units daily. Her PRN medications include diphenhydramine 25 mg PRN for itching and/or sleep (started 2 weeks ago and given an average of two times per day) and albuterol HFA PRN for shortness of breath. Among other concerns, you recommend discontinuation of diphenhydramine due to its anticholinergic effects and trial of moisturizing, fragrance-free lotions for Ms. Smith's itching (American Geriatrics Society [AGS], 2019). You educate Ms. Smith's daughter on the typical progression of dementia and non-pharmacological therapies recommended for behavioral disturbances (see Dementia/Delirium Chapter 20, Central Nervous System Impairments).

Significant Drug–Drug Interaction

Example Case 5

Mrs. Jones is a 78-year-old female who presents for a follow-up appointment. She reports that she recently saw a neurologist who diagnosed her with essential tremor. She brings her records, which include a new medication, "primidone 50 mg once daily for essential tremor." Her past medical history includes atrial fibrillation (CHA2DS2-VASc of 4) and hypertension. Her estimated creatinine clearance is >60 mL/min. Her other medications include an over-the-counter (OTC) vitamin D/calcium supplement, rivaroxaban 20 mg daily with evening meal for stroke prevention, and lisinopril 5 mg daily for blood pressure. When you add her new prescription to your electronic record, a "critical interaction" alert pops up.

Example Case 5 Discussion

Primidone is a potent cytochrome P450 3A4 (CYP3A4) inducer, which can significantly reduce the concentrations of CYP3A4 substrates. Rivaroxaban is a CYP3A4 substrate. Therefore, the concentration and clinical effects of rivaroxaban may be significantly reduced by concomitant primidone use, which may lead to adverse effects as severe as a stroke. The package insert for rivaroxaban indicates that concomitant use of CYP3A4 inducers should be avoided. As her primary care provider, you contact her neurologist to discuss the interaction. They agree to discontinue primidone and trial propranolol for her essential tremor.

Example Case 6

Mr. Jones is a 75-year-old male who presents for his yearly physical exam. His past medical history includes coronary artery disease (coronary artery bypass grafting [CABG] ×2 at age 67) and hypertension. His labs from today are mostly within normal limits, with elevated triglycerides of 300 mg/dL. His current medications include atorvastatin 80 mg daily for cholesterol, lisinopril 40 mg daily for blood pressure, and aspirin 81 mg daily. You decide to prescribe gemfibrozil for his elevated triglycerides, but receive a "critical interaction" alert.

Example Case 6 Discussion

Gemfibrozil is contraindicated with atorvastatin, and the interaction extends to the entire statin class. Concomitant use of fibrates, such as gemfibrozil, with statin therapy increases the risk of myopathy and rhabdomyolysis. Additionally, gemfibrozil is poorly tolerated in many patients even when used alone for myopathy and rhabdomyolysis.

Adverse Reaction

Older adults are more prone to adverse drug reactions (ADRs) due to polypharmacy, changes in pharmacokinetics and pharmacodynamics, and multiple comorbidities. A recent study of nationwide Veterans Affairs adverse event reporting noted the most common ADRs and the most common severe ADRs by age group. As predicted, the percentage of severe ADRs has increased with age (3% in adults 20–29 years of age compared to 6% in adults 90 years and older; Moore et al., 2019). Table 27.1 describes the common and severe adverse reactions in older adults.

TABLE 27.1 Most Common Adverse Reactions and Most Common Severe Adverse Reactions Reported in Older Adults

	A. Top 10 Most Common Adverse Reactions Reported			
Rank	60 to 69 Years	70 to 79 Years	80 to 89 Years	≥90 Years
1	Lisinopril	Lisinopril	Lisinopril	Lisinopril
2	Simvastatin	Simvastatin	Simvastatin	Terazosin
3	Atorvastatin	Atorvastatin	Terazosin	Warfarin
4	Pravastatin	Terazosin	Warfarin	SMX/TMP
5	Metformin	Pravastatin	Atorvastatin	Simvastatin
6	Rosuvastatin	Warfarin	Pravastatin	Donepezil
7	Gabapentin	Rosuvastatin	SMX/TMP	Amlodipine
8	Amlodipine	Metformin	Amlodipine	Ciprofloxacin
9	Terazosin	Amlodipine	HCTZ	Tramadol
10	HCTZ	HCTZ	Donepezil	Tamsulosin
Relevant others	SMX/TMP #11 HCTZ/lisinopril #13 Ciprofloxacin #17	SMX/TMP #11 Ciprofloxacin #14 Tramadol #18 Oxybutynin #20	Oxybutynin #13 Ciprofloxacin #15 Tramadol #18	HCTZ #11 Levofloxacin #20
	B. Top 10 Most Common Severe Adverse Reactions Reported			
1	Lisinopril	Warfarin	Warfarin	Warfarin
2	Warfarin	Lisinopril	Lisinopril	Lisinopril
3	SMX/TMP	SMX/TMP	SMX/TMP	SMX/TMP
4	Heparin	Heparin	Simvastatin	Aspirin
5	HCTZ/lisinopril	Simvastatin	Heparin	Simvastatin

(continued)

TABLE 27.1 Most Common Adverse Reactions and Most Common Severe Adverse Reactions Reported in Older Adults (*continued*)

	B. Top 10 Most Common Severe Adverse Reactions Reported			
6	Simvastatin	Enoxaparin	Clopidogrel	Clopidogrel
7	Vancomycin	Clopidogrel	Dabigatran	Furosemide
8	Enoxaparin	Aspirin	Metoprolol	Metoprolol
9	Morphine	Dabigatran	Enoxaparin	Heparin
10	Ibuprofen	Vancomycin	Aspirin	Glipizide
Relevant others	HCTZ #15 Amiodarone #19 Ciprofloxacin #20	Amiodarone #14 HCTZ/lisinopril #18 HCTZ #19 Ciprofloxacin #20	Ciprofloxacin #11 Digoxin #13 Amiodarone #16 HCTZ #19 Atenolol #20	Dabigatran #11 Digoxin #12 HCTZ #14 Hydrocodone/APAP #17

APAP, acetaminophen; HCTZ, hydrochlorothiazide; SMX/TMP, sulfamethoxazole/trimethoprim.

Source: Data from Moore, V. R., Glassman, P. A., Au, A., Good, C. B., Leadholm, T. C., & Cunningham, F. E. (2019). ADRs in the Veterans Affairs healthcare system: Frequency, severity, and causative medications analyzed by patient age. *American Journal of Health-System Pharmacy, 76*(5), 312–319. doi:10.1093/ajhp/zxy059

Example Case 7

Mr. Thompson is a 76-year-old White male who presents to your clinic after a 4-day hospitalization for heart failure exacerbation. His past medical history includes heart failure (ejection fraction [EF] 30%–35%), colon cancer in remission, coronary artery disease, depression, benign prostatic hypertrophy (BPH), and atrial fibrillation. His medication list prior to the recent hospitalization included furosemide 40 mg daily, metoprolol succinate 50 mg daily, potassium chloride 10 mEq Sustained Action (SA) daily, pravastatin 40 mg daily, sertraline 100 mg daily, terazosin 10 mg daily, and warfarin as directed by the clinic for stroke prevention. After discharge, his relevant medications changed/started including furosemide 80 mg BID, losartan 25 mg daily, metoprolol succinate 200 mg daily, potassium chloride 20 mEq SA daily, and terazosin 10 mg daily. His blood pressure today in the clinic is 104/52 mmHg after drinking a soda, but his wife noted his blood pressure this morning before any medications to be 88/56 mmHg. She states that most mornings over the past week since discharge, his blood pressure runs 90s/60s mmHg and HR runs 50s to 60s bpm. She relays her concern that the patient may be overmedicated due to the changes on his hospitalization, and that he has had dizziness and fatigue that has significantly affected his quality of life. His symptoms are suggestive of some orthostasis. Mrs. Thompson reports he "passed out" and fell 3 days ago, and that she reduced his metoprolol succinate dose to 100 mg daily at this time. She also reports that he has had to stop losartan in the past because of low blood pressures. Patient's labs from today are within normal limits, except for a low potassium of 3.1 mmol/L. His weights have been stable since discharge, indicating he is at his "dry weight." Due to his symptoms and hypotension, you agree with his wife's reduction in the metoprolol dose. You recommend that the wife hold his losartan and continue to monitor his blood pressure until she receives a follow-up nurse visit with repeat basic metabolic panel (BMP) next week. Since terazosin can contribute to orthostasis, you change his terazosin to tamsulosin 0.4 mg QHS for his BPH. Finally, you increase his potassium supplement to 40 mEq SA BID because it was not increased proportionately to his furosemide dose increase.

At Mr. Thompson's 1-week follow-up, his serum potassium has improved and is now within normal limits at 3.8 mmol/L. Mr. Thompson reports that he is "doing better than he has in years" and is much more functional since losartan has been held. His home blood pressures off of losartan over the past week have ranged from 105 to 135/57 to 67 mmHg. Given his symptomatic improvement and low to normotensive blood pressure readings, you discontinue his losartan prescription order and enter an adverse reaction to this medication.

When titrated too quickly, metformin can cause significant diarrhea. For this reason, slow titration or trial of sustained-release metformin should be used to prevent refusal of retrial of metformin. This medication remains first line for diabetes mellitus type 2 and its use should be preserved as long as possible.

Unnecessary Drug Therapy

Example Case 8

A 73-year-old African American female presents to your clinic for a post-hospitalization follow-up. She was hospitalized for an acute exacerbation of her chronic obstructive pulmonary disease (COPD) due to influenza A infection and spent one night in the ICU. You review her post-discharge summary dated 1 week ago today and note her new medications include "azithromycin 250 mg on Monday, Wednesday, and Friday, omeprazole 20 mg QAM, and prednisone 20 mg for three additional days." She reports she has completed the prednisone course and is taking her azithromycin as prescribed. Her past medical history on your records include COPD, tobacco use disorder, hypertension, and depression. She has been stable on her medication regimen, with the exception of the recent COPD exacerbation. When asked why she was prescribed omeprazole, she states she is not sure. She denies acid reflux, recent ulcer, or history of hernia or Barrett's esophagitis. You review her hospitalization records in greater detail and it appears the omeprazole was started in the ICU for "stress ulcer prophylaxis."

Example Case 8 Discussion

PPIs are commonly prescribed in the critical care setting to reduce the risk of stress ulcers, but this practice is somewhat controversial. Regardless, prophylaxis for stress ulcers is not needed once on a general medical floor (Grube & May, 2007). This is a commonly continued medication at transfer and discharge in many hospitals, and some patients may continue on this medication for years without questioning its indication. Recommended duration of PPI use in most patients is 4 to 8 weeks for gastroesophageal reflux disease and peptic ulcer disease. Some indications, such as Zollinger–Ellison and Barrett's esophagitis, require extended durations of treatment with PPIs (Bez, 2013).

Example Case 9

A 72-year-old African American female recently diagnosed with non-small cell lung cancer (NSCLC) and likely brain metastases presents to your clinic for follow-up. She is undergoing treatment for the cancer and was prescribed megestrol for appetite 1 year ago by another provider. She was diagnosed with an upper extremity deep vein thrombosis (DVT) 3 months ago and started on apixaban for the clot above. Her daughter relays that the brain metastases have been affecting her memory and mood, and tearfully indicates that she has been referred to palliative care due to her poor prognosis. In clinic today, the patient is 62 inches and 64 kg. Megestrol is associated with increased risk of clots and no significant clinical benefit has been shown when used in older adults for appetite stimulation without cancer or AIDS (Reuben, Hirsch, Zhou, & Greendale, 2005). After discussion of risks and benefits of continued megestrol therapy, particularly with the patient's recent upper extremity DVT, the patient and her daughter would like to discontinue this medication and plan to discuss alternative agents for symptom management at initial palliative care appointment next week.

SUMMARY

Adverse effects from medications increase with age, polypharmacy, and multiple comorbidities. These examples of inappropriate prescribing provide tips to avoid adverse medication-related events.

REFERENCES

American Geriatrics Society. (2019). Updated AGS Beers Criteria® for potentially inappropriate medication use in older adults. *Journal of the American Geriatrics Society, 67*(4), 674–694. doi:10.1111/jgs.15767

Backonja, M., & Glanzman, R. L. (2003). Gabapentin dosing for neuropathic pain: Evidence from randomized, placebo-controlled. *Clinical Therapeutics, 25*(1), 81–104. doi:10.1016/s0149-2918(03)90011-7

Bez, C., Perrottet, N., Zingg, T., Leung Ki, E., Demartines, N., & Pannatier, A. (2013). Stress ulcer prophylaxis in non-critically ill patients: A prospective evaluation of current practice in a general surgery department. *Journal of Evaluation in Clinical Practice, 19*(2), 374–378. doi:10.1111/j.1365-2753.2012.01838.x

Grube, R. R. A., & May, D. B. (2007). Stress ulcer prophylaxis in hospitalized patients not in intensive care units. *American Journal of Health-System Pharmacy, 64*(13), 1396–1400. doi:10.2146/ajhp060393

Moore, V. R., Glassman, P. A., Au, A., Good, C. B., Leadholm, T. C., & Cunningham, F. E. (2019). Adverse drug reactions in the Veterans Affairs healthcare system: Frequency, severity, and causative medications analyzed by patient age. *American Journal of Health-System Pharmacy, 76*(5), 312–319. doi:10.1093/ajhp/zxy059

Pérez, T., Moriarty, F., Wallace, E., McDowell, R., Redmond, P., & Fahey, T. (2018). Prevalence of potentially inappropriate prescribing in older people in primary care and its association with hospital admission: longitudinal study. *British Medical Journal, 363*, k4524. doi:10.1136/bmj.k4524

Reuben, D. B., Hirsch, S. H., Zhou, K., & Greendale, G. A. (2005). The effects of megestrol acetate suspension for elderly patients with reduced appetite after hospitalization: A phase II randomized clinical trial. *Journal of the American Geriatrics Society, 53*(6), 970–975. doi:10.1111/j.1532-5415.2005.53307.x

Testa, G., Cacciatore, F., Della-Morte, D., Mazzella, F., Mastrobuoni, C., Galizia, G., . . . Abete, P. (2014). Atenolol use is associated with long-term mortality in community-dwelling older adults with hypertension. *Geriatrics & Gerontology International, 14*(1), 153–158. doi:10.1111/ggi.1207

28 Polypharmacy and Nonadherence/Patient Education Tips

Megan Hebdon

OBJECTIVES
1. Define and describe polypharmacy and its implications in older adults
2. Identify the factors contributing to medication adherence in older adults
3. Outline the process for deprescribing in the geriatric patient

INTRODUCTION
Adverse events related to pharmacotherapy increase in the presence of polypharmacy (U.S. Pharmacist, 2017). There are no concrete definitions of polypharmacy, although it is considered a major medical issue in the elderly. This is due to higher rates of comorbid health conditions in the elderly, a complex medical system, and treatment guidelines that recommend multiple medications to manage chronic conditions such as diabetes mellitus, hypertension, chronic obstructive pulmonary disease, and cardiovascular disease (U.S. Pharmacist, 2017). These same issues, along with healthcare access and prescription costs, may also contribute to issues with medication adherence in the elderly. Patient education and deprescribing are two essential approaches for nurse practitioners to address polypharmacy and medication adherence in all patients, including geriatric patients.

POLYPHARMACY
Polypharmacy is a significant issue in aging patients due to increased rates of comorbid health conditions requiring medications, changes in drug metabolism with age, increased risk of hospitalization due to adverse drug events, and decreased functional status following hospitalizations (Ayaz, Sahin, Sahin, Bilir, & Rakici, 2014; Rochon, 2019). The risk of polypharmacy increases with age, and the rate of patients over the age of 65 taking five or more medications has increased (U.S. Pharmacist, 2017). Additionally, adverse drug events related to polypharmacy are one of the most common, preventable reasons for hospital admission in aging patients (Abe, Tamiya, Kitahara, & Tokuda, 2016). Research has demonstrated that geriatric patients experience greater cognitive and functional decline in the presence of polypharmacy, independent of disease burden (Rochon, 2019). Finally, the risk of hip fracture is increased with polypharmacy, especially central nervous system (CNS) depressants or medications with high anticholinergic activity (Rochon, 2019).

Traditionally, "polypharmacy" has been described as greater than five medications for one patient, but a more apt definition for geriatric patients is taking more medication than is medically necessary (Maher, Hanlon, & Hajjar, 2014). Many aging patients will have five or more medical diagnoses; so, prescribing in these patients should emphasize modifying the natural history of disease, concomitant behavioral and non-pharmacologic treatments, and ongoing conversations about the goals of care with patients and families (Boyd et al., 2019). Nurse practitioners are responsible for understanding why patients are taking medications and whether medications are appropriate based on age, health status, comorbidities, other medications, and goals of care (U.S. Pharmacist, 2017).

One of the challenges related to prescribing for older patients is the prescribing cascade, where side effects of one medication are mistaken for a medical condition, and more medications are prescribed to treat side effects (Hueftle & Fellow, n.d.; Rochon, 2019). To complicate the matter of prescription medications is the use of over-the-counter and herbal supplements, which is becoming increasingly common in the elderly population (Rochon, 2019). Multiple medications, providers, and medical conditions may also contribute to poor medication adherence, especially in patients with sensory deficits (Rochon, 2019).

MEDICATION ADHERENCE

Medication adherence is an issue encountered frequently by nurse practitioners with all patients, but there are unique issues that affect adherence in the elderly. As previously discussed, polypharmacy can make medication regimens so complex that they are difficult for patients to manage. In addition, polypharmacy may result in greater side effects for patients, so they may be less willing to take the prescribed medications. The complications related to poor medication adherence may include subtherapeutic medication levels, unintentional overtreatment, increased healthcare costs, more frequent hospitalizations, and overall poorer health outcomes (Yap, Thirumoorthy, & Kwan, 2016).

A key aspect of determining medication adherence is the use of medication review or medication reconciliation with each appointment and transfer of care (Northwestern Memorial Hospital, 2012). This is often conducted by pharmacists in the inpatient setting, but often nurse practitioners do not have on-site access to pharmacist team members in the outpatient setting. So, they may be responsible to conduct the review with the collaboration of supportive care staff. In settings where team management of medications can be accomplished with nurse practitioners and pharmacists, this should be a priority of care. In the primary care setting, an effective starting point for medication review or reconciliation is having patients bring all prescription, over-the-counter, and herbal medications to appointments. This provides healthcare team members, patients, and family members with tangible items to review for medication names, dosage, frequency, reason, cost, and accessibility. This can be compared to the existing medication list in the healthcare record, and discrepancies can be reviewed and addressed.

Sometimes medication adherence can be attributed solely to the patient and family, but it is important to remember that all team members and patient contexts contribute to medication adherence issues. There may be patient-specific issues such as cognition, past and present health, social determinants of health, behavior and attitudes, and knowledge and beliefs about medications or self-care (Yap et al., 2016). Elderly patients may have physical barriers such as poor eyesight, tremors, fine motor weakness, or mobility issues that impact their ability to open bottles, blister packs, or administer injections. Additionally, aging patients with cognitive impairments may not be able to track multiple medications given at multiple times of day (Yap et al., 2016). Complex dosing regimens are challenging for patients of any age, but more so for those who have memory deficits. In addition to cognition, literacy level, especially health literacy, is an integral factor in medication adherence (Lee, Yu, You, & Son, 2017).

Medication issues may interact with patient-specific issues including cost, mode of delivery, labeling, side effects or drug interactions, and ease of use (Yap et al., 2016). Providers may affect patient adherence through communication barriers, lack of trusting relationships, and poor practices related to medication review. The system itself may contribute to medication adherence due to timing of visits that prevent patient education, poor follow-up plans, short prescription durations, and lack of community-based nursing support to help patients navigate barriers to medication use (Yap et al., 2016). Family members are often the source of informal caregiving, so they are key to medication adherence. Providers need to remember the importance of both educating caregivers on medication administration and providing them with tools and support for their caregiving role (Yap et al., 2016).

Every time a new medication is being considered for a geriatric patient, the nurse practitioner should evaluate whether it is necessary, accessible, formulated for ease of use, and aligns with the patient's medical history and current medications. This can be addressed only if the nurse practitioner knows and understands the patient and family caregivers and has conducted a thorough medication review. Finally, it is essential that clear patient education has been provided and patient and caregiver understanding has been elicited. If there are health literacy or communication issues, the nurse practitioner may need additional support through translation services, health literacy educational programs, home health or community nursing, and short-term follow-up with patients to ensure patients have the tools they need to be successful with their medications.

PATIENT EDUCATION

"Patient education" has been described as a method to promote medication adherence for individuals with chronic illness (Kini & Ho, 2018). This may be done during office visits with providers, nurses, and other trained healthcare staff, or through telephone, home-based, or telemedicine counseling (Kini & Ho, 2018). For elderly patients, nurse practitioners must remember patient-specific issues related to vision, hearing, and cognition that might impact how they receive or understand health-related education. A one-size-fits-all approach to patient education is rarely adequate to accommodate literacy levels, patient motivation, physical or social barriers to learning, and beliefs regarding medications or chronic disease care (Speros, 2009). An additional consideration for nurse practitioners should be the inclusion of informal and family caregivers in patient education whenever possible.

Age-appropriate strategies for providing health education to geriatric patients include the following (Speros, 2009):

- Promote an environment that is respectful, supportive, and allows for patients to communicate what they do not understand.
- Schedule multiple, brief teaching sessions in mid-morning to limit patient fatigue.
- Provide additional time for processing, and assess understanding through the teach-back method before moving on to new information.
- Connect knowledge and skills to past experiences through storytelling or reminiscing.
- Identify practical and relevant strategies that coincide with safety, independence, and the older adult's routine schedule.

- Minimize distractions and limit education to five or less main points.
- Face the patient, speak slowly, articulate clearly, and avoid large words or medical jargon. Sit at the patient level.
- Provide written material written in large print and readable at a fifth-grade level or below.
- Use simple visual aids that are relevant for the patient.
- Encourage the use of journal or file to keep written information accessible.
- Provide specific instructions regarding recommended behaviors, such as "eat three cups of vegetables per day" versus "increase vegetable intake."
- Engage the older adult in active learning through demonstration and practice of new skills. Repeat essential points and ask patient to recall those points periodically during the session.
- Evaluate the patient's daily activities and connect behaviors to existing cues in the patient's routine.

DEPRESCRIBING

Deprescribing is another method to address polypharmacy, prevent adverse drug reactions, and promote medication adherence. This can be a complicated process due to multiple chronic health conditions requiring guideline-directed therapy. Another challenge in deprescribing is fragmentation of care among multiple specialists and primary care providers, where communication regarding medical necessity of medications may be lacking. Coordination of care through provider notes, provider-to-provider consultations, and team meetings may help with this barrier. Additionally, electronic health records that are interoperable can support care and information coordination. Overall, the number of providers involved in prescribing for a patient should be limited to prevent adverse drug events (Rochon, 2019). The culture of medicine in the United States promotes diagnosing and prescribing, and often the support for deprescribing is limited. In general, benzodiazepines, atypical antipsychotics, statins, tricyclic antidepressants, and proton pump inhibitors are all higher-risk drugs in elderly patients, yet there is limited evidence for appropriate deprescribing practice (Farrell et al., 2015).

Deprescribing involves the identification and discontinuation of unnecessary medications due to lack of efficacy, need, or appropriateness. This should be a collaborative process among providers, patients, and family members to ensure that benefits and harms have been addressed, patient goals are being respected, and the level of functioning is optimized (McGrath, Hajjar, Kumar, Hwang, & Salzman, 2017). First, the medication review should be conducted to assess what the patient is taking. Then, efficacy and side effects of medications should be evaluated. Drug–drug interactions should be identified, and geriatric syndromes such as delirium, falls, urinary incontinence, orthostasis, weight loss, and constipation should be addressed (McGrath et al., 2017). Once medications have been identified that may be causing harm and may not be benefiting the patient, then a discussion regarding the deprescribing process should occur. Medications to be discontinued should be prioritized based on the level of harm and need, cost and access, and patient goals of care. Consultation with a pharmacist will support this decision-making process (McGrath et al., 2017). There are also several tools and resources such as the Beers criteria, STOPP/START criteria, Deprescribing.org, Medication Management Instrument for Deficiencies in the Elderly (MedMaIDE), Medi-Cog, Appropriate Medications for Older people

(AMO)-Tool, and Good Palliative-Geriatric Practice Algorithm that can support this decision-making process (McGrath et al., 2017).

When deprescribing, one medication should be discontinued at a time. Short-term follow-up by phone, in-office, or with nurse consultation will help allay patient and provider fears about withdrawal symptoms or disease relapse. Some drug classes such as antianginal agents, anticonvulsants, benzodiazepines, beta-blockers, and corticosteroids increase the risk of discontinuation effects, so providers should have a clear plan for patients and caregivers regarding symptoms to watch for and plans to address the symptoms (Frank & Weir, 2014). Communication with specialist providers regarding medication issues such as adverse effects, limited efficacy, adherence issues, and access will contribute to coordinated, patient-centered care (McGrath et al., 2017). While the deprescribing process is occurring, symptoms or disease severity may increase, necessitating reintroduction of medication. When this is the case, considering the optimal drug in the class for geriatric patients can optimize therapy while decreasing the risk. Finally, ongoing medication review should occur, so that providers, patients, and family members have a clear understanding regarding the plan of care.

FUTURE DIRECTIONS FOR PHARMACOLOGIC THERAPY IN THE ELDERLY

There are many developments on the horizon that have the potential to improve care and prevent adverse drug events in the elderly. The use of Big Data to understand the prescribing patterns, hospitalizations related to adverse drug events, and the interactions of drug therapy with patient disease has the potential to promote better prescribing decisions. In addition, increased uptake of telemedicine may provide an avenue for more frequent follow-up, patient support, and opportunities for patient assessment and education, so that adverse drug events can be prevented and deprescribing can be facilitated. Wearable devices may be an avenue for medication reminders and health monitoring. Precision medicine, where pharmacogenomic factors are applied to prescribing decisions, may prevent the use of inappropriate medications in individuals based on genetic factors. Additionally, certain medications optimize outcomes based on a patient's genotype. Finally, greater uptake of palliative care support services for aging patients with chronic disease will facilitate better health outcomes in the context of beliefs and desires of patients and families.

SUMMARY

Prescribing in the elderly is complex and challenging due to patient and family, provider, and healthcare factors. These factors may affect the burden of polypharmacy, medication adherence, and overall health outcomes for aging patients. Nurse practitioners can address these issues through medication review, educational interventions, and deprescribing practices. Clinical pharmacists are a key resource with these activities. Patient and family goals should be at the forefront of decision-making for either prescribing or deprescribing with quality of life being a guiding value of care.

REFERENCES

Abe, T., Tamiya, N., Kitahara, T., & Tokuda, Y. (2016). Polypharmacy as a risk factor for hospital admission among ambulance transported old-old patients. *Acute Medicine & Surgery, 3*(2), 107–113. doi:10.1002/ams2.153

Ayaz, T., Sahin, S. B., Sahin, O. Z., Bilir, O., & Rakici, H. (2014). Factors affecting mortality in elderly patients hospitalized for nonmalignant reasons. *Journal of Aging Research, 2014*, 1–7. doi:10.1155/2014/584315

Boyd, C., Smith, C. D., Masoudi, F. A., Blaum, C. S., Dodson, J. A., Green, A. R., . . . Tinetti, M. E. (2019). Decision making for older adults with multiple chronic conditions: Executive summary for the American Geriatrics Society guiding principles on the care of older adults with multimorbidity. *Journal of the American Geriatrics Society, 67*(4), 665–673. doi:10.1111/jgs.15809

Farrell, B., Tsang, C., Raman-Wilms, L., Irving, H., Conklin, J., & Pottie, K. (2015). What are priorities for deprescribing for elderly patients? Capturing the voice of practitioners: A modified Delphi process. *PLOS One, 10*(4), e0122246. doi: 10.1371/journal.pone.0122246

Frank, C., & Weir, E. (2014). Deprescribing for older patients. *Canadian Medical Association Journal, 186*(18), 1369–1376. doi:10.1503/cmaj.131873

Hueftle, K., & Fellow, P. (n.d.). *Polypharmacy and deprescribing: A guide for hospitalists* [Powerpoint]. Retrieved from https://www.acponline.org/system/files/documents/about_acp/chapters/mt/bigsky17/polypharmacy_hueftle.pdf

Kini, V., & Ho, P. M. (2018). Interventions to improve medication adherence: A review. *Journal of the American Medical Association, 320*(23), 2461–2473. doi:10.1001/jama.2018.19271

Lee, Y.-M., Yu, H. Y., You, M.-A., & Son, Y.-J. (2017). Impact of health literacy on medication adherence in older people with chronic diseases. *Collegian, 24*(1), 11–18. doi:10.1016/j.colegn.2015.08.003

Maher, R. L., Hanlon, J. T., & Hajjar, E. R. (2014). Clinical consequences of polypharmacy in elderly. *Expert Opinions on Drug Safety, 13*(1), 57–65. doi:10.1517/14740338.2013.827660

McGrath, K., Hajjar, E. R., Kumar, C., Hwang, C., & Salzman, B. (2017). Deprescribing: A simple method for reducing polypharmacy. *The Journal of Family Practice, 66*(7), 436–445. Retrieved from https://mdedge-files-live.s3.us-east-2.amazonaws.com/files/s3fs-public/Document/June-2017/JFP06607436.PDF

Northwestern Memorial Hospital. (2012). *Medications at transitions and clinical handoffs (MATCH) toolkit for medication reconciliation.* Retrieved from https://www.ahrq.gov/professionals/quality-patient-safety/patient-safety-resources/resources/match/index.html

Rochon, P. A. (2019). Drug prescribing for older adults. In K. E. Schmader & J. Givens (Eds.), *UpToDate*. Retrieved from https://www.uptodate.com/contents/drug-prescribing-for-older-adults

Speros, C. I. (2009). More than words: Promoting health literacy in older adults. *The Online Journal of Issues in Nursing, 14*(3), 5. Retrieved from http://ojin.nursingworld.org/MainMenuCategories/ANAMarketplace/ANAPeriodicals/OJIN/TableofContents/Vol142009/No3Sept09/Health-Literacy-in-Older-Adults.aspx

U.S. Pharmacist. (2017). *Polypharmacy.* Retrieved from https://www.uspharmacist.com/article/polypharmacy

Yap, A. F., Thirumoorthy, T., & Kwan, Y. H. (2016). Medication adherence in the elderly. *Journal of Clinical Gerontology & Geriatrics, 7*(2), 64–67. doi:10.1016/j.jcgg.2015.05.001

Index

ACD. *See* anemia of chronic disease
acetaminophen, 204, 212
acetylcholine, 162
acetylcholinesterase inhibitors (ACIs), 169, 171
ACIs. *See* acetylcholinesterase inhibitors
ACOVE quality measurement. *See* Assessing Care Of Vulnerable Elders quality measurement
acute sinusitis
  analgesics, 129
  antihistamines, 129
  antimicrobial therapy, 130
  corticosteroids, 129–130
  decongestants, 129
  mucolytics, 129
  natural history, 128
  saline nasal irrigation, 129
acyclovir, 231
adjuvant pain medications, 215–216
advanced practice nurse (APRN), 3
agonist, 24
Alcohol, Smoking, and Substance Involvement Screening Test (ASSIST), 188
Alcohol Use Disorders Identification Test (AUDIT), 188
alditols, 145
alendronate, 200
alfuzosin, 249
allergic rhinitis, 134–135
alosetron, 150
alpha-glucosidase inhibitor, 94
Alzheimer's disease, 68–69
  medications, 169–171
  nonpharmacologic measures, 169
  prevalence and risk factors, 166–167
  prevention and treatment, 168–169
  screening tools and diagnosis, 167–168
amantadine, 233
American Urological Association Symptom Index (AUA-SI), 248

aminoglycosides, 229
aminosalicylates, 151
amoxicillin/clavulanate, 260
anemia, 72–74, 73–74
anemia of chronic disease (ACD), 73–74
antagonism, 24
antagonist, 24
antibiotic therapies
  chronic obstructive pulmonary disease, 136
  inflammatory bowel disorder, 151
antihistamines, 46, 128
antispasmodics, 150
antitussives, 132
anxiety disorders, 183–188
apolipoprotein B (apoB), 107
aripiprazole, 182
ASB. *See* asymptomatic bacteriuria
ASCVD. *See* atherosclerotic cardiovascular disease
ASCVD Risk Estimator tool, 110
Assessing Care Of Vulnerable Elders (ACOVE) quality measurement, 32
Assessment of Underutilization of Medication, 32
ASSIST. *See* Alcohol, Smoking, and Substance Involvement Screening Test
asthma, 137–138
asymptomatic bacteriuria (ASB), 259, 264–265
atenolol, 232
atherosclerotic cardiovascular disease (ASCVD)
  exercise recommendations, 111
  ezetimibe, 111
  hypertriglyceridemia, 113
  lifestyle interventions, 111
  niacin and fibrates, 111
  PCSK9 inhibitors, 111
  risk-enhancing factors, 109
  screening and diagnosis, 108–110
  statin therapy, 111–113

AUA-SI. *See* American Urological Association Symptom Index
AUDIT. *See* Alcohol Use Disorders Identification Test
auditory disorders
  hearing loss, 59–62
  interprofessional case study, 62–64
avanafil, 252

bacterial pneumonia, 132–133
Beers criteria, 31
  clinical application, 294
  drug–drug interactions, 284–287
  expert panel and Delphi system, 277
  history, 277–278
  potentially inappropriate medication use, 278–285
  reduced kidney function, 287–288
  strong anticholinergic properties drugs, 288–289
behavioral and psychological symptoms of dementia (BPSD), 171–172
benign prostatic hyperplasia
  assessment and evaluation, 248
  definition and pathophysiology, 247
  guidelines, 248
  nonpharmacological treatment, 248–249
  pharmacotherapy, 249–253
benzodiazepines, 46
biguanides, 92
bile acid sequestrants, 150
bipolar depression, 179–183
bisacodyl, 145
bisphosphonates, 101–102, 202
bone mineral testing, 202
BPSD. *See* behavioral and psychological symptoms of dementia
bronchitis
  acute, 130–132
  chronic, 135
bronchodilators, 131
bupropion, 182
buspirone, 186

caffeine, 190
calcitonin, 200
CAM. *See* Confusion Assessment Method
capsaicin, 216
cardiovascular disease (CVD)
  coronary heart disease, 120
  incidence, 119
  interprofessional case study, 122–124
  primary prevention, 121
  primordial prevention, 120–121
  risk factors, 119
  secondary prevention, 121
cardiovascular system changes, 4
CARET. *See* Comorbidity-Alcohol Risk Evaluation Tool
CD. *See* Crohn's disease
cefdinir, 260
Center for Epidemiologic Studies Depression Scale, 181
central hearing loss, 61
central nervous system impairments
  aging brain, 161–162
  delirium, 162–166
  interprofessional case study, 173–175
  MCI and dementia, 166–171
cephalexin, 260
cephalosporins, 229
chronic bronchitis, 135
chronic conditions, 43–44
chronic obstructive pulmonary disease (COPD)
  adjunctive treatments, 137
  antibiotic therapies, 136
  chronic bronchitis, 135
  corticosteroids, 136
  emphysema, 135
  methylxanthines, 137
  mucolytic agents, 136
  nonmedicine interventions, 137
  nonreversible asthma, 135
  pharmacological interventions, 136
chronic sinusitis, 128, 130
ciprofloxacin, 261
citalopram, 182
cognition and memory assessment, 13
Comorbidity-Alcohol Risk Evaluation Tool (CARET), 188
competitive antagonist, 24
conductive and sensorineural hearing loss, 13
conductive hearing loss, 60–61
Confusion Assessment Method (CAM), 163
constipation
  complicating factors, 143
  diagnosis, 144
  lifestyle changes, 144
  medications, 144–146
  Rome criteria, 143
  secondary causes, 144
COPD. *See* chronic obstructive pulmonary disease
Cornell Scale for Depression in Dementia, 181
coronary heart disease (CHD), 120
corticosteroids

chronic obstructive pulmonary disease, 136
IBD, 151
Crohn's disease (CD), 151
cromolyn, 128
CVD. *See* cardiovascular disease
cyclosporine, 152

dabigatran, 232
darifenacin, 250
DDIs. *See* drug–drug interactions
delirium, 8
   medications, 165–166
   nonpharmacologic measures, 165
   prevention, 165
   screening tools and diagnosis, 163–165
dementia
   behavioral and psychological symptoms of dementia, 171–173
   definition, 166
   medications, 169–171
   nonpharmacologic measures, 169
   prevalence and risk factors, 166–167
   prevention and treatment, 168–169
   screening tools and diagnosis, 167–168
   sexual function, 268
denosumab, 102, 200, 202
deprescribing, 308–309
depressive disorders
   diagnostic criteria, 180–181
   predisposing issues, 180
   treatment, 181–183
dermatology interprofessional case study, 55–56
diarrhea, 146–147
digital hearing aids, 61
digital rectal exam (DRE), 248
digoxin, 232
disaccharides, 145
diverticulitis, 148
diverticulosis, 148
dizziness, 9
docusate sodium, 145
donepezil, 169
dopamine receptors, 162
dosing guidelines
   chronic illnesses, 51
   chronic kidney disease, 51–52
   dermatology interprofessional case study, 55–56
   drug class considerations, 52–53
   goal of, 54
   inappropriate drug prescribing, 53
   medication subsets, 53–54
   pharmacokinetic changes, 53

   polypharmacy, 53
Down syndrome, 167
doxazosin, 249
DPP-4 inhibitors, 93
DRE. *See* digital rectal exam
driving status, 14
drug absorption, 22
drug therapies
   adverse effects, 46
   antihistamines, 46
   benzodiazepines, 46
   challenges, 47
   medicine prescribing, 45
   principles, 45
drug–drug interactions (DDIs)
   in geriatric population, 35–36
   pharmacodynamics, 36
   pharmacokinetics, 35
   probability, 35
drug–food interactions
   acetaminophen and alcohol, 40
   antibiotics and dairy products, 40
   antithyroid drugs and iodine foods rich, 40
   calcium channel blockers and grapefruit juice, 40
   digoxin and dietary fiber, 40
   monoamine oxidase inhibitors and smoked food, 40–41
   oral diabetic agents and alcohol, 39
   statins and grapefruit juice, 40
   warfarin and vitamin K, 39
drug/receptor interaction, 23
duloxetine, 186
dutasteride, 250
dyslipidemia, 107, 108
dyspareunia, 267

ECRP. *See* endoscopic cholangiopancreatography
Elder Assessment Instrument, 14
electroconvulsive therapy, 182
eluxadoline, 150
emphysema, 135
endocrine disorders
   diabetes mellitus, 89–96
   interprofessional case study, 102–104
   osteoporosis, 100–102
   parathyroid disease, 98–99
   thyroid disease, 97–98
endocrine system, 6
endoscopic cholangiopancreatography (ECRP), 154
enoxaparin, 232
Epworth Sleepiness Scale, 190

erectile dysfunction, 265–267
ertapenem, 261
escitalopram, 182
exenatide, 231
ezetimibe, 112

falls, 8
familial hypercholesterolemia (FH), 108
FAST. *See* Functional Assessment Staging tool
fatigue, 9
fesoterodine, 251
FH. *See* familial hypercholesterolemia
finasteride, 250
fluoroquinolones, 230
fluoxetine, 182
fluvoxamine, 182
fosfomycin, 261
Fracture Risk Assessment Tool (FRAX), 100
fractures, 197. *See also* osteoporosis
frailty, 8
Framingham General CVD Risk Profile, 110
FRAX. *See* Fracture Risk Assessment Tool
Fulmer SPICES tool, 7
Functional Assessment Staging tool (FAST), 168
functional decline, 8
functional gallbladder disease, 154
functional status assessment, 12–13

GAD. *See* generalized anxiety disorder
gait disorders, 8
galantamine, 169
gallbladder disease, 153–154
gastrointestinal disorders
  constipation, 143–146
  diarrhea, 146–147
  diverticulitis, 148
  diverticulosis, 148
  false-positive cholescintigraphy, 155
  gallbladder disease, 153–154
  inflammatory bowel conditions, 149, 151–152
  interprofessional case study, 155–157
  irritable bowel syndrome, 148–150
  pancreatitis, 152–153
generalized anxiety disorder (GAD)
  clinical manifestations, 183
  diagnosis, 184
  risk factors, 183
  treatment, 184–188
Generalized Anxiety Disorder 7-item (GAD-7), 184

genetic mutations, 4
genitourinary pharmacotherapy
  interprofessional case study, 269–271
  sexual function, 265–269
  urinary tract infections (*see* urinary tract infections)
geriatric care, 3
Geriatric Depression Scale, 13, 181
geriatric examination
  environment, 12
  interprofessional team, 11
  medical history, 12
  physical exam, 12–16
  preparation, 11–12
geriatric syndromes, 7–9
Get Up and Go test, 13
Global Initiative for Chronic Obstructive Lung Disease (GOLD), 136
glyburide, 231
GOLD. *See* Global Initiative for Chronic Obstructive Lung Disease
gray matter, 161
guanylate cyclase agonists, 150

HADS. *See* Hospital Anxiety and Depression Scale
head-to-toe exam, 15–16
hearing loss
  causes of, 59
  conductive, 60–61
  definition, 59
  listening difficulties, 60
  management, 61–62
  mental health aspect, 61
  sensorineural, 61
hearing process, 60
hematologic and immune systems, 6–7
hematologic disorders
  age-related assessment findings, 75
  anemia, 73–74
  interprofessional case study, 75–77
Hospital Anxiety and Depression Scale (HADS), 184
hyperglycemia
  behavioral changes, 91
  life expectancy, 91
  medications, 91–96
  treatment response, 96
hyperlipidemia
  atherosclerotic cardiovascular disease, 108–113
  interprofessional case study, 113–115
hyperparathyroidism, 99
hyperthyroidism, 97
hypertriglyceridemia, 108, 110, 113

hypoparathyroidism, 98–99
hypothyroidism, 97–98

ibandronate, 102, 200
IBS. *See* irritable bowel syndrome
inappropriate medication prescribing
   adverse drug reactions, 300–302
   Beers criteria, 278–285
   dose changes, 297–298
   drug–drug interaction, 299
   medication changes, 298
   medication discontinued, 298–303
   unnecessary drug therapy, 302
inflammatory bowel conditions, 149, 151–152
influenza, 133–134
insomnia, 190
insulin therapy, 96
integrins, 152
integumentary system, 6
intra-articular steroid injections, 204
ipratropium bromide, 128
iron deficiency anemia, 74
irritable bowel syndrome (IBS), 148–149

Katz Index of Independence in Activities of Daily Living, 12

Lawton Instrumental Activities of Daily Living scale, 12–13
levetiracetam, 231
levofloxacin, 261
lidocaine, 216
linaclotide, 145
lipid disorders, 108
lipophilic drugs, 29
lipoprotein disorder, 108
lipoproteins, 107, 108
lithium, 233
loperamide, 150
lower urinary tract symptoms (LUTS), 247
lubiprostone, 146, 150
LUTS. *See* lower urinary tract symptoms

macrocytic anemia, 74
malnourished older adults, 83–84
malnutrition, 79
MAST-G. *See* Michigan Alcohol Screening Test-Geriatric version
MCI. *See* mild cognitive impairment
medical history, 12
medication adherence, 306–307
Medication Appropriateness Index, 32
medications
   adverse effects, 44

reconciliation and screening, 14
memantine, 171
mental disorders
   anxiety disorders, 183–188
   depressive disorders, 179–183
   interprofessional case study, 192–194
   psychosis, 188–189
   sleep disorders, 189–192
   substance use disorders, 188
menthol/methyl salicylate, 216
metabolic syndrome, 120
methotrexate, 152
methylcellulose, 145
methylnaltrexone, 146
methylxanthines, 137
metoclopramide, 231
Michigan Alcohol Screening Test-Geriatric version (MAST-G), 188
microcytic anemia, 74
mild cognitive impairment (MCI)
   definition, 166
   medications, 169–171
   nonpharmacologic measures, 169
   prevalence and risk factors, 166–167
   prevention and treatment, 168–169
   screening tools and diagnosis, 167–168
Mini-Mental State Exam (MMSE), 13, 167
mirtazapine, 186
mixed hyperlipidemia, 108
MMSE. *See* Mini-Mental State Exam
MoCA. *See* Montreal Cognitive Assessment
Montreal Cognitive Assessment (MoCA), 167
mood disorders, 13
mucolytic agents, 136
musculoskeletal disorders
   interprofessional case study, 206–208
   osteoarthritis, 202–206
   osteoporosis and fractures, 197–202
   pathophysiology, 197

neurologic disorders
   adverse health outcomes, 67
   Alzheimer's disease, 68–69
   interprofessional case study, 69–71
   Parkinson's disease, 67–68
   stroke, 67
neurologic system, 6
neurons, 162
neuropathic pain, 154
neurotransmitters, 162
nicotine, 190
nociceptive pain, 154
nonreversible asthma, 135

nonsteroidal anti-inflammatory drugs (NSAIDs), 203, 204, 212–213
normal aging changes, 3
normocytic anemia, 74
NSAIDs. *See* nonsteroidal anti-inflammatory drugs
NuDESC. *See* Nursing Delirium Symptom Checklist
Nursing Delirium Symptom Checklist (NuDESC), 163
nutrient imbalances, 8
nutritional issues
   adequate nutritional content, 81
   aging process, 79–81
   body mass index, 82–83
   deficiencies, 79
   digestive system, 80
   food intake, 81
   fruits and vegetable consumption, 80
   interprofessional case study, 84–86
   malnourished older adults, 83–84
   malnutrition, 79, 80
   nutritional screening, 82
   nutritional support, 83
   risk factors, 81–82
   undernutrition, 83
nutritional status assessment, 13

open-ended questions, 12
opioids, 144, 213–215
osmotic laxatives, 145
osteoarthritis
   definitions, 202
   diagnosis and treatment, 203
   medications, 204, 205
   nonpharmacologic measures, 203–204
   prevalence and risk factors, 203
   screening tools and diagnosis, 203
osteopenia, 100–102
osteoporosis
   definition, 198
   diagnostic criteria, 101
   pharmacologic agents, 199–202
   prevalence, 198
   prevention and treatment, 198–199
   risk factors, 198
   screening and diagnosis, 100–101
   screening tools and diagnosis, 198
   treatment, 101–102
oxymetazoline, 128

pain
   assessment, 211–212
   interprofessional case study, 221–223
   neuropathic, 154
   nociceptive, 154
   nonpharmacological therapy, 216–221
   pharmacological therapy, 212–216
paliperidone, 233
pancreatitis, 152–153
panic disorder, 183
parathyroid disease, 98–99
parathyroidectomy, 99
parenteral nutrition, 84
Parkinson's disease, 67–68
paroxetine, 182
patient education, 307–308
Patient Health Questionnaire-9 (PHQ-9), 13, 181
PCE. *See* Pooled Cohort Equation
PCSK9 inhibitors, 111
penicillins, 229
Penn State Worry Questionnaire, 184
periodic limb movements in sleep (PLMS), 190
pharmacodynamics, 23–24, 47
pharmacokinetics, 47
   age-related processes, 27
   and aging impact, 27–29
   distribution equilibrium, 22–23
   drug absorption, 22
   excretion, 23
   LADME scheme, 21–22
   metabolism, 23
   pharmacotherapeutic plan, 27–29
pharmacotherapeutic plan, 27–29
phobia-related disorder, 183
PHQ-9. *See* Patient Health Questionnaire-9
physical exam, 12–16
physiologic changes
   advanced practice nurse, 3
   cardiovascular system, 4
   endocrine system, 6
   geriatric syndromes, 7
   hematologic and immune systems, 6–7
   integumentary system, 6
   musculoskeletal system, 5
   neurologic system, 6
   respiratory system changes, 4–5
   theories of aging, 3–4
   urologic system, 4
PIM. *See* potentially inappropriate medication
PLISSIT model, 269
PLMS. *See* periodic limb movements in sleep
polyethylene glycol, 145
polypharmacy, 305–306
Pooled Cohort Equation (PCE), 110

potentially inappropriate medication (PIM), 31. *See also* inappropriate medication prescribing
pregabalin, 186
pressure injuries, 8
probiotics, 144, 150
programmed senescence, 3–4
protussives, 132
psychosis, 188–189
psyllium, 145

quetiapine, 187

raloxifene, 102, 200, 202
renal anatomy, 227
renal impairments
    categories, 228
    chemotherapeutic agents, 234–239
    disorders, 228
    geriatric population, 227–228
    interprofessional case study, 240–242
    renally adjusted drugs, 228–233
    renin–angiotensin system drugs, 229–234
renin–angiotensin system drugs, 229–234
respiratory disorders
    interprofessional case study, 138–140
    upper respiratory tract infections (*see* upper respiratory tract infections)
respiratory system changes, 4–5
restless legs syndrome (RLS), 190
Reynolds Risk Score, 110
ribavirin, 231
rifaximin, 150
risedronate, 200
risperidone, 233

Saint Louis University Mental Status (SLUMS) Examination, 167
saxagliptin/sitagliptin, 231
SBIRT. *See* Screening, Brief Intervention, and Referral to Treatment
Screening, Brief Intervention, and Referral to Treatment (SBIRT), 14, 188
Screening Tool of Older Persons' potentially inappropriate Prescriptions/Screening Tool to Alert doctors to the Right Treatment (STOPP/START) criteria, 32
    clinical application, 284
    content validity, 289
    history, 278, 289
    version 2, 290–294
senna, 145
sensorineural hearing loss, 61
sensory deficits, 8

serotonin and norepinephrine reuptake inhibitor (SNRI), 182
serotonin reuptake inhibitor (SSRI), 182
sertraline, 182
sexual function
    barriers to expression, 268
    dementia, 268
    dyspareunia, 267
    educational resources, 269
    erectile dysfunction, 265–267
    PLISSIT model, 269
    sexual interest and activity, 267–268
    women's health, 267
sexual health, 13
sildenafil, 252
silodosin, 249
skin breakdown, 8
sleep apnea, 189–190
sleep disorders, 8
    chronic diseases, 191
    chronic pain, 191
    insomnia, 190
    medications, 190
    periodic limb movements in sleep (PLMS), 190
    pharmacologic therapies, 191–192
    sleep apnea, 189–190
    sleep hygiene, 191
    substance use, 190
sleep hygiene, 191
SLUMS Examination. *See* Saint Louis University Mental Status Examination
smoking cessation, COPD, 137
SNRI. *See* serotonin and norepinephrine reuptake inhibitor
social assessment, 14
solifenacin, 251
soluble fiber, 150
sotalol, 233
SSRI. *See* serotonin reuptake inhibitor
statin therapy
    high-intensity statins, 111, 112
    intensity levels, 111
    moderate-intensity statin, 111, 112
    PCSK9 inhibitor, 112
    side effects, 112
STOPP/START criteria. *See* Screening Tool of Older Persons' potentially inappropriate Prescriptions/Screening Tool to Alert doctors to the Right Treatment criteria
stroke, 67
substance use disorders, 188
substance use screening, 14
sulfonylurea, 91, 92

tadalafil, 252
tamsulosin, 250
terazosin, 250
teriparatide, 102, 201
theophylline, 137
theories of aging, 3–4
therapeutic drug selection
    Beers criteria, 31
    potentially inappropriate medication, 31, 32
    STOPP/START criteria, 32
thiazolidinediones, 92
thiopurines, 152
thyroid disease
    hyperthyroidism, 97
    hypothyroidism, 97–98
Tinetti Balance and Gait evaluation tool, 13
tissue plasminogen activator, 67
topical agents, 216, 220
topiramate, 232
trazodone, 182
type 2 diabetes mellitus
    diagnostic criteria, 90
    hyperglycemia, 91–96
    screening and diagnosis, 89–90

ulcerative colitis (UC), 151
undernutrition, 83
unipolar depression, 179–183
upper respiratory tract infections (URTIs)
    acute bronchitis, 130–132
    acute sinusitis, 128–130
    allergic rhinitis, 134–135
    antihistamines, 128
    asthma, 137–138
    bacterial pneumonia, 132–133
    chronic obstructive pulmonary disease, 135–137
    chronic sinusitis, 128, 130
    cromolyn, 128
    influenza, 133–134
    ipratropium bromide, 128
    nonmedicine interventions, 128
    oxymetazoline, 128
    pseudoephedrine/phenylephrine, 127
urinary incontinence, 8, 13
urinary tract infections (UTIs)
    asymptomatic bacteriuria, 259, 264–265
    benign prostatic hyperplasia, 247–253
    causative organisms, 255
    definition, 254
    guidelines, 255
    medications, 259–263
    nonpharmacological changes and prevention, 255–259
    prevalence, 254
    risk factors, 255
    symptoms, 254
urologic system, 4
URTIs. *See* upper respiratory tract infections
UTIs. *See* urinary tract infections

vaginal atrophy, 267
vancomycin, 229
vardenafil, 253
venlafaxine, 182, 186, 233
vision assessment, 13
vitamin D, 198

Weber and Rinne tests, 62
weight loss, 8

zoledronate, 233
zoledronic acid, 201

www.ingramcontent.com/pod-product-compliance
Ingram Content Group UK Ltd.
Pitfield, Milton Keynes, MK11 3LW, UK
UKHW022324240125
454187UK00022B/333